The Life-Giving Gift of Acknowledgment

Philosophy/Communication
Ramsey Eric Ramsey, Series Editor

The Life-Giving Gift of Acknowledgment

(A Philosophical and Rhetorical Inquiry)

Michael J. Hyde

Purdue University Press
West Lafayette, Indiana

Printed in the United States of America.

Library of Congress Cataloging-in-Publication Data
Hyde, Michael J., 1950-
  The life-giving gift of acknowledgment : a philosophical and
rhetorical inquiry / Michael J. Hyde.
     p. cm. -- (Philosophy/communication)
  Includes bibliographical references and index.
  ISBN 1-55753-402-0 (pbk.)
  1. Conduct of life. 2. Recognition (Philosophy)--Moral and
ethical aspects. 3. Gratitude. I. Title. II. Series.
  BJ1531.H93 2005
  128'.4--dc22
                                             2005005572

*F*or my wife, Bobette
A Life-Giving Gift

*A*nd for Calvin O. Schrag
Teacher, Scholar, Colleague, and Friend

Contents

Acknowledgments

Acknowledging others in a book on the life-giving gift of acknowledgment is a joy, especially since my understanding of this gift makes much of the notion of reciprocity. Our moral well-being is cultivated by our ability to receive acknowledgment *and* to offer it to others.

I am indebted to a host of colleagues who read earlier drafts of some of my chapters and who provided me with encouragement, intellectual stimulation, and instructive feedback: Pat Arneson, Anne Bishop, Jason Black, Connie Chesner, Gregory Clark, Rod Heintz, Denise Jodlowski, Spoma Jovanovic, Walter Jost, Claudia Kairoff, Deepa Kumar, Tripp Lumpkin, Martin Medhurst, Rebecca Meisenbach, Ananda Mitra, Christopher Poulos, Randall Rogan, Kenneth Rufo, Calvin Schrag, Craig R. Smith, Betsy Taylor, Shepard Wallace, Eric Watts, Roy Wood, and David Zarefsky. I also thank those groups who heard pieces of this project at the Universities of Amsterdam, Denver, and North Carolina, Greensboro; Denison, Duquesne, Purdue, and Wake Forest University. The project was supported by teaching and research grants from Wake Forest University and the Lilly Foundation. Very special thanks is owed to Carrie Anne Platt, who served as my graduate student assistant and whose professionalism was unprecedented. Hats off, too, to Ramsey Eric Ramsey, the series editor, for his support and direction. I also wish to thank those from whom I received help in working with Purdue University Press: Thomas Bacher, Margaret Hunt, Pamela Judd, and Donna Van Leer.

Chapters 1, 3, 4, 8, and 10 contain portions of my previously published essays: "The Gift of Acknowledgment," in *Experiences Between Philosophy and Communication: Engaging the Philosophical Contributions of Calvin O. Schrag*, ed. Ramsey Eric Ramsey and David James Miller (Albany: State University of New York Press, 2003), 109–124; "The Ontological Workings of Dialogue and Acknowledgment," in *Dialogue: Theorizing Difference in Communication Studies*, ed. Rob Anderson, Leslie A. Baxter, and Kenneth N. Cissna (Thousand Oaks, CA: Sage, 2004), 57–73; "Acknowledgment, Conscience, Rhetoric, and Teaching: The Case of *Tuesdays with Morrie*," *Rhetoric Society Quarterly* 35:2 (Spring 2005): 23–46; "The Rhetor as Hero and the Pursuit of Truth: The Case of 9/11," *Rhetoric & Public Affairs* 8:1 (Spring 2005): 1–30. Grateful acknowledgment is made to the editors and publishers of these books and journals for their permission to use the material in question. Its present adaptation represents various degrees of revision and expansion of those first versions.

Foreword: Drawing from Many Wells

It is becoming increasingly apparent that the university of the new millennium will have as one of its features an unprecedented emphasis on the multidisciplinary character of human knowledge. Recent developments in the exponential growth and globalization of knowledge have attuned us to a realization that the world of our experience does not come to us in the pieces that our insular institutionalized departments within academe have been carving out. The maps of knowledge in the arts and the sciences alike are being refigured in response to the hyper-specialization within the sundry disciplines that has led to self-isolating vocabularies that impede communication not only across the disciplines but also veritably within the disciplines themselves. We have now become aware that our academic genres are more blurred and open-textured than we have traditionally assumed. Such is particularly the case when the discourses of philosophy and communication studies are at issue. It may indeed become a requirement of the times to problematize the very idea of disciplinarity and conduct thought experiments on postdisciplinary research and learning.

The ancient Greeks had already come upon the insight that the tasks of philosophy and rhetoric are entwined. This insight informed the institution of the medieval trivium, in which logic, rhetoric, and grammar were viewed as intercalating disciplines. Throughout the course of the development of the modem university, however, these three disciplines began to go their own way, occluding the requirement to attend to an inescapable overlap of issues and vocabulary. This was particularly accented in the development of modem philosophy, in which rhetoric was marginalized at best, and relegated to the dustbin of sham wisdom at the worst. Modernity's efforts to ground all knowledge on a criteriological concept of rationality, oriented towards unimpeachable truth conditions, left little room for the function of a praxis-oriented rationality that has always been the hallmark of rhetorical understanding.

With the development of departments of communication studies across North America and Europe, a new challenge has emerged. A relatively new kid in the academic neighborhood, communication encompasses a multiplicity of disciplinary foci, intensifying the requirement for multidisciplinary study and research, and affording opportunities for new alliances with the field of philosophy. A manifold of challenges are issued from the side of communication studies, including investigations of the social sources of human knowledge, strategies of argumentation, relation of theory and practice, and the implications of all these for ethics.

These considerations, as even the novice of philosophical discourse quickly recognizes, are considerations that have preoccupied philosophers since the beginning of their discipline. Indeed, to know and to communicate are not as neatly separable as some of the architects of modem philosophy had assumed.

The Purdue University Press Series in Philosophy/Communication provides opportunities for explorations, deliberations, and investigations across the terrains of those disciplines that deal with issues concerning the intersections of philosophical and communicative practice. It seems unlikely that major new advances could be made in either field without considerations drawn from what each offers the other.

There are well-worn paths for familiar professional studies that remain inside historical and institutionalized boundaries. This series is on a different route, one that takes its new direction at a multidisciplinary intersection that might well lead to post-disciplinary destinations fitting to the university in particular and the larger intellectual life in general at the dawn of the millennium.

—Calvin O. Schrag
George Ade Distinguished Professor of
Philosophy Emeritus, Purdue University

—Ramsey Eric Ramsey
Philosophy/Communication Series Editor

Preface

The idea for this book came to mind while I was completing its predecessor, *The Call of Conscience: Heidegger and Levinas, Rhetoric and the Euthanasia Debate.*[1] There, in light of a critical assessment of Martin Heidegger's and Emmanuel Levinas's respective phenomenological investigations of the workings of conscience, I examined the relationship between this phenomenon and the practice of rhetoric. I then went on to analyze how the relationship shows itself in the ongoing debate in the United States over the justifiability and social acceptability of euthanasia and physician-assisted suicide. In this debate, no matter whether people are on the side of the "right to die" or the "right to life," the issue of acknowledgment is right in one's face.

The ontological assault of a life-threatening illness or accident disrupts a person's conditioned and typical ways of understanding and inhabiting the world. This disruption, in turn, incites anxiety over the question of the person's Being—his or her *ability to be.* In anxiety one stands face-to-face with the not-yet of the future, trying to decide about what is to become of his or her existence now that it is no longer what it used to be and perhaps may never be again. This is what makes the experience of anxiety so disquieting and so dreadful, and thus quite distinctive: More than any other emotion, anxiety reveals the ontological fact that one's ability to be is finite and thus fated to breakdown. With life comes death—the ultimate source of anxiety. Situations of life and death emit a "call of conscience"—a call that summons a person (qua patient) and his or her loved ones and caretakers to assume the ethical responsibility of affirming their freedom through resolute choice in order to reestablish a sense of meaning, order, and control in their lives. The patient's pain, suffering, and expressed desire to live or to die enhance the call's moral urgency: "Where art thou?" The euthanasia debate is informed by the rhetoric of those who come into conflict as they argue for the most "humane" way to attend to the patient's circumstances and requests, to say "Here I am!" to one who is in desperate need of help and whose wounded presence is likely to make others wonder anxiously about what life would be like if nobody cared enough to acknowledge their existence.

My involvement in and study of the euthanasia debate confirmed time and again the importance of what I will continue to term here the life-giving gift of acknowledgment. Being all alone when you are sick and dying is a terrible way to live and a terrible way to go. Such is the case whether the patient's call of "Where art thou?" is intended as a plea for life or for death. Although it may sound strange to speak of the life-giving gift of acknowledgment when considering the second alternative, the rhetoric of the euthanasia debate, especially as it comes from the advocates of the right to die, emphasizes the existential legitimacy of the juxtaposition. Hence, the argument that helping one to die with dignity does not merely put an end to dignity; rather, it also may help both to demonstrate and to serve as a reminder of this virtue's essential worth. Being the ultimate sacrifice, dying with dignity can define a holy act (*sacer facere*, "to make holy")—one that not only allows a patient a last chance for taking some control over the final chapter of his or her life-story before it is too late, but also one that pays homage to the "good life" of others and their need for stories that, as much as possible, have a good ending. Self-respecting human beings who hold a loving concern for others have an interest in the kind of memories that will survive after death. When they call out "Where art thou?" and request release, we owe it to them to say "Here I am!" It is a matter of mercy, not murder; a matter that calls for the life-giving gift of acknowledgment as a way of being for others who want to be remembered for the way they lived and died with dignity rather then for the way they ended up suffering in a prolonged and abject state of "living death." Human beings have a desire to *live on* in the *fond* memories of others.

Although I am not one who favors the legalization of euthanasia and physician-assisted suicide, at least at the present time, I am taken with the above argument. For the various ways the argument is made known in the rhetoric of the euthanasia debate attests to the *ontological significance* of acknowledgment. I write about this phenomenon here not only because there is more to say about it than I have said in the past, but also because in talking about it with students, colleagues, family, other close friends, and members of academic and non-academic audiences, I became convinced that, despite the crucial role acknowledgment plays in our lives, it remains a topic that is all too easily taken for granted, forgotten, and even forsaken until the lack of it in our lives threatens our well-being—and then it sometimes is too late to fix all (or any) of the hurt.

We need acknowledgment as much as we need such other easily taken for granted things as air, blood, and a beating heart. Without the life-giving gift of acknowledgment, we are destined to exist in ways that are marked by the loneliness of what I describe as "social death." One senses the presence of this state of being, for example, in the lives of college students who "don't fit in with the crowd" or who are suffering from a disturbance brought on by breaking up with their girlfriend or boyfriend. "Where art thou?" Not hearing a familiar "Here I am!" can sometimes even lead a young person to admit that he or she "feels like dying." Like their teachers who publish so as not to *perish* and who then worry incessantly over who, if anyone, is even reading their work, students are an especially vulnerable population when it comes to dealing with the hurt of being unacknowledged by their peers (*and*, to be sure, their teachers).

The life-giving gift of acknowledgment reveals itself in the midst of everyday existential disturbances that, even if they are less powerful and anxiety provoking than a serious illness or accident, are still "death-like" in how they bring something in our lives to at least a momentary end and thereby call into question our well-being. As creatures whose evolutionary progress remains at the point where death and its approximations give rise to the dreaded emotion of anxiety, it is not "unnatural" for us to want to avoid thinking about the ontological significance and workings of acknowledgment. The euthanasia debate provides a constant reminder of how such "uncourageous" behavior can prove to be disastrous at a moment's notice.

What I have to say here about the scope and function of acknowledgment is intended to extend both the depth and breadth of the observations that I made about the phenomenon when considering the role it plays in the rhetoric of the euthanasia debate. I thus will have more to say about the origins of acknowledgment; how it operates as a form of consciousness that transforms time and space into dwelling places where people can feel at home; how this transformation is facilitated by the rhetorical competence of human beings; how an appropriate use of such competence happens as an acknowledging caress; how the refusal to engage in this caress contributes to the disease of social death; how postmodern culture, with its computer revolution, offers itself as a *pharmakon* in the treatment of this specific ailment; and how the rhetorical accomplishment of acknowledgment, especially in times of crisis, speaks of the importance of humankind's ability to have a way with words dedicated to showing-forth the truth of matters of importance. When all is said and done, the reader will have been told a story about the life-giving capacity of the workings of acknowledgment. There is "hope" to be found in this story—the very thing that such noteworthy intellectuals as George Steiner, in his *Grammars of Creation*, maintains has been made "problematic" by sociopolitical, scientific, and philosophical developments happening throughout the twentieth century.[2] More will be said about Steiner's position in chapter 1.

Both Heidegger and Levinas once again provide philosophical direction for the narrative. Rhetorical theory, religion, and science continue to be sources of inspiration. I also occasionally draw insights from the literatures of architectural design and evolutionary psychology. The various case studies that are presented to illustrate in a concrete way all the theory going on here are drawn from nonfictional and fictional literature, poetry, film, history, politics, the world of computer technology, and the hellish happenings of terrorism. With these case studies I also will be offering rhetorical artifacts that both display and speak to the importance of the specific type of competence that facilitates the giving and receiving of the gift of acknowledgment.

I realize, of course, that with such a wide range of sources of inspiration and case studies I risk telling a story that is unwieldy. This risk, however, is worth it. Acknowledgment warrants respect as a robust phenomenon that brings life to people and their social and political relationships. This way of thinking about acknowledgment aligns the phenomenon with such key terms in communication and rhetorical theory as "affirmation" and "validation." Gregory Bateson's general theory of communication, for example, which culminated in the double-bind theory of schizophrenia, in effect describes what happens when a child repeatedly is not affirmed, validated, or acknowledged.[3] Another highly influential orientation towards acknowledgment employed by communication and rhetorical scholars is found in Martin Buber's theory of "confirmation":

> The basis of a man's life with man is twofold, and it is one—the wish of every man to be confirmed as what he is, even as what he can become, by men; and the innate capacity in man to confirm his fellow men in this way. That this capacity lies so immeasurably fallow constitutes the real weakness and questionableness of the human race: actual humanity exists only where this capacity unfolds. On the other hand, of course, an empty claim for confirmation, without devotion for being and becoming, again and again mars the truth of the life between man and man.[4]

Psychological researchers R. D. Laing, Paul Watzlawick, and Evelyn Sieburg bring together the work of Bateson and Buber in their respective examinations of the various nuances of the human need for confirmation. For example, some people, given their particular "psychological makeup" and family situations, need validation more than others; some actions can be affirmed on one level while being simultaneously disconfirmed on another; some people are more, some less, sensitive to not being acknowledged.[5] Buber's theory is especially prominent in the writings of communication theorists Kenneth Cissna, Rob Anderson, and Ronald Arnett, who all emphasize how confirmation informs and is informed by our everyday "dialogical" interactions.[6]

With their various research projects, all of these authors help to address the problem referred to above by Buber regarding how the capacity for confirmation "lies so immeasurably fallow." I agree with this observation; I am thus supportive of the theory and research offered by these authors. I believe, however, that more can be specified about the fundamental workings of acknowledgment than what one finds in these authors' writings. The capacity of "confirmation" or "affirmation" or "validation" retains something of a "fallow" character as long as its essential (ontological) nature remains under-theorized and thus un-clarified. An ontological assessment of the life-giving gift of acknowledgment is thus warranted.[7] Such an assessment emphasizes how acknowledgment is something that should never be taken for granted, forgotten, or forsaken for too long of a time. To make such a mistake is to put others and ourselves in uncomfortable, if not dangerous, situations. Granted, the lesson is at least as old as the biblical story of Adam and Eve and their anxious response to One who, with a simple question ("Where art thou?"), demanded acknowledgment. I believe, however, that we are still in need of learning how to improve our ability to offer a genuine response for the sake of others as well as ourselves. Evolution continues and so must the ethics and rhetoric that help guide its moral direction.

Based on reactions I have received from academic and nonacademic audiences who have heard some of what can be read here, I suspect that there will be certain observations about acknowledgment that strike readers as being "obvious." I certainly hope that this is the case, especially given my claim about the ontological significance of the phenomenon. The reader who comes away from this book "dazzled" by all that it has to offer will have to admit that he or she is *really* lacking in an understanding of something that is essential to the good health of humanity. I would find such a person to be a bit "scary." The smiles, chuckles, and nervous laughter that I have perceived coming from audiences who have heard me admit as much is reassuring. Is there anyone out there who has *no* appreciation for the life-giving capacity of acknowledgment? Is there anyone out there who is certain that he or she knows *everything* there is to know about the phenomenon? I possess no such wisdom. Still, I hope that at least some of what I have to say about acknowledgment is enlightening—even to those who take great pride in knowing themselves to be the kind of people who are *always* there to say "Here I am!" when they hear a call for help.

Chapter One

Introduction

The Question of Acknowledgment

What would life be like if no one *acknowledged* your existence? The question confronts one with the possibility of being isolated, marginalized, ignored, and forgotten by others. The unacknowledged find themselves in an "out-of-the-way" place where it is hard for human beings, given their social instinct, to feel at home. The suffering that can accompany this way of being-in-the-world is known to bring about fear, anxiety, sadness, anger, and sometimes even death in the form of suicide or retaliation against those who are rightly or wrongly accused of making one's life so lonely, miserable, and unbearable.

Acknowledgment provides an opening out of such a distressful situation, for the act of acknowledging is a communicative behavior that grants attention to others and thereby makes room for them in our lives. With this added living space comes the opportunity for a new beginning, a "second chance" whereby one might improve his or her lot in life. There is hope to be found with this transformation of space and time as people of conscience opt to go out of their way to make us feel wanted and needed, to praise our presence and actions, and thus to acknowledge the worthiness of our existence. Offering positive acknowledgment is a moral thing to do.

Granted, such acknowledgment may embarrass us, and it might even make us feel guilty if we know that our presence and actions have something deceitful about them or, at least in our humble opinion, are not really that great. But generally speaking, positive acknowledgment makes us feel good, as it recognizes something about our being that is felt by others to be worthy of praise and perhaps even remembrance after we are gone. Indeed, have you ever thought about your own death, your funeral, and who might show up to pay their respects? And when thinking about this last matter, have you ever become upset with those people who you believe should have attended the ceremony but did not? Even when we have passed to the most out-of-the-way place there is, we still crave the goodness of positive acknowledgment—the way it brings us to mind and thus, in a sense, keeps us "alive." Following Ernest Becker, then, one might say that acknowledgment provides a way to satisfy a human being's "urge to immortality"—an urge that "is not a simple reflex of the death anxiety but a reaching out by one's whole being toward life . . . , a reaching-out for a plenitude of meaning. . . . It seems that the life force reaches naturally even beyond the earth itself, which is one reason why man has always placed God in the heavens."[1]

Of course, not all acknowledgment that comes our way is positive. For example, hearing someone say "Looking good" to you in a certain situation may be understood correctly as a compliment. In a different situation, however, these same words, coming from someone with whom you have never gotten along, might also be legitimately heard as a sarcasm, a slight, an articulation whose tone of voice speaks ridicule, disrespect, and dislike. Such negative acknowledgment is also at work whenever we call people "stupid" or "worthless," thereby opening and exposing them to the further ridicule of others. Like its opposite, negative acknowledgment creates a place for being noticed. But the space created here, even if it is made with the best of intentions—as when a parent, trying to provide careful guidance, scolds a child for being "naughty"—more often than not makes us feel bad.[2]

Acknowledgment is a significant and powerful form of behavior, one that can bring joy to a person's heart and also drive a stake through it. Acknowledgment functions as both a life-giving gift and a life-draining force. Moving from its positive to negative form and then to a state of no acknowledgment at all, we find ourselves in a place that is hard-pressed to support life because it is so barren of the nourishment provided by the caring concern of others. Institutionalized forms of negative acknowledgment such as racism, sexism, and ageism expose people to this fate. Certain rituals of culture, on the other hand, are meant to protect us from it. Proper decorum dictates, for example, that we say "hello" and "goodbye" to people so that they feel noticed; that we make them feel important and respected by simply holding open a door and saying "after you"; or that we send them a birthday or condolence card to assure them that, at a moment of great joy or great distress, they are in our thoughts and perhaps our prayers. The presence of people in need of acknowledgment sounds a call of conscience: "Where art thou?" Good manners encourage us to say, "Here I am!" Knowing or at least believing that this response truly "comes from the heart," others are likely to feel better than if they know or believe that what they are receiving is mostly some ritualized behavior steeped in the shallows of unthinking habit rather than in the depths of genuine care.

The difference in "feeling" being noted here corresponds to what I take to be the essential difference that exists between the phenomena of acknowledgment and simple "recognition." People often speak of these two phenomena as if they were one in the same. For the purposes of the current project, however, their difference must be kept in mind.[3] Consider the following example, which describes an interaction that I suspect most readers have had in their lives.

Acknowledgment and Recognition

While walking down the street, John notices a person approaching him whom he recognizes to be an old acquaintance, Mary. She notices and recognizes John, too, and they greet each other with "heys!" and some gentle pats on the back. "Long time no see. How've you been? What's going on?" asks Mary. John's reply is simple: "Great! Nothing much. I am just heading to my office." John then asks Mary the same questions as a way of being polite, hoping that her reply will be equally economical, for John has many things to do today at the office and he is not much in the mood for conversation.

Not having made this point clear to Mary, however, John begins to hear answers that he senses might be too involved and time-consuming for his immediate purposes. John displays some non-verbal cues (looking away from Mary's face and shifting his body from side to side) that, as far as he is concerned, are commonsensical enough to be read as a clear but still polite indication that "now is not the time to get into all of this stuff." For whatever reason, however, Mary is determined to share with John what is on her mind, and, therefore, she disregards or perhaps remains oblivious to his cues. After another fifteen seconds of "listening" to her speak, John feels compelled to interrupt at an "appropriate" moment with a not entirely truthful excuse: "Mary, I'm sorry, but I have an appointment that I can't miss. How about if I try to give you a call later this week and maybe we can arrange to do lunch." "Of course," says Mary. "I look forward to hearing from you. Really, let's get together."

Mary is being genuine with this last request. She is seeking more than the recognition that John has given her so far; she is looking forward to the added space and time, the openness, that comes with John's acknowledgment of her and that provides a "dwelling place" (*ethos*) for developing a more caring conversation. This *ethos* of acknowledgment establishes an environment wherein people can take the time to "know together" (*con-scientia*) some topic of interest and, in the process, perhaps gain a more authentic understanding of those who are willing to contribute to its development. Recognition is only a preliminary step in this process of attuning one's consciousness toward another and his or her expression of a topic in order to facilitate the development of such existential knowledge and personal understanding. Acknowledgment requires a sustained openness to others even if, at times, things become boring or troublesome.[4]

Such openness is what Mary wanted and was willing to give. John, on the other hand, opted to keep the relationship in a state of simple recognition—a state that at least gives the impression that one is being noticed and that genuine acknowledgment is thus a possibility. If this possibility is negated by John's decision not to call Mary later in the week, then she has evidence that might rightly lead her to think that the extent of John's acknowledgment of her was more of a ruse than anything else. "Where art thou?" John offers no "Here I am!"

In his related investigations of the nature of skepticism and the dynamics of tragedy, Stanley Cavell teaches that "the alternative to my acknowledgment of the other is not my ignorance of him but my avoidance of him, call it my denial of him." Moreover, Cavell contends that acknowledgment, and not just mere recognition, is "something owed another simply as a human being, the failure of which reveals the failure of one's own humanity."[5] I agree with both of these statements. John's behavior is an affront to Mary's being. He owes her an apology: "I know I was wrong not to get back in touch with you, Mary." As Cavell points out, to say "I know" in this case "is to admit, confess, *acknowledge*."[6] With his apology John *opens* himself to Mary, *reveals* that he *knows* himself to be guilty of a wrongdoing that most likely was harmful to her well-being, and thereby acknowledges and *affirms* Mary's existence—"Here I am!"—by granting her the time and space, the dwelling place, that is needed for her to offer an "appropriate" response. Following Cavell, one could now describe John as a person who has "shown his humanity."

Mary, of course, will be the judge of this display of humanity as she decides whether John's apology does in fact "come from the heart," whether he is truly sorry, and whether this time he is, indeed, offering her the life-giving gift of acknowledgment and not just another mere moment of manipulating recognition. For Cavell, our everyday understanding of the world stabilizes itself in our "agreements of judgment" about the authenticity of acknowledgments that are offered by ourselves and others for the purpose of giving meaningful and moral direction to all that we say and do. In other words, the stability of any given symbolic order presupposes a process of people working together to acknowledge their acknowledgments and to agree on or question the "truth" of these acknowledgments. Ludwig Wittgenstein, whose philosophical investigations of language-use informs Cavell's take on the matter, puts it this way: "Knowledge is in the end based on acknowledgments."[7] Cavell writes in the hope that readers will acknowledge the sensibleness of his stance on acknowledgment and thereby agree with his earlier quoted claim that, in the name of humanity, acknowledgment is "something owed another simply as a human being."

Indeed, acknowledgment *is* a life-giving gift; it makes possible the moral development of recognition. This different way of stating the claim is significant for my purposes. Throughout this book I attempt to go further than Cavell in acknowledging the scope and function of acknowledgment by focusing on its life-giving capacity—a capacity that enables us to be open to the world of people, places, and things such that we can "admit" (Middle English: *acknow*) its wonders into our minds and then "admit" (Middle English: *knowlechen*) to others the understanding we have gained and that we believe is worth sharing.[8] *The project is undertaken with the belief that the phenomenon of acknowledgment ought to warrant careful and continual attention from anyone whose life would suffer without it.* This belief is certainly affirmed, for example, by social scientific research dealing with the therapeutic effects of "supportive communication" in healthcare, family, and organizational settings.[9] I, too, am interested in such effects, although my appreciation of them follows from a phenomenological understanding of acknowledgment. What is revealed here about the phenomenon is thus directed toward certain of its essential (ontological) aspects whose existential robustness is too often left unacknowledged and thus unappreciated when the measurement of effects is given priority in the scientific study of the phenomenon. I have pointed to certain of these aspects in the discussion so far. They include such things as time, space, openness, emotion, discourse, conscience, and the alterity or otherness of others that necessarily is a part of social existence. All of these things and acknowledgment go hand in hand; the "evolution" of the relationship is essential to the communal spirit and moral well-being of humankind.[10]

In developing this last point throughout the book, I, at the same time, will be making an argument for the importance of people becoming ever more "competent" in the practice of acknowledgment. I thus must be clear at the outset about my understanding and use of this term.

Acknowledgment and Rhetoric

Beginning at least with the ancient Sophists, the study and the teaching of such competence has been associated with the "art of rhetoric"—a practical art that, once Socrates, Plato, Aristotle, and Cicero all had their say about it, was appreciated as a type of "know how," a complex competence that gives expression to our ability to inspire critical judgment about contestable matters, to encourage collaborative deliberation, and to be persuasive. Rhetoric is at work whenever language is being employed to *open* people to ideas, positions, and circumstances that, if rightly understood, stand a better than even chance of getting people to think and act wisely. Orators are forever attempting to create these openings, for this is how they maximize the chance that the members of some audience will take an interest in what is being said. Neither persuasion nor collaborative deliberation can take place without the formation of this joint interest. "We interest a man by dealing with his interests," writes Kenneth Burke.[11] Indeed, and acknowledgment happens as such dealing takes place. The "good" speaker is always seeking acknowledgment from some audience whose "good" members are also waiting for the speaker to acknowledge their interests in some meaningful way. In short, rhetorical competence has a significant role to play in providing places (openings) where a life-giving gift can be received.

For those who are in the habit of thinking about rhetoric in only a pejorative way—that is, for example, as it was used by John to deceive Mary—the present project may seem to be, to say the least, a bit wrongheaded. I hope, however, that when all is said and done I am not merely understood to be claiming something akin to what Gorgias supposedly once said about the power and importance of rhetoric when defending his "craft" to Socrates: ". . . if a rhetorician and a doctor visited any city you like to name and they had to contend in argument before the Assembly or any other gathering as to which of the two should be chosen as doctor, the doctor would be nowhere, but the man who could speak would be chosen, if he so wished."[12] Such a claim, to be sure, is sophistry gone too far, an unfortunate burst of egoism coming from a theorist, teacher, and practitioner of an art that was then, and still is now, in need of positive acknowledgment from its detractors. The art of rhetoric is fated to admit a defensive posture as long as its material is used in unethical ways and for immoral purposes. Still, I think it warrants praise for its potential for creating places where acknowledgment can happen and flourish.

Gorgias was a master when it came to putting to use this inventive capacity of rhetoric. And so was Abraham Lincoln, although, unlike Gorgias, Lincoln did believe in the importance and legitimacy of seeking, finding, and articulating the truth about matters of importance. Consider, for example, his Gettysburg Address, a short piece of oratory whose 272 words are now widely recognized as having "remade America."[13] Lincoln performed this rhetorical feat by creating a particular opening where his present and ever-growing future audience could recognize and know together the honorable deeds of others. The opening that is created in the Address allows for the appropriate amount of aesthetic distance to form between Lincoln's subject matter and his audience. Commenting on this specific artistic and rhetorical happening, Richard Weaver notes: "If one sees an object from too close, one sees only its irregularities and protuberances. To see an object right or to see it as a whole, one has to have a proportioned distance from it." Weaver then goes on to claim that "at Gettysburg, Lincoln spoke in terms so 'generic' that it is almost impossible to show that the speech is not a eulogy of the men in grey as well as the men in blue, inasmuch as both made up 'those who struggled here.' Lincoln's faculty of transcending an occasion [like Gettysburg] is in fact only this ability to view it [rhetorically] from the right distance, or to be wisely generic about it."[14]

I agree with Weaver's assessment of Lincoln. Moreover, like Weaver and many others, I think of Lincoln as exemplifying what the orator is obligated to be: "the ethical teacher of society," or what Weaver elsewhere describes as a "doctor of culture."[15] Lincoln was and remains such a person because he possessed the requisite rhetorical competence needed to create the openings of places where the "truth" and thus the awesomeness of objects, events, and people could be rightly acknowledged. This is the standard of competence that I will have in mind when discussing the particular communicative behavior in question here. Be it positive or negative, the genuine expression of acknowledgment must always make at least some use of the human capacity of rhetorical competence. That this fact of life has long been and will continue to be taken advantage of by people with evil intentions defines yet another good reason for investigating the nature of acknowledgment—what it is and how it functions. I hope to show that genuine acknowledgment is informed by an ontological impulse that points people in the direction of "the good and the just." I also hope to make clear how rhetoric that fails to serve this end is not being true to its essence, which consists of being a tool for acknowledgment—something that is necessary for the well-being of humankind.

Acknowledgment, Creation, and Hope

The story I have to tell about the ontological and rhetorical workings of acknowledgment speaks of creation and hope. Acknowledgment is a moral act; it functions to transform space and time, to *create* openings wherein people can dwell, deliberate, and know together what is right, good, just, and truthful. Acknowledgment thereby grants people *hope*, the opportunity for a new beginning, a second chance, whereby they might improve their lot in life. In developing these points throughout the remaining chapters of this book, I will thus be addressing the concerns of and offering a critical response to those who, like the literary theorist, critic, and philosopher George Steiner, contend that

> The twentieth century has put in doubt the theological, the philosophical and the political-material insurance for hope. It queries the rationale and credibility of future tenses. . . .Who except fundamentalists now awaits the actual coming of a Messiah? Who except literalists of a lost communism or anarcho-socialist Arcadia now awaits the actual re-birth of history? . . . Grammars of nihilism flicker . . . on the horizon.[16]

Steiner takes "grammar" to mean "the articulate organization of perception, reflections and experience, the nerve structure of consciousness when it communicates with itself and with others" (*GC* 6). The "grammar" of the Judeo-Christian theory of creation provides the most well-known and hopeful world-view. Steiner emphasizes, however, that this grammar has been called into question by the "violence, oppression, economic enslavement and social irrationality" that have transpired over the last century. Moreover, he notes, the "grammar" of science offered by the "new cosmologies regard 'creation' as being ambiguous, mythological, and even taboo. To ask what preceded the Big Bang and the primal nanoseconds of the

compaction and expansion of our universe is, we are instructed, to talk gibberish"
(*GC* 336). Steiner also identifies the "postmodern" literary and philosophical projects of "deconstruction" that seek direction from such thinkers as Jacques Derrida
to be additional sources of discontent when it comes to an appreciation of "origins" and "beginnings" made possible by the presence of some Supreme reason or
by the genius of creative artists. "Deconstruction, in today's critical theories of
meaning, is . . . an 'un-building' of those classical models of meaning which assumed the existence of a precedent *auctoritas*, of a master-builder. There are in
Derridean deconstruction neither 'fathers' nor beginnings" (*GC* 22–23).

Of these two grammars of nihilism, Steiner objects most strenuously to the
first. Near the end of his work he thus does not hesitate to claim that

> Both elementary logic and common sense should tell us that [sci-
> ence's] ruling [about the "nothingness" that came before the Big
> Bang] is arrogant bluff. The simple fact that we can phrase the ques-
> tion, that we can engage it with normal thought processes, gives it
> meaning and legitimacy. The postulate of unquestionable ("not to
> be questioned") nothingness and intemporality now made dogma
> by astrophysicists is as arbitrary, is in many regards more of a mys-
> tique, than are creation narratives in Genesis and elsewhere. The
> reasoned intuition of a coming into being which we do not under-
> stand, but whose efficacy suggests itself via the analogies of human
> creativity [as seen in the arts, for example], has lost none of its chal-
> lenge. . . . The God-hypothesis will not be mocked without cost.
> (*GC* 336)

Steiner wrote his book to substantiate and dramatize this last point—one
that is phrased in an especially self-revealing way in the book's final sentences: "We
have long been, I believe that we still are, guests of creation. We owe to our host
the courtesy of questioning" (*GC* 338). This assertion harkens back in a challenging, albeit indirect, manner to the book's first sentence, which records the author's
assessment of our present-day postmodern condition: "We have no more beginnings" (*GC* 2). The assertion also reflects Steiner's Judaic heritage and its teachings
on the importance of hearing and responding to "the Word" uttered "in the beginning." Steiner puts it this way:

> Speech demands a listener and, if possible, a respondent. To whom
> does God say, in Genesis I, 26, *naase adam*—"let us make man"? To
> His own solitude at the very hour in which that solitude is to be
> broken by the creation of man-the-listener, of man-the-respondent
> and gainsayer. In echoing turn, human speech declares its origins in
> transcendent dialogue. We speak because we were called upon to
> answer; language is, in the root sense, a "vocation." (*GC* 34)

Caught up in this vocation, human beings show themselves to be, among other things, the questioning animal—"*homo quaerens*, the animal that asks and asks" and, in so doing, affirms the presence, the "otherness," of what is "out there," something that needs to be understood for the purpose of making the world as meaningful and as moral as possible (*GC* 20). The "God-hypothesis"—which comes to us from religion and which, as Steiner sees it, is granted feasibility in the wondrous, creative accomplishments of human beings—treats this otherness with the highest reverence.

> [The great] poet, playwright, or novelist names his characters as Adam names the animals around him; in either case, nomination entails both truth and "real" existence. The successful dramatist or story-teller or painter is "God" in large miniature. He or she ushers into the world agents out of the imaginary, out of some dust of pre-existence, whose subsequent fate, whose freedom of action can, precisely as in the mystery of free will accorded by God to His creations, challenge the maker. (*GC* 173)

As he continues to develop this analogy between religion and aesthetics, Steiner also would have us grant that, as is the case with "the Word,"

> It is the production and reception of works of art, in the widest sense, which enables us to share in the experiencing of duration, of time unbounded. Without the arts, the human psyche would stand naked in the face of personal extinction. Wherein would lie the logic of madness and despair. It is (again together with transcendent religious faith and, often, in a certain relation to it) *poiesis* which authorizes the unreason of hope.
>
> In that immensely significant sense, the arts are more indispensable to men and women than even the best of science and technology (innumerable societies have long endured without these). Creativity in the arts and in philosophic proposal is, in respect of the survival of consciousness, of another order than is invention in the sciences. We are an animal whose life-breath is that of spoken, painted, sculptured, sung dreams. . . . Truth is, indeed, with the equation and the axiom; but it is a lesser truth. (*GC* 259)

As *homo quaerens*, who perhaps has yet to abandon all hope for a better world, Steiner would have us keep in mind and once again learn to appreciate the greater truth—if not for God's sake then at least for the sake of the arts and humanities and whatever is left of their "grammars of creation."

The story I have to tell about the ontological and rhetorical workings of acknowledgment contains its own grammar of creation, wherein lies the story's sense of hope. Acknowledgment *is* a conscious act of creation that marks an origin, a beginning, an opening in space-time where people can feel at home as they dwell, deliberate, and know together. Emotion and discourse play a fundamental role in the creation and maintenance of this moral place of being-with-and-for-others, a place where the giving and receiving of a caring word and heartfelt caress can grant a sense of hope to all concerned. With the workings of acknowledgment at hand it is incorrect to say, contrary to Steiner's contention, that "We have no more beginnings." In fact, as I hope to show, these workings are so much a part of the ontological structure of human existence that no "grammar of nihilism"—be it of the scientific or deconstructive kind—can deny their life-giving capacity. On the contrary, the doing of "good" science and "good" deconstruction presupposes the presence and vitality of acknowledgment.[17]

In differing with Steiner on these matters, I will have occasion, as he does, to introduce Western religion into the unfolding story of acknowledgment. For this specific phenomenon, being what it is and doing what it does, necessarily brings to mind a central question of religion regarding what it means to be a "beginning" arising from a creative act. How is acknowledgment possible? How can it be that human beings are capable of opening themselves to others, of responding "Here I am" to a call for help ("Where art thou?")? My phenomenological treatment of these questions will require that I, as much as possible, keep my nose to the empirical grindstone. In so doing, I will discuss how the ontological structure of existence that makes possible acknowledgment—*and thus its use by any institutionalized religion*—is also an originating force for the human propensity to wonder about "who we really are" and "where we really came from."[18] Scientists who are interested in the occurrence of the Big Bang and related phenomena (e.g., singularities, black holes) take us a *long* way in answering these questions, for they are trained to be expert acknowledgers, and if they have a tolerance for the metaphysical, they may even end up contributing to the grammar and rhetoric of what has come to be called "theistic science" or the theory of "intelligent design." Steiner omits any discussion of this field of study, which contests the bifurcation between science and religion that one finds in his work. A phenomenological assessment of acknowledgment, however, encourages one not only to take an interest in this field but also *to try to keep the conversation going* between science and religion—even when their respective advocates have had enough and are fed up with their interlocutors' ways of thinking. Remember, the story of acknowledgment speaks of creation and hope.

Chapter Outline

In chapter 2, I begin developing a phenomenological appreciation of acknowledgment by focusing on how the phenomenon itself *begins* as an act that transforms space and time with the creation of its openings, its places *to be*. A discussion of a short story by Annie Dillard initiates the inquiry. I then have occasion to consider certain theories of the "beginning" drawn from religion and science as a way of clarifying the "origin" and "awesomeness" of the phenomenon of acknowledgment. Here I speculate on the relationship that might exist between acknowledgment, God, and the Big Bang—a relationship that invites consideration as a way of explaining how it is that the evolution of the universe allows for beings whose capacity for consciousness enables them to acknowledge and to be awed by its wonders.

When considering the possibility of this relationship I will have occasion to discuss briefly such scientific matters as the evolution of stars and their demise into "black holes" in order to help readers comprehend the complexity and vastness of the universe in which we live. Despite the counterclaims made by scientists, the awesomeness of the universe is alleged by religious souls to have initially materialized with the acknowledging Word of One, who also demands acknowledgment. Please note, however, that the guidance I seek from science is not intended to dismiss religion but rather to help to ensure that the "Mystery" that informs and guides its teachings is thought about in a rigorous and respectful way. This is not to say that my assessment of acknowledgment is designed to set readers on a path toward an ultimate metaphysical realm or kingdom where "the truth will set you free." Although I am interested in the truth of acknowledgment, this interest does not necessarily make one a "true believer." It does, however, require that I remain open to both religion and science and the stories that each has to tell us about how it *all* began. As will be emphasized and clarified throughout this book, acknowledgment demands such openness on the part of those who wish to comprehend its scope and function. Such openness defines the act of consciousness that is at work when one is awestruck by the wonder of it all. Neither "honest to goodness" religion nor "honest to goodness" science could exist without the workings of this act.

In chapter 3, I continue to address this matter by focusing more closely on the consciousness that prevails when acknowledgment is at work and that converts "seeing" (recognition) into "observation." Here I am guided primarily by Martin Heidegger's phenomenological investigations of the meaning and truth of Being. With these investigations, Heidegger helps to make clear that the question of Being is one that necessitates giving serious consideration to the nature and function of acknowledgment, especially its "emotional" workings and the way they "attune" us to our surroundings.

Chapter 4 offers an examination of how the production of discourse that gives expression to such attunement helps to construct and secure "dwelling places" wherein human beings can seek and find the life-giving gift of acknowledgment. In developing this topic I also make much of the role played by the "appropriateness" of rhetoric—especially its "epideictic" form—in the creation, maintenance, and reconstruction of these dwelling places. The topics of religion and science will once again be referenced as resources that can provide direction for thinking about the scope and function of epideictic rhetoric and its relationship with the workings of acknowledgment.

Chapter 5 extends the consideration of this matter with a specific assessment of how the workings of acknowledgment function rhetorically to transform a dwelling place into a "home." The home is where acknowledgment should thrive; it is, or at least it should be, a moral environment. I develop this point with the help of architectural design theory and by way of a rhetorical assessment of Robert Frost's "The Death of the Hired Man." When Frost ends this poem the reader is left to ponder, among other things, how the human "caress" facilitates the workings of acknowledgment, making us feel at home.

Chapter 6 presents a detailed assessment of the ontological, metaphysical, and rhetorical nature of the caress. The assessment is grounded primarily in Emmanuel Levinas's phenomenological investigations of the phenomenon. I consider Levinas's philosophy of the caress to be most instructive when it comes to revealing the way in which acknowledgment defines a particular interpersonal transaction wherein a question is raised—"Where art thou?"—and an answer is expected: "Here I am!" The ethical workings of this transaction emphasize how the "self" has an obligation "to be for others." As is seen in Levinas's philosophy of the "caress," this obligation announces itself as a hallmark of "postmodern" philosophy, with its emphasis on the importance of the "otherness" or "alterity" that characterizes the fundamental nature of human existence. What Levinas fails to clarify with his philosophy of the caress, however, is an issue of significant rhetorical and practical importance: the "appropriateness" of actually engaging in a caress.

I attend to this issue in chapter 7 by offering a case study of the award-winning film *Ordinary People*—a work of art that holds its audience in a rhetorically designed caress while at the same time telling a true-to-life and moving story about the existential workings of the phenomenon and its relationship with the life-giving gift of acknowledgment. In assessing this work of art, I will also begin making a case for the value of "entertainment" as a pedagogical device that can enhance an appreciation of the pragmatics of acknowledgment. The instructive capacity of entertainment helps one to see how the rhetorically informed art of teaching and acknowledgment ought to go hand in hand.

Chapter 8 expands on this point with a discussion of how the essence of teaching *is* acknowledgment, how this essence grants teaching a "religious" quality, and how the teacher should thus be at one and the same time both a giver and a receiver of this particular life-giving gift. Standing in front of his or her students, the teacher is one who is always in the position of having to answer and raise a question: "Where art thou?" This exchange between teacher and student, I argue, encourages the realization that teaching, both inside and outside the classroom, is a life and death experience. As a way of appreciating the rhetorical dynamics of this experience and the acknowledgment that goes with it, I offer a critical reading of Mitch Albom's best-selling book *Tuesdays with Morrie*, which tells the true story of a much loved teacher who is dying and a student who attends the teacher's last course.

Chapter 9 is also concerned with the relationship between acknowledgment, teaching, and death. But here my attention is directed primarily toward a phenomenon—social death—that is not mentioned in Albom's book and that describes a state of being that materializes with what was described earlier as institutionalized forms of negative acknowledgment such a racism, sexism, and ageism. Social death and the rhetoric that sustains it marginalizes people and defaces the human spirit. The specific rhetoric of social death that will serve as a case study is found in the much publicized and ongoing controversy about the flying and the removal of the Confederate Battle Flag over the Statehouse in Columbia, South Carolina. This controversy not only illustrates the lingering disease of race relations in this country but also provides a case whose troublesome character is seen in how opposing groups of people, committed to teaching others about their respective positions, both do and say things to receive the life-giving gift of acknowledgment as well as to prevent the giving of this gift to the opposition. The desire for acknowledgment, which instructs us about the importance of being-for-others, can nevertheless encourage selfish behavior.

Chapter 10 extends a consideration of this predicament by offering a discussion of how acknowledgment is faring in today's postmodern, computer-oriented culture. Although academics are known for writing about postmodernity in a host of highly specialized and jargonized ways, the "meaning" of the term, when all is said and done, typically points to the need for people to be tolerant of personal differences, especially when these differences (as in the case of the Confederate Flag controversy) call into question well-rehearsed standards of taste, temperament, and truth. Such tolerance is praised for its open-mindedness and hence for the way it encourages acknowledgment. The computer revolution is attuned to this outlook. No technology in the history of humankind allows for and facilitates acknowledgment more than the personal computer. Cyberspace is teeming with rhetorically fashioned utterances and presentations from people who are searching for others who might be willing to answer a call—"Where art thou?"—with a welcoming response: "Here I am!" Would it thus be fair to describe the evolving computer revolution as being itself a life-giving gift? Many people and corporations would have us think so. I, however, will be a bit more cautious in addressing the question, as I provide various examples of how the computer is affecting humankind's need for acknowledgment. Here, too, I offer a brief case study of my university's involvement in the computer revolution to lend additional focus to the matter at hand.

Chapter 11 offers a discussion of how worthwhile it is to have a way with words that bring with them a life-giving gift. Acknowledgment and rhetorical competence go hand in hand. The evolution of moral consciousness, whereby selfishness is called into question, depends on the cultivation of this relationship. The rhetorical situation arising from the terrorist attack on the United States on September 11, 2001, will serve as my final illustration of this point, which I develop with the notion of the "rhetor as hero" in mind.

As should be clear with all that has been said so far, the treatment of acknowledgment offered here develops with the help of a wide range of resources: philosophy and rhetorical theory, to be sure; but also religion, science/cosmology, literature, poetry, architectural design theory, film, history and politics, the social and communicative dynamics of today's ongoing computer revolution, and an act of war. The way in which I weave these resources together as a narrative is intended to provide a robust appreciation of the life-giving gift of acknowledgment and the rhetorical competence that helps to make it happen. This gift certainly warrants such appreciation. Think about it: What would life be like if no one cared enough to take the time to acknowledge your existence and thereby to make a place for you in his or her life?

Chapter Two

In the Beginning

The Pulitzer Prize–winning author Annie Dillard writes of her encounter with someone who was in need of acknowledgment: a "little boy" who "looked to be about eight," whom she met while on a walk through the countryside near her Virginia home. It was January. Cold. She had a leg of lamb in the oven. "The idea was to exercise my limbs and rest my mind, but these things rarely work out as I plan."[1]

Dillard spotted the child from a hilltop lined with a barbed-wire fence. He was playing in his yard, pretending to write with a stone. His canvas was the tool shed wall. He alternated between this activity and fooling with the two family dogs from outside their pen. "The dogs were going crazy at their fence because of me, and I wondered why the boy didn't turn around; he must be too little to know much about dogs. When he did see me, by accident, his eyebrows shot up. I smiled and hollered and he came over to the barbed wire" (96).

They talked about the dogs and the dun mare and her new foal who stood outside the fenced horse barn. The child

> was formal and articulate; he spoke in whole sentences, choosing his words. "I haven't yet settled on a name for the foal, although Father says he is mine." When he spoke this way, he gazed up at me through meeting eyebrows. His dark lips made a projecting circle. He looked like a nineteenth century cartoon of an Earnest Child. This kid is a fraud, I thought. Who calls his father "Father"? But at other times his face would loosen; I could see then that the accustomed gesture of his lips resembled that of a person trying not to cry. Or he would smile, or look away shyly . . . (96–97)

Dillard wondered why she had allowed herself the encounter. "Wasn't there something I should be reading?" she asked herself. This question was interrupted as the boy asked another one: 'Do you know the Lord as your personal savior?' The question sparked a connecting memory in Dillard's mind; hence, she could reply with a bit of humor: 'Not only that,' she said, 'I know your mother.' The two had met about a year ago when Dillard visited the woman's house seeking permission to explore the land on her property: "The driveway made a circle in front of the house, and in the circle stood an eight-foot aluminum cross with a sign underneath it reading CHRIST THE LORD IS OUR SALVATION. Spotlights in the circle's honeysuckle were trained up at the cross and the sign" (97). When the woman met Dillard at the door she appeared nervous, displaying "the same trembling lashes as the boy. She wore a black dress and one brush roller in the front of her hair. She did not ask me in" (98).

The woman gave Dillard permission to walk the property and then, after an awkward pause, asked: "Do you know the Lord as your personal savior?" "My heart went out to her," writes Dillard. "No wonder she had been so nervous. She must have to ask this of everyone, absolutely everyone, she meets. That is Christian witness. It makes sense, given its premises. I wanted to make her as happy as possible, reward her courage, and run." Dillard reports that the woman

> was stunned that I knew the Lord, and clearly uncertain whether we were referring to the same third party. But she had done her bit, bumped over the hump, and now she could relax. She told me about her church, her face brightening. She was part of the Reverend Jerry Falwell's congregation . . . in Lynchburg, Virginia . . . . She drove, I inferred, 120 miles round trip to go to church. While I waited behind the screen door she fetched pamphlets, each a different color. I thanked her kindly; I read them later. The one on the Holy Spirit I thought was good. (98)

The child was glad to hear that Dillard had met his mother; it made him more comfortable, although each time she smiled or laughed he looked at her in a bewildered way. But he continued to talk. He never played at the nearby creek "because he might be down there, and Father might come home not knowing he was there, and let all the horses out, and the horses would trample him." He also told of the snakes he thought were in the creek. "Caution passes for wisdom around here," writes Dillard, "and this kid knew all the pitfalls" (99).

Dillard found herself trying to persuade the boy that the creek was worth exploring, at least in *her* opinion. Noticing that the boy's lips were turning blue from the cold, however, Dillard told him that she had to go. The boy pretended not to hear her. He asked Dillard if she knew how to fish. They chatted a little about fishing. Dillard again noted that she had to go. But as soon as she tried to turn away another question came forth: 'One more thing! . . . Did you ever step on a big old snake?' Dillard then admits to the reader: "All right, then, I thanked God for the sisters and friends I had had when I was little; I have not been lonely yet, but it could come at any time" (100).

The boy described the one time he had stepped on a snake: "We were walking through the field beneath the cemetery. I called. Wait, Father, wait! I couldn't lift my foot.' Dillard "wondered what they let him read; he spoke in prose, like a *le bourgeois gentilhomme.*" She asked him if he was scared when he stepped on the snake. He admitted that he was knee-deep in honeysuckle at the time and thus never really saw the creature. Dillard was now a bit skeptical and realized that "there was no way now to respond to his story all over again, identically but sincerely" (100). No matter, however, it *was* time to go. "We parted sadly. . . . The boy lowered his enormous, lighted eyes, lifted his shoulders, and went into a classic trudge. He had tried again to keep me there. But I simply had to go. It was dark, it was cold, and I had a roast in the oven, lamb, and I don't like it too well done" (101).

Annie Dillard is renowned for her way with words, especially when it comes to describing and interpreting things she has witnessed and keenly observed while dwelling in nature and with other people. I have hardly done her justice with my recounting of her story. I hope, however, that I have said enough to justify what I take to be her "meaning." She tells a story that prompts one to think about various related questions that are part of a larger one: What would life be like if no one acknowledged your existence, if no one took the time to open themselves to *you*, *your* situation, *your* concerns and needs? Fortunately, the little boy's situation is not that extreme. From afar he seems to be content pretending he is an artist, or a teller of tales, or at least a sign painter. He has the company of two dogs and two horses. His parents are alive, married, and together with God. He has been raised in an environment that has conditioned him to be an "Earnest Child" who listens not just to his father, but to his Father!—who, perhaps with his mother, put up an eight-foot spot lit aluminum cross in their front yard.

This is a very Christian family, one whose members cannot let a meeting with a stranger go too far before they ask a question: "Do you know the Lord as your personal savior?" The little boy, whose accustomed gesture of his lips made him look sad, asked the question soon after Dillard smiled at him and hollered hello. Her verbal and non-verbal response suggested a friendly acknowledgment, one that opened a space for some conversation that, as Dillard would soon realize, would go on too long for her purposes if this "lonely" little boy had his way.

Dillard was uncomfortable with such loneliness; she thanked God for a childhood filled with sisters and friends who helped prevent the feeling from having a place in her life. The boy's mother was remembered as also looking lonely, nervous, and cautious. She, too, had Dillard's attention once when she asked a holy question shortly after they had met. Dillard was moved and impressed with the mother's courage, but still she wanted to run—not away from religion per se, but away from another whose question posed an extreme test in acknowledgment. The mother was up for this test everyday. The more she asked the question the more she acknowledged One who was always there to acknowledge her. She need never feel lonely. Nervous and cautious, yes, but never lonely.

Dillard, it seems, has a hard time with this way of thinking. It is not right for her; and perhaps the same could be said about a boy who could be a kid (once?) again if only he thought differently, for example, about a creek, its wonders and inhabitants, and played there for a while. For the time being, however, Dillard had to provide an outlet with her presence and words of acknowledgment, creating a place where two strangers could become acquainted with each other.

Hence, Dillard's problem. She perceives the child's questions and tales to be functioning also as a call that reaches beyond religious doctrine and a barb-wired fence: Where art thou? Coming from this little boy, the call will necessarily have a religious aspect to it. But it is not all religion. He is not his Father or mother. He is only a kid whose imagination and need for human company have yet to be tamed completely. Yes, he "knows" the Lord is his savior, but that is not enough. He wants Dillard to stay with him. He welcomes the added living space that came with Dillard's taking the time to go out of her way and say hello. Her acknowledgment transforms the everyday spatial and temporal dimensions of his religiously oriented world. Somebody was there, outside the barbed wire, somebody who provided a break in his routines. This child was not alone, but still acted lonely, still asked "Where art thou?" And Dillard said "Here I am!"

But the space that opened with this acknowledgment was not a gift without conditions. As she began to think of the boy as a possible "fraud," Dillard's mind wandered to such things as reading material, the weather, and properly prepared food. Dillard certainly had the boy's welfare in mind, but not totally. The time and space that was needed by the child exceeded the constraints of Dillard's own situation and needs. Dillard created an opening that, owing to specific cultural, environmental, and other practical factors, was destined to shrink instead of grow. The end was sad. As Dillard headed home to attend to a leg of lamb, she left alone a little boy whose dwelling place in the world was now a bit smaller than it was only a short time ago.

Acknowledgment presupposes, at least to some degree, the attention of consciousness. We can only say "Here I am!" to something or someone we have brought to mind or otherwise have in view and can touch with our presence and words. Dillard's writings have the cultivation and education of such obliging and respectful attunement as one of their goals. She speaks of the importance of being a "perfect witness" (94) to the matters and mysteries of everyday life. She is convinced that being wide awake is a prerequisite for good health and advancement.

We teach our children one thing only, as we were taught: to wake up. We teach our children to look alive there, to join by words and activities the life of human culture on the planet's crust. As adults we are almost all adept at waking up. We have so mastered the transition we have forgotten we ever learned it. Yet it is a transition we make a hundred times a day, as, like so many will-less dolphins, we plunge and surface, lapse and emerge. We live half our waking lives and all of our sleeping lives in some private, useless, and insensible waters we never mention or recall. Useless, I say. Valueless, I might add, until someone hauls their wealth up to the surface and into the wide-awake city, in a form that people can use. (22–23)

Acknowledgment displays the wealth of wakefulness, for with this behavior comes the attunement of consciousness and the openings it makes possible by way of the strength and discipline of its attunement. When such attunement wavers and wanes, the openings begin to disappear. Dillard's story of the little boy offers an illustration of how this is so. The beginning is different than the ending: a lonely little boy who, through an act of acknowledgment, is given the opportunity to open up to another whose attunement with the child is not strong enough to last as long as the boy would like. Dillard becomes more mindful of a leg of lamb than of a strange (but not so strange) little boy. Of course, Dillard was mindful enough of the whole experience that she could later write about it and thus, in a way, bring it back to life. The boy was not simply forgotten. Out of sight, yes; but not out of mind. He is remembered in a story of and about acknowledgment.

It might seem, then, that the life-giving gift that concerns us here begins with an act of consciousness, of attunement, of mindfulness that transforms space and time and thereby provides openings and thus more living room for people in the thickets of existence. The whole process defines a specific act of "response" which, for my purposes, must not be taken for granted. As Joan Stambaugh reminds us:

> Response is nothing passive or reactive; it is the essential human deed. People with severe depression are in what is perhaps the most unbearable state there is, because they are utterly unable to respond to anything at all. Even pain or suffering can be preferable to that since they are, after all, some sort of response. Without some kind of response, no poet would write a poem, no composer would write a symphony, nobody would fall in love, no one would find a friend. We need to ponder more deeply what it means to respond.[2]

Indeed, for the response of acknowledgment requires more than an attuning and transforming act of consciousness to begin its work; acknowledgment, too, needs what it brings into being for the sake of ourselves and others: a space, a place, the planet's crust, at the very least. Acknowledgment does not materialize out of nothing. It needs somewhere to happen. Edward Casey points to the primordial support that allows acknowledgment to happen when he writes:

> Can you imagine what it would be like if there were no places in the world? None whatsoever! An utter, placeless void! I suspect that you will not succeed in this thought-experiment, which is not just difficult to perform (can you really eliminate any trace of place from your experience of *things*?) but also disturbing (can you really picture yourself in a *world* without places?). Our lives are so place-oriented and place-saturated that we cannot begin to comprehend, much less face up to, what sheer placelessness would be like.[3]

Hence, the importance of acknowledgment, which, in truth, begins with something other than itself and the places it opens for us.

Fine, you say. "We grant you the planet's crust. The earth is a given." Yes, but that does not necessarily put an end to the matter of *where to begin* when trying to understand the nature and function of acknowledgment. Recall, for example, one of the essential ingredients of Dillard's story: religion—which, as recorded in the Bible, tells how the greatest act of acknowledgment ever performed took place long before human beings could return the favor: "In the beginning God created the heaven and the earth" (Genesis 1:1). Or, if you will, "In the beginning was the Word, and the Word was with God, and the Word was God" (John 1:1). Only after God "spoke" and created the largest opening there is—the universe—could life begin. The Word (*Logos*) at work here was the ultimate *avowal*, coming as it did from One uttering declarative speech ("Let there be light!") whose function was "to bring and show forth" (*epideixis*) at the appropriate moment (*kairos*) the truth of what was on One's mind (some object of consciousness, such as "heaven" and "earth").[4] God is the Great Avower: the One who declares most assuredly, openly, bluntly, and without shame. Such an open declaration or avowal is, of course, also known as a instance of "acknowledgment."

By way of acknowledgment, God created the place where all other acts of acknowledgment could happen. A more scientific appreciation of this event is commonly known as the "Big Bang," an event which, according to many scientists, may or may not have anything to do with God's genius, generosity, and grace. Moreover, argue these scientists, the notion of God need not be called upon in order to acquire an empirically based and extremely precise mathematical understanding of an event that, despite its complexity, can still be put into words for the non-expert. Thus, the Astronomer Royal of Great Britain, Sir Michael Rees, tells us that "Our universe sprouted from an initial event, the 'big bang' or 'fireball.' It expanded and cooled; the intricate pattern of stars and galaxies we see around us emerged thousands of millions of years later; on at least one planet around at least one star, atoms have assembled into creatures complex enough to ponder how they evolved."[5]

God and the Big Bang: two "beginnings" credited with making acknowledgment possible by giving those who would perform this behavior a place to stand. In the remainder of this chapter, I offer a more detailed discussion and comparison of these two beginnings and the ways in which they would have one understand the nature and function of acknowledgment. Although various religious and scientific works address the issue of the relationship (or non-relationship) between God and the Big Bang, I am unaware of anyone who has made the phenomenon of acknowledgment their primary focus in discussing the complementarity or incommensurability of the topics. With what I have to say about these topics, I also intend to highlight further the other matters (i.e., time, space, openness, emotion, discourse, conscience, otherness, rhetoric) that need to be considered in a phenomenological assessment of acknowledgment.

First Things First

Religion.[6] From beginning to end, the Bible tells the story of the One Supreme Being who time and again demands acknowledgment from the creatures who were brought into being by way of such an act and who thereby possess the capability of continuing its practice for the good of all concerned—God included: the One who heard and responded to the cries of the children of Israel suffering under Pharaoh's rule; the One who made possible an exodus; the One who promised a living place that One's children could call their own; the One who allowed One's "Son" to die a horrible death so that others might then be moved enough to see the light and be saved. In the wilderness of Sinai, God told Moses of commandments that must be followed: "I am the Lord thy God, which hath brought thee out of the land of Egypt, out of the house of bondage. Thou shalt have no other gods before me. . . . Thou shalt not bow down thyself to them, nor serve them: for I the Lord thy God am a jealous God . . ." (Exodus 20: 1–5). God made Oneself known in a way that left no doubt about what was expected in return: genuine positive acknowledgment. This expectation was meant to inspire fear, but for a good reason; hence, Moses' words to his people: "Fear not: for God is come to prove you, and that his fear may be before your face, that ye sin not" (Exodus 20: 20).

A jealous God, One who gave the gift of life and who wants the favor returned. God demands acknowledgment. Moreover, as in the case of Job, for example, the Lord allows for the evil of great suffering to occur as a way of testing humankind's faith, integrity, and the genuineness of its acknowledgment. Job, of course, passed the test, but not before his many misfortunes stimulated a host of questions about God and his ways. Why, asks Job, do you "hide your face," remain "silent" when I beg for understanding, and treat me like an "enemy"? (Job 13: 24). Silence can be crushing to people in desperate need of help; its presence might even encourage those in dire straits to think of life as being but a game controlled by One who, short of annihilating all players, will do anything to receive the acknowledgment that One *will* have, come hell or high water.

The people prayed: "Keep not thou silence, O God: hold not thy peace, and be not still" (Psalms 83: 2). The prophet Isaiah gave much consideration to the problem of God's self-concealment and silence (Isaiah 45: 15). He, however, perceived this concealment and reticence in a positive way: God is actually present in God's absence, something which comes about as a sign for humankind to keep searching for the One who promises: "I have taken out of thine hand the cup of trembling, even the dregs of the cup of my fury; thou shalt no more drink it again. But I will put it into the hand of them that afflict thee" (Isaiah 51: 22). So, yes, it might have seemed all along that God is mischievous, spiteful, inattentive, and inappropriately reticent, but this, in truth, is not the case. Hidden within all the craziness and cruelty of everyday existence there lies a Mystery that perhaps someday will be understood, but only after we have taken to heart the obligation to be "God-fearing" (Hebrew: *yire shamayim*) creatures who are willing to acknowledge with undying faith God's almighty status and infinite wisdom.

God uses fear appeals to demand God's due, but God also sustains God's creation in grace, loving-kindness, and mercy (Hebrew: *hesed*): "Thou shalt not hate thy brother in thine heart. . . . Thou shalt not avenge, nor bear angry grudge against the children of thy people, but thou shalt love thy neighbor as thyself" (Leviticus 19: 17–18; also Hosea 6: 6, where "mercy," not "sacrifice," is called for). God built the world on *hesed* (Psalms 89–2) and needs it enacted in our daily lives in order to secure this habitat as a place that invites the opening act of love back again and again. This emotion, more than any other one, opens us to others and even keeps us close to loved ones who are far away in time and space. Out of God's love arose the original home of Adam and Eve, "a garden eastward in Eden" (Genesis 2: 8) that was safe and secure, unstained by anxiety, shame, and guilt, but where, at a particular apple-eating moment, God's word was not properly acknowledged, thereby causing God to sound a powerful question to a knowingly naked and hiding Adam and Eve: "Where art thou?" (Genesis 3: 9).

This question, to be sure, is rhetorical. God, being who God is, certainly must have known what Adam and Eve did and where they were. With the question, love takes on the tone of anger. Adam and Eve broke the law: they ate from the tree of knowledge, became self-aware, and were right to feel the heretofore unknown discomforts of anxiety, shame, and guilt. God's rhetorical question is a call to confession, judgment, and action. Adam and Eve must therefore acknowledge their sin and then suffer the further consequences of having to deal from now on with the finitude of their new mortal nature: "for dust thou art, and unto dust shalt thou return" (Genesis 3: 19).

Where art thou? Here I am! In the Christian tradition, this exchange between God and Adam and Eve is associated, of course, with the doctrine of

"Original Sin." In the Hebrew (and especially its Kabbalistic) tradition, however, the exchange is seen as more than that fearful moment marking "the fall of man." The self-consciousness that accompanies Adam's and Eve's transformation marks the moment when humankind is born and set free to develop spiritual awareness along with the grace, loving-kindness, and mercy toward others that such awareness inspires. Warren Zev Harvey summarizes the matter this way:

> God built this universe on *hesed*, but whether the universe is at any moment a true arena of grace and loving-kindness depends ultimately on the free deeds of man. Having created man free, God is now at man's mercy. By acts of cruelty toward others, we cause him anguish. By acts of *hesed* toward others, we give him cause to rejoice, thereby helping him to "ride upon the heavens" [Deut. 33: 26]. In other words, we do an act of *hesed* for God.[7]

Such an act returns God's favor of positive acknowledgment. Although fear may still play a role in the performance of this act, more often than not the life-giving gift being exchanged makes the situation an occasion of good tidings and joy as we open ourselves to the needs of others. The question "Where art thou?" comes not only from God but also from God's creations. Rabbi Abraham Heschel thus tells us that "All of human history as described in the Bible may be summarized in one phrase: *God is in search of man.*"[8]

With the first line on its opening page, the Bible indicates when this search was initiated: "In the beginning . . ." (Genesis 1: 1). And before the first chapter is over, we know that the search *really* began to take form on the "sixth day" when God "created man in his own image" (Genesis 1: 27). A world built on and in need of acknowledgment was now set in order. And when the related capacities of human consciousness and self-awareness kicked in, the world became a place of time and space where some of its inhabitants could display their "gift" of desiring to know when and where it all began, what exactly the structure and the meaning of life is, and how it might all end.

Acknowledgment, time, space, consciousness, emotion, rhetorical language: the Bible tells of these related things with its story of creation and recounting of the early development of the Hebrew and Christian traditions. Although I am not yet done gathering "evidence" from the Bible that can shed further light on the nature and function of my primary topic, I now want to turn my attention to another domain of knowledge that, like Western religion, is known for its commitment to making good use of the human desire to understand the truth of where and who we are and what the future has in store for us. In this other domain, the vocation that rules the day is that of science—a vocation whose precise measurements of the universe have added much fuel to the long-standing controversy over what it really means to speak of a Creator who is unsurpassed in the ability to grant acknowledgment. Please note, however, that these same measurements have also inspired hope in religious souls who read them as clues for learning about "the Truth": "Study astronomy and physics," writes the twelfth-century rabbinic authority and physician, Moses Maimonides, "if you desire to comprehend the relation between the world and God's management of it."[9] Hence, the emergence of what is today referred to as "theistic science," which "postulates that the universe was created by a personal God a finite time ago and that it was intelligently designed with the arrival of human life in mind."[10] I deal with this specific matter more fully when concluding the present chapter.

Science.[11] The vocation of scientist is a difficult one; some might even say that it is sadomasochistic: the conscientious scientist is forever engaged in discovery, creating theory, testing it out, and inviting others to show that what he or she has accomplished is basically *insignificant.* This procedure is often painful: it hurts to have one's hard work called into question because it's "not right," "wrongheaded," "misdirected," "unfounded," or otherwise "a waste of time." For those who raise the questions in all seriousness, however, the procedure can still be fun and rewarding. There is something pleasurable in finding a chink in the armor, especially if it does not belong to you. Now they, too, can be credited for making a discovery that might initiate a new beginning for a line of research. In the scientist's constant quest for the truth, such an accomplishment warrants positive acknowledgment. Moreover, the ethical standards of "pure" science require such acknowledgment to come even from those who have been proven wrong and who are thus presently in the harsh limelight of negative acknowledgment. The importance of "turning the other cheek" is never to be underestimated by scientists.[12]

It has taken centuries for the science of cosmology to formulate its present and widely accepted understanding of the beginning, of how our place in the cosmos is a result of the Big Bang—that primordial explosion of a *highly* compact universe, whereby it began to expand and evolve into what it supposedly is now. I say "supposedly" because the conscientious scientist would have it no other way. Yes, the creation story put together by cosmologists is presently so well established that it is generally referred to as the "Standard Model." But, as will be discussed below, this empirically tested and verified model can only go so far before it must admit a fair amount of speculation in its formulations and predictions. With some of this speculation, scientists acknowledge the possibilities of a Creator and this Being's initial act of acknowledgment that brought everything into existence. According to these scientists, approaching the issue of God the Great Avower from the findings of science rather than from the assumptions of religion allows for *a more empirically precise and detailed understanding* of when and how the first act of acknowledgment took place.[13]

Cosmology is the study of the entire observable universe, treated as a single entity. With powerful technologies (e.g., telescopes, computers) and highly sophisticated mathematical theory at hand, cosmologists look to the sky to study "fossils" (e.g., old stars, synthesized chemical elements) that tell of how the universe is expanding. To speak of an expanding universe is to admit the possibility that the process had a starting point, a beginning that was there before the process itself began with a Big Bang. "Using well-established physics," writes cosmologist Martin Rees, "we can extrapolate cosmic evolution back to the stage when the universe was a millisecond old (10^{-3} seconds); the most powerful particle accelerators can generate the conditions that prevailed at 10^{-14} seconds; earlier than that, energies would have been higher still."[14] The awesomeness of such calculations is clear when one realizes that they also allow cosmologists to claim with mathematical "certainty" that the Big Bang took place "approximately" 15 billion years ago and that the entire universe is at least 10 billion light-years across and growing. In writing about how "our Solar System stretches our conception of *time*scales to an extent that is hard to relate to human (or even historical) perspectives," Rees provides a wonderful analogy from which to grasp in more simple and vivid terms the space and time involved here.

> Suppose America had existed forever, and you were walking across it, starting on the East coast when the Earth formed, and ending up in California when the Sun was about to die. To make this journey, you'd have to take *one step every two thousand years*. A mere three or four steps would represent all recorded history. . . . Our Sun is less than halfway [4.5 billion years] through its life; we are still near the "simple beginning" of the evolutionary story.[15]

With the science of cosmology as our guide we must realize that from "the beginning" to the sixth day when God created and acknowledged "man" marks a period of billions of years. Taking a closer look at what was happening during this evolutionary period can add to one's sense of awe, as can what cosmologists have to say about what immediately preceded the Big Bang.

Before the Big Bang blasted everything in the universe into being (space, matter, time), there existed what cosmologists term a "singularity." According to the theoretical physicist Paul Davies, "A singularity is the nearest thing that science has found to a supernatural agent."[16] At a singularity, one finds a state of infinite temperature, infinite density, and infinite energy all condensed into a point the size of an infinitesimal speck of dust, where space-time as we know it does not exist. A singularity exists outside of space-time, or what cosmologists sometimes describe as a state of "nothingness." Before the Big Bang there *was* something that *was* nothing, a presence of absence that exploded and thereby set forth (created) all the material of the universe that will ever exist. The Big Bang was not an explosion *in* space, but an explosion of *all* space, an explosion whose echo is still detectable as long-wavelength radiation or what is also called the "cosmic microwave background."

A singularity and then the Big Bang. If one assumes that God is behind this creation story, then the topic of acknowledgment must be appreciated as having, at the very least, a very long history. The conscious and conscientious performance of acknowledgment is directed toward the transformation of space and time and thus the creation of a place wherein people can dwell together. God is the Great Avower—the One whose first act of acknowledgment brought about the greatest transformation of space and time and hence the biggest place (the universe) known to humankind. On the other hand, if one eliminates God from the story, then the topic loses something that makes it all the more wondrous.

Stephen Hawking speaks of this "something" as a "theoretical concept" that may show itself to be true once cosmologists and their fellow scientists figure out all there is to know about the universe and its ancient singularity.[17] Following Hawking and his colleagues, it is hard not to believe that science offers a more concrete and thus surer path than religion in the search for God. Indeed, as Davies notes: "Our ignorance of the origin of life [and the universe] leaves plenty of scope for divine explanations, but that is a purely negative attitude, invoking 'the God-of-the-gaps' only to risk retreat at a later date in the face of scientific advance." Hence, "To invoke God as a blanket explanation of the unexplained is to invite eventual falsification, and make God the friend of ignorance. If God is to be found, it must surely be through what we discover about the world, not what we fail to discover."[18]

Notice that with this way of thinking, scientists do God a favor by acknowledging the possibility of the Creator while at the same time saying that the best way to do this is to not acknowledge this possibility because it gets in the way of and undercuts the scientific endeavor. I will have more to say about this paradox shortly. First, however, I want to return to the matter of the Big Bang, its founding singularity, and its evolution; for with some additional understanding of these related matters, my comments about this paradox should prove more useful in appreciating the nature, function, and scope of acknowledgment.

A singularity, the Big Bang, an expanding universe: scientists have learned much about this evolutionary process by studying the life and death of stars. Stars, like everything else in the universe, are residues of what emerged and happened with the Big Bang; they form from giant molecular clouds composed of dust and gas (primarily 90 percent hydrogen and 9 percent helium). These clouds are subject to a pair of opposing forces: gravity (which pulls the matter of clouds inward, causing it to collapse and coalesce) and the pressure of fusion-produced and expansion-causing heat (which results as the constituent atoms of the cloud come together due to gravitational pull). When these two forces achieve and maintain a balance, the cloud remains in equilibrium. When, however, the cloud becomes gravitationally unstable, it begins to collapse and breaks into stellar fragments; hence, the birth of stars whose particular masses are determined by the size of the fragment from which they take form. These fragments also are subject to the forces of gravity and fusion-produced heat. Once the fragment's core temperature reaches 10 million Kelvin, the evolving star begins to fuse hydrogen into helium and thereby generates enough outward moving radiation (and thus energy) to balance the force of gravity.

Stars begin to die as their core fuel burns out and they start to collapse under their own gravity. If the core is massive enough (more than three solar masses) the collapse is unstoppable and will continue "forever"—disappearing into the singularity of what is commonly referred to as a "black hole." I have already discussed what such a singularity is. It existed "before" the Big Bang happened and shows itself again as a dying star reaches its end. A black hole is a massive star collapsing into infinity with such force that, with the exception of a generic form of radiation that it emits back into the universe, not even light can escape its gravitational pull. The infinitely dense result (a singularity) of such a limitless collapse is incalculable. Cosmologists can say, however, that once something crosses the boundary or "event horizon" of a black hole and is propelled towards its singularity, there is no turning back. The object or creature is fated to be stretched like spaghetti and torn apart by the forces at work.[19]

What exactly is going on at the bottom of a black hole? Does the word "bottom" make any sense in the world of quantum theory and mechanics? Might there be an exit from a black hole on the "other side" of its singularity? Would such a place be another universe that perhaps dwarfs the universe that scientists now call "home"? Would the "laws" of physics that presently affect our material existence be the same in this other universe? Cosmologists can only speculate about answers to such questions.[20] Neither the physical bodies nor the cognitive abilities of human beings are strong enough to withstand and comprehend the "nothingness" of a black hole's singularity. According to the physicist Gerald Schroeder, all that we can say about the matter with "almost" complete certainty is that from "that ethereal mass of pure energy and exquisitely thin substance [that came with the first instant of creation], stones and galaxies and humans were . . . formed. We are products of the Big Bang. We are, in fact, made of star dust. The material aspects of man are totally rooted in the universe."[21] From the strict scientific standpoint, then, it would be appropriate to say the following words to one who was about to end his or her life by stepping into a black hole: "From dust thou art, and unto dust shalt thou return."

With all this in mind, I now return to the paradox of acknowledgment that arises when the scientific mentality confronts the question of where such dust might have originated. Recall the paradox coming from science's claim that the most appropriate way of acknowledging the One who is "known" to have said, "I am that I am," is to avoid acknowledging this Being while investigating all that It "supposedly" created. I do not intend to argue for or against the logic at work here; instead, I want only to keep a focus on the phenomenon of acknowledgment—that type of human behavior that opens places where things and people can dwell together.

The "doing" of science presupposes the happening of such behavior; without it and the way it can and must be trained in order to ensure the most "objective" results possible, scientists could not do their job. Science is a way of being conscious of the world; it exists, at least as it sees itself, in order to provide the clearest and most accurate openings to things, others, and ourselves so that those who care to look and listen can understand the truth of the matters at hand. Science lives and breathes with the help of acknowledgment; it follows, then, that the same can be said about practitioners of science, although in this case acknowledgment can easily take on a selfish attitude. Being the human beings that they are, scientists have egos; they want to be read and listened to so that they might experience the joy of being acknowledged in a positive way. There is nothing necessarily wrong with that. Wanting to be someone who is worthy of praise is a desire that helps bring passion and commitment to the scientist's work. And yes, I know, the committed scientist still might insist: "Wait a minute! There is no need to bring 'passion' into the discussion. Science should be done by dedicated professionals who are unselfish and altruistic and whose only genuine motivation is to produce the most objective assessment possible." Indeed, this is the supreme ethic of scientists, one that guards against the dismissal of their work by requiring research designs and statistical tests that help them engage in self-effacing behavior directed toward the production of valid and reliable results that can advance knowledge and sustain progress.

This ideal certainly warrants praise; it is nevertheless an ideal that presupposes acknowledgment. Scientists must open themselves to the awesome wonders of the world. Even if one grants the argument that there are scientists who embody the ideal, the issue of acknowledgment still remains; for no matter how rigid and reductionistic scientists might be, they cannot avoid being both witnesses to and avowers of whatever matter of interest stimulates their attention, their consciousness, their mind. Human beings must offer that which they also need if they want to know anything about what is going on in their particular lives and in the universe in general. Scientists are no exception; acknowledgment is essential to their lives. And, of course, one need not necessarily appeal to the "mind of God" to explain why this is so. Rather, as Rees points out, one need only try to find a way to explain why it is that the evolution of our universe allows for it to be "'cognizable,' in the sense that it permitted some kind of conscious entity or 'observer' to evolve within it."[22]

Theistic Science. A "cognizable" universe; a place where acknowledgment was bound to happen. Cognitive scientists have much to tell us about the biological and chemical bases of consciousness and the inquiring and acknowledging mind. They leave it to astrophysicists and cosmologists, however, to discover the workings of some universal "mind-stuff" that came with a singularity and a Big Bang, that accounts for the laws of physics, and that, at the appropriate moment in the universe's evolution, saw fit to make itself known, at least, on planet Earth. "What is it that breathes fire into the equations and makes a universe for them to describe?" asks Stephen Hawking. "Why does the Universe go to all the bother of existing?"[23] And I would add: *Why does it allow for creatures who can be awed by and acknowledge its wonders?* Does the universe itself really call for such acknowledgment? Is that truly part of its logic and laws? Is there an Intelligent Designer behind all the chaos and order that appears before us, or is it all merely chance and accident?[24]

Cosmology has certainly come to realize the importance of trying to account for the role of "the participant observer" in the evolution of the universe. Hence, for example, the thinking of physicist John Wheeler, who maintains that the "system of shared experience which we call the world is viewed as building itself out of elementary quantum phenomena, elementary acts of observer-participancy. In other words, the questions that the participants put—and the answers they get—by their observing devices, plus the communication of their findings, take part in creating the impressions which we call the system: that whole great system which to a superficial look is time and space, particles and fields."[25] Is this to suggest that the "elementary quantum phenomena" being referred to here were somehow coded in the singularity that founded the Big Bang? It would appear so.

For someone like Rees, allowing this participatory view of the universe to play a role in the work of cosmologists is asking for trouble: "The 'participatory universe' seems hard to accept—hard, even, to take seriously. What sort of observer must be invoked to 'bring the universe into being': a mouse? a human? or a Ph.D. physicist?"[26] The fact that God is not asked of here is the result of Rees staying true to the reductionistic and cautious ways of science: "Scientists' incursions into theology or philosophy can be embarrassingly naive or dogmatic."[27] Rees would thus have his colleagues accept and defend their limits. There is acknowledgment going on in the universe that cosmologists and other interested scientists should recognize and speak of, but without jumping to conclusions that invoke "the God of the gaps." If a scientist wants to think about the One who might have started it all with an act of acknowledgment, so be it, says Rees; but let not the actual work of the scientist go beyond what he or she can observe, theorize about, and test out mathematically.[28]

This way of handling the phenomenon of acknowledgment does not, however, eliminate the paradox that concerns us here. Scientists are still in the position of acknowledging something that the laws of physics have yet to explain and that, according to the ethics of science, ought therefore to remain out of the picture. For the devoted scientist, the best way to recognize God is not to recognize God. Acknowledgment without acknowledgment.

Admittedly, there is a way to relieve some of the strain of this paradox. Scientists need only point out that I am stacking the deck: "You are focusing on a phenomenon that is all too easily associated with existential and spiritual concerns. Such concerns are fine, but the vocabulary that prevails here is too subjective. We study the laws of nature, physics, the universe. Indeed, that makes us 'acknowledgers.' But it doesn't necessarily follow from this that hidden within or beyond or behind the laws themselves is some Supreme Being, Mind, or Consciousness whose 'logic' entails a primordial form of acknowledgment." Granted, and I am not here to maintain otherwise. Yet, given how much acknowledgment means to the well-being of people, I still think it wise to press for an understanding of the phenomenon that allows for a robust appreciation of both its actual and potential status. Such an appreciation must be weary of the limitations of reductionism. With respect to the topic of acknowledgment, the history of Western science, it must be noted, helps to make this point.

Beginning at least with the ancient Greeks, scientists have long emphasized the essential "wondrous" nature of their vocation; the training of scientists is geared toward having them experience the "awesomeness" of what they are doing and studying. What this training typically excludes, however, is the development of some formal appreciation (beyond the body's biology and chemistry) of how human beings are even capable of being awed. Although I would in no way deny that acknowledgment is inextricably tied to human physiology, I do not believe that the existential and communicative workings of the phenomenon can be fully appreciated when reduced to this level of "life." Hence, for example, the ethical standard operating in medicine that dictates how the "personhood" of patients should never be treated only "by the numbers." Be they ill or well, human beings should remain a source of awe, especially for those whose ancient Hippocratic Oath demands that they "do no harm."[29]

Awe, of course, presupposes acknowledgment: it is an act of consciousness that is exceptionally taken with (if not totally overwhelmed by) what stands before it. Awe is a state of highly attuned consciousness that allows an opening to take place between an observer and something observed—an opening that allows this something to be perceived in a heretofore unknown and thus exciting or shocking way. Any study of acknowledgment must take the topic of awe seriously, for the phenomenon of acknowledgment is never more alive and robust than when it unfolds in a moment of being awestruck by some object's or person's presence.

The Judeo-Christian tradition of religion has more to say about this happening than science does. Rabbi Abraham Heschel, for example, tells us that awe "is the cardinal attitude" in the Old Testament. Awe draws one near to the object that inspires; it is "evoked not in moments of calculation but in moments of being in rapport" with what is being witnessed.[30] In a moment of awe, one's orientation toward the world assumes a way of being whose watchword is this: *Let there be!* The moment is "holy," for now the manner in which one experiences the presence of things is most like the "saying" that first acknowledged life by calling it into being: "And God said, Let there be light . . ." (Genesis 1: 3). In moments of awe, things "speak" in mysterious ways. The experience is humbling. It is a time of wonder, of finding oneself in a place for acquiring wisdom. Heschel writes: "There is . . . only one way to wisdom: awe. Forfeit your sense of awe, let your conceit diminish your ability to revere, and the universe becomes a market place for you. The loss of awe is the great block to insight."[31]

I know of no scientist or academic who would disagree with these claims, although many scientists might feel more comfortable if Heschel admitted that awe can also be evoked in moments of calculation. Cosmologists are certainly awed by the universe, and their calculations of this immense place provide a lot of evidence for why they and everybody else should be overwhelmed by its dimensions and workings. Science speaks of the wonder and awesomeness of such things as singularities, black holes, stars, planets, and the molecular structures of things and creatures that live on these rocks. Religion, on the other hand, would have the scientist understand that when caught up in wonder and awe, we are in the "the state of being asked," the state where we are addressed and acknowledged ("Where art thou!" Genesis 3: 8–9), where one is thereby given the opportunity to respond and be accountable ("God . . . said unto him, Abraham: and he said, Behold, here I am." Genesis 22: 1), and where our capacity for moral feeling is called forth and directed ("And now . . . what doth the Lord thy God require of thee, but to fear the Lord thy God, to walk in all His ways, and to love Him, and to serve the Lord thy God with all thy heart . . ." Deuteronomy 10: 12). Science makes use of wonder and awe but religion goes a step further by offering an account of their related workings.

One learns from Western religion that there is something moral going on here, something that is related to the "heart," which is a "gift": "I will give them a heart to know Me, that I am the Lord" (Jeremiah 24: 7). In the Old Testament, the use of the term "heart" is generally associated by rabbinic scholars with moral consciousness or "conscience" and the emotions such as fear, guilt, joy, and love that oftentimes come with it.[32] In returning God's favor of acknowledgment, we ought to be, at the very least, conscientious. No scientist worth his or her salt would deny the importance of this state of being for doing good research. Even at its "dispassionate" best, science is not an activity void of emotion and moral responsibility.

Please keep in mind that my intention here is not to belittle science, nor to preach religion. I am interested in the workings of acknowledgment. Acknowledgment needs a place to happen—at the very least it needs the planet's crust. I have spoken of Western religion and science because they both have much to say about this place and where it came from. Taken together, these not necessarily "conflicting" perspectives provide a compelling account of some of the history and complexity of acknowledgment.[33] Was this phenomenon at work with the Big Bang? Does it make sense to believe that somewhere—in the infinity of a singularity—there existed a code or a law for developing a being who, at a certain moment of self-awareness, could ask a question that goes right to the heart of this being's existence: What would life be like if nobody acknowledged one's presence on earth? I, of course, think it is correct to say that without acknowledgment human beings would not be, as Stuart Kauffman puts it, "at home in the universe."[34]

In his book whose title contains these words, Kauffman—a highly acclaimed biologist, physicist, MacArthur Fellow, and pioneer of the new "science of complexity"—presents a rich and scientifically based argument regarding how, amidst all the chaos going on in the cosmos, there still exist "deep and beautiful laws [of 'self-organization'] governing that unpredictable flow."[35] Kauffman seeks and writes about these laws while "holding the hope that . . . the new science of complexity may help us find anew our place in the universe, that through this new science, we may recover our sense of worth, our sense of the sacred"—a sense that Kauffman acknowledges as being worn away by the reductionist teachings and habits of modern science. He writes:

> Once, a scant few centuries ago, we of the West believed ourselves the chosen of God, made in his image, keeping his world in a creation wrought by his love for us. Now, only 400 years later, we find ourselves on a tiny planet, on the edge of a humdrum galaxy among billions like it scattered across vast megaparsecs, around the curvature of space-time back to the Big Bang. We are but accidents, we're told. Purpose and value are ours alone to make. Without Satan and God, the universe now appears the neutral home of matter, dark and light, and is utterly indifferent. We bustle, but are no longer at home in the ancient sense.[36]

Kauffman would have his colleagues and readers open themselves to scientific evidence that speaks of the importance of another way of being and of seeing ourselves. We are part of a cosmic process, he argues, "created by it, creating it. In the beginning was the Word—the Law. The rest follows, and we participate." By way of this participation, we are able to witness a universe that exhibits the beauty of order and that thereby warrants the utmost "awe and respect"—things that Kauffman believes "have become powerfully unfashionable in our confused postmodern society" but that he still maintains can be recovered with the help of science and the Law from which it evolved.[37] This Law commends self-organization and order in the midst of complexity and chaos. Science abides by this Law as its practitioners enact that capacity that must be at work if they are to see, observe, and understand all that stands before them. Kauffman, in other words, calls for what is being studied here: the life-giving and life-ordering act of acknowledgment.

Although he never employs the term in his book, Kauffman's position is supportive of what was defined above as theistic science. I was led to consider this matter by way of my interest in the workings of acknowledgment. Theistic science would have one think of these workings in a most rigorous and robust way and thus with the highest reverence. I think that the challenge here is worthwhile, although, to emphasize once again, my inquiry is not the result of having a particular religious or scientific axe to grind. Rather, if anything, the "tool" I intend to employ as I continue the present inquiry has more of a philosophical edge to it. Remember, I am attempting a phenomenology of acknowledgment here in order to understand the existential nature and function of this act. With the discussion so far I have pointed to a host of related matters—creation, the time and space of dwelling places, otherness, emotion, discourse, rhetoric, conscience, and the attunement of consciousness—that also come into play with a phenomenological assessment of the act and that therefore warrant attention when attempting to comprehend the phenomenon in question. The *being* of acknowledgment is a complex event. In the next chapter I continue to unravel and clarify this event by focusing more closely on the consciousness that prevails when acknowledgment is at work. Phenomenology is a fitting way to approach the task because, with its investigative bent, the related matters of consciousness and acknowledgment take center stage and, at the same time, encourage an openness to the additional matters mentioned above.

Chapter Three

The Attunement of Consciousness

Seeing and Observing

Acknowledgment presupposes the workings of consciousness. Consciousness is what first attunes us to our surroundings so that they can be both *seen and observed with care.* The attunement of consciousness grows as seeing something evolves into observing what this something truly is. A person surfing the World Wide Web, for example, may or may not demonstrate this degree of attunement. For although this person may have been recorded as a "visitor" on any number of websites, these visits might have actually been nothing more than a momentary and forgettable experience wherein consciousness was operating only at the level of a not particularly perceptive glance. A hit on a website counter can be misleading, especially when it has nothing to do with someone taking the time to open themselves to all that a site has to offer.

The term "spacey" is often used to describe a person who, for one reason or another, appears to have difficulty with maintaining the concentration that is needed for the attunement of consciousness to develop. There are, of course, people whose spaciness is sometimes due to their ability to concentrate so hard and diligently on some matter of interest that they become oblivious to the rest of the world. With Sir Arthur Conan Doyle's famous detective, Sherlock Holmes, for example, one finds a character whose attunement of consciousness is so powerful that, no matter how spacey he might appear to be, nevertheless warrants praise for being what his friend and colleague, Dr. Watson, describes as "the most perfect reasoning and observing machine that the world has seen."[1]

In Doyle's first story of the famous detective, "A Scandal in Bohemia," a conversation between Watson and Holmes reveals what the detective considers to be the key to his extraordinary powers of consciousness, acknowledgment, and deduction. After being dazzled by a demonstration of Holmes's powers, Watson says: "When I hear you give your reasons [regarding a specific deduction] the thing always appears to me to be so ridiculously simple that I could easily do it myself, though at each successive instance of your reasoning I am baffled, until you explain your process. And yet I believe that my eyes are as good as yours" (12). Holmes agrees, but only to make a point:

> "Quite so . . . . You see, but you do not observe. The distinction is clear. For example, you have frequently seen the steps which lead up from the hall to this room."
>
> "Frequently."
>
> "How often?"
>
> "Well, some hundreds of times."
>
> "Then how many are there?"
>
> "How many! I don't know."
>
> "Quite so! You have not observed. And yet you have seen. That is just my point. Now, I know that there are seventeen steps, because I have both seen and observed." (12–13)

Here, again, the distinction between seeing and observing is being made as a way of explaining what the attunement of consciousness entails. The distinction is also implied in Annie Dillard's notion of the "perfect witness" that was introduced in the beginning of the last chapter. Because Dillard's and Holmes's powers of observation are, in their own particular ways, directed toward uncovering some truth for the benefit of humankind, one might begin to think (with these two souls in mind) that the ability to both see and observe is more of virtue than anything else.

Let us think about this for a moment. The question has been posed: What would life be like if no one took the time to acknowledge your existence? Now consider this question: What would life be like if everyone you knew and happened to meet was as keen an observer as either Dillard or Holmes? When reading Dillard, one gets the sense that here is a woman who is as caring as she is perceptive and who would go to great lengths to protect another's feelings. Holmes, on the other hand, is a different story. According to Watson, Holmes's powers of observation and deduction were in great part due to his ability to halt the "intrusions" of emotion when doing his job: "Grit in a sensitive instrument, or a crack in one of his own high power lenses, would not be more disturbing than a strong emotion in a nature such as his" (11). Indeed, when not injecting cocaine to combat the *ennui* that tortured him whenever he was not on a case, Holmes was the consummate scientist and logician who would let nothing get in the way of his pursuit of the truth.

Living in a world where your friends, neighbors, and everyday acquaintances were more like Holmes than Dillard, you would most likely be subjected to many uncensored observations. While talking to your boss, for example, you might hear him say: "That piece of dry, green mucus under your fingernail tells me that you have been picking your nose recently." Be it right or wrong, this observation would most likely bring about an uncomfortable and embarrassing situation. A life filled with such situations would be maddening. Imagine how much time, energy, and money it would take to create a presence that was perfect enough to prevent such negative acknowledgment from coming your way. Would it be worth it? Do you think you would ever get tired of being told how ravishing, attractive, smart, and morally upstanding you are? Does positive acknowledgment ever get old in the way negative acknowledgment does? Is acknowledgment thereby something that is best practiced within the boundaries of decorum? Are we not in fact talking about a realm of decorum when referring to a Holmesian world where stating the truth in an uncensored way is the rule of the day?

Such questions encourage one to think about the ethics of the attunement of consciousness and the acknowledgment it makes possible. I will be addressing this matter throughout the current chapter as I continue to discuss how the attunement of consciousness allows people to both see and observe their surroundings. The specific phenomenological perspective employed here is informed primarily by the writings of Martin Heidegger. As originally established by Heidegger's teacher, Edmund Husserl, phenomenology defines a procedure of returning to the immediate content of experience in order to analyze and describe this content as it actually presents itself to one's consciousness. With Husserl, the ultimate goal is to develop a "pure descriptive science of essential being."[2] Heidegger adheres to the basic phenomenological impulse of his teacher by striving to return to the data of immediate experience whereby he can circumvent the obscuring preconceptions of what he terms the "Being of beings." Heidegger is an ontologist; he seeks to disclose the meaning and truth of Being; thus he, too, is a thinker taken with an "essential" aspect of existence.

For Heidegger, however, the task at hand requires a phenomenology that has a more robust, existential appreciation of consciousness than that found in Husserl. With Husserl's early and middle writings, one learns to think of consciousness primarily as a "cognitive" operation and thus as an act (*noesis*) of "intentionality" that is always directed toward some specific object of thought (*noema*). Heidegger, on the other hand, grants the intentional structure of consciousness but insists that it is not primarily a cognitive and theoretical operation geared to *knowing what* something is. Rather, the intentional structure of consciousness, argues Heidegger, shows itself first and foremost as a pre-cognitive relatedness to a world of existential concerns (for example, being able to fix breakfast without giving it much thought). Here consciousness works to attune us emotionally to our environment whereby we can learn and demonstrate a competence of *knowing how* to deal with the immediacy of our everyday, goal-directed activities. Before it is employed reflectively to convert human understanding into the abstract and formal rules, logics, and laws of theoretical knowledge, with its penchant for knowing what something is, consciousness assumes the more primordial and performance-based function of facilitating a person's knowing how to get along successfully in everyday life.

Heidegger begins his investigation into the meaning of Being by offering a phenomenological assessment of how Being typically shows itself in the practical and instrumental world of know how. Being and consciousness are related; consciousness opens us to the reality of our environments, to the *existence* of things and others, to the *happening*, the "it is" or "givenness" (*es gibt*), of Being. In the world of know how, however, the relationship between Being and consciousness operates more in terms of a "seeing" than an "observing" of whatever presents itself to us. For example, having an egg for breakfast does not require you to know all there is to know about eggs; rather, all you need to know is that what you are breaking, scrambling, and eating *is* an egg. In the world of know how, the meaning of an egg need go no further than "something that is eatable."

With his interest in the meaning of Being, Heidegger, of course, does not concern himself with advancing a phenomenological appreciation of eggs. An egg, to be sure, has being, but it certainly is not Being itself. The same can be said about all things (including human beings) that exist in the world: they have being but are not themselves Being. Heidegger is after the meaning of Being, not merely the meaning of *some* being. Yet, as a phenomenologist, the only way he can approach his particular topic is by seeing and observing how Being manifests itself in that which it needs (i.e., beings) in order to be noticed at all. The existence of beings presupposes Being, but Being needs beings so that it can show itself and have *its* presence affirmed. "Every affirmation consists in acknowledgment," writes Heidegger—which is to say that every affirmation presupposes the attunement of consciousness. Heidegger also puts it this way: "Acknowledgment lets that toward which it goes come toward it."[3]

With this claim, Heidegger is associating acknowledgment with the particular attunement of consciousness that must be at work in the doing of phenomenology, an attunement that is always moving from seeing to observing. This attunement presupposes the emotional capacity of "awe," which in moments of anxiety, joy, and love, for example, opens us most powerfully to what is other than ourselves. Within this opening, space and time are transformed and we find ourselves inhabiting a place where our living space has begun to expand. In chapter 2 I examined this phenomenon with the help of Western religion and science. I discussed how any act of acknowledgment requires what it, itself, creates—a "beginning," a time and a place where things can happen; hence my interest in how the universe and our planet's crust came into being. In the beginning was the Word,

God, the Big Bang. Heidegger, however, thinks of the matter differently: "Being," he claims, "is the beginning."[4]

Beginning with Being

Listen for a moment to how Heidegger speaks of Being: "'Being' . . . is not God and not a cosmic ground. Being is farther than all beings and is yet nearer to man than every being, be it a rock, a beast, a work of art, a machine, be it an angel or God. Being is the nearest. Yet the near remains farthest from man."[5] Heidegger would have us think about this "mystery" of Being without making an appeal to religion or science; for religion takes too much for granted in its appreciation of the phenomenon, while science, in attempting to avoid "the-God-of-the-gaps" problem, is too reductionistic in its view of the matter. This is not to say that Heidegger would have us dismiss any and all insights that the two enterprises could offer about the truth in question. As a phenomenologist, however, he is committed to investigating his topic by allowing *it*, as much as possible, to speak for itself.

But is it not the case that without God, or the Big Bang, or perhaps both, Being would be a moot issue? Heidegger answers this question with the first option primarily in mind:

> Only from the truth of Being can the essence of the holy be thought. Only from the essence of the holy is the essence of divinity to be thought. Only in light of the essence of divinity can it be thought or said what the word "God" is to signify. . . . How can man at the present stage of world history ask at all seriously and rigorously whether the god nears or withdraws, when he has above all neglected to think into the dimension in which alone that question can be asked.[6]

The truth of Being is everywhere to be seen and observed. Being *is* wherever the existence of anything shows itself. The truth of Being is an empirical question and, for Heidegger, this truth is most apparent in the existence of that being whose consciousness is most advanced in its related capacities of reflection (critical thinking) and articulation (symbolic expression). Heidegger initially puts it this way: Human being "is an entity which does not just occur among other entities. Rather it is ontically distinguished by the fact that, in its very Being, that Being is an *issue* for it."[7] In other words, what Heidegger designates as the "special distinctiveness" of human being—that differentiates it from other entities—is that this entity is *concerned with* its existence, its Being, its way of becoming what it is. This concern for Being is constantly demonstrated in our everyday involvements with things and with others. Reflecting on the meaningfulness of what is being demonstrated, we can, and often do (especially in times of personal crisis), raise the question of what it means to be. The question makes explicit human being's concern for Being. Only human being is *consciously* concerned enough to do this. And because it is also capable of understanding (to various degrees) what it is doing out of concern for its Being, human being can provide an answer to the question. Heidegger thus tells us that, "man should be understood, within the question of being, as *the* site which being requires in order to disclose itself. Man is the site of openness, the there," the place within all of existence where Being finds a "clearing" and whereby it can be seen and observed with rigor and care.[8] Human being, in other words, is "gifted" with the ability of acknowledgment.

Heidegger investigates this gift throughout his philosophy. Here, for example, is Heidegger once again speaking of its presence in his later writings:

> Man obviously is a being. As such he belongs to the totality of Being—just like the stone, the tree, or the eagle. To "belong" here still means to be in the order of Being. But man's distinctive feature lies in this, that he, as the being who thinks, is open to Being, face to face with Being; thus man remains referred to Being and so answers to it. Man *is* essentially this relationship of responding to Being. . . . Being is present to man neither incidentally nor only on rare occasions. Being is present and abides only as it concerns man through the claim it makes on him. For it is man, open toward Being, who alone lets Being arrive as presence. Such becoming present needs the openness of a clearing, and by this need remains appropriated to human being.[9]

With this way of speaking about the gift of acknowledgment, Heidegger is developing his thinking on human being beyond what he explicitly established in his early work, especially *Being and Time*. There we are told that human being ("*Dasein*") is that place, the "there" (*Da*), where Being (*Sein*) can show itself to a consciousness that can not only feel, see, and hear its presence in the materials of everyday life, but can also reflect on and articulate an understanding of the perceived event. Being, the gift of acknowledgment, and language go hand in hand.

It is this specific relationship that Heidegger has in mind when he claims, as noted above, that human being "*is* essentially this relationship of responding to Being." As long as we live and breathe, we are open to the truth of Being, a truth that we must deal with if we intend to exist in a meaningful and moral way. The space and time of this opening defines the basis of human responsibility; it is the place where human being first hears and responds to what Heidegger, in his early writings, designates as the "call of conscience." We are "fated" to hear this call, which comes to us out of the uncertainty and contingency of human existence, with its "futural" orientation. The call of conscience, which is ever present as part of our temporality, "summons" us to the challenge of assuming the ethical responsibility of affirming our freedom through resolute choice such that we can structure and live our existence in a meaningful and moral way.[10] This challenging summons is what Heidegger eventually speaks of as "the claim" that Being makes on us. In the beginning, and forever after, is the happening of this claim: "the call of Being"—a call that "needs" to be acknowledged for the benefit of humankind and for everything else that *is*. Remember, in order to show itself, Being needs that which it makes possible: beings, especially those who can speak of what it means to be and understand what Being calls us to think and to do.

By the time I end this chapter it should be clear that, at least for Heidegger, there is no more reverent way of responding to this call than to grant it positive acknowledgment. Before discussing in greater detail what such a response entails, it will be helpful if I first offer a concrete illustration of how human beings can (without the help of a professional philosopher) learn something of the special relationship they hold with Being—a relationship that houses the tension between seeing and observing the world. Remember, Heidegger's understanding of this relationship emerged with his initial investigation of how the attunement of consciousness takes shape in the everyday world of know how. The following illustration is drawn from such a world of practice; I thus speak of what might be termed a specific day in the life of Being—a day where, like it or not, people were forced to come face to face with the question of the meaning of (their) Being.

Coming Face-to-Face with Being

The day begins; 6 a.m., Tuesday. A radio alarm clock automatically turns on. You wake, listen, and remain mostly still. A song is playing or people are talking, chattering about some topic or perhaps reporting the news. It doesn't really matter, for unless there is something special about the day that is on your mind and immediately affects your outlook, the sound of the radio marks only the start of another typical day in your life—a day that will most likely be controlled by the well-rehearsed habits and routines that help you to be the purposive and pragmatic person that you are.

For example, you know how to move your hand with little effort to the place where the radio sits near the bed and where one of its buttons, when pushed, turns it off. You wake not merely in physical space but also in a room designed by you to be a user-friendly environment. In other words, you wake to a ready-made world filled with familiar objects that can be handled in familiar ways. Hence, the everyday world of know how: a habitat for habits and routines. The bedroom is such a habitat, complete with its own routines: turning alarms and lights on and off; putting on clothing; moving toward yet another place, the bathroom, in order to engage in other habits and routines (e.g., going to the toilet, brushing your teeth) that you have programmed yourself to follow so that you can move on to still other places, like the kitchen, where different but still old habits and routines take over and guide you along throughout the rest of the day.

The day marks out a world of practice, of knowing where you are and where you have to be throughout the minutes and hours of the day, and of knowing how to get things done so that you can go to bed at night with some sense of accomplishment. Perhaps you keep a checklist: kids to school, pick up Mary and go to work, send e-mails to customers, grocery shopping, call mother and dad, finish painting the guest room . . . The day is filled with people and places and tools for getting things done. The more smoothly your activities proceed, the more unobtrusively these people, places, and tools present themselves and disappear back into their working environments, and thus the less they present themselves as material substances that get in the way of progress, like a car with a flat tire. The everyday world of know-how operates best when matters at hand are going well, remain transparent, and can thus be easily taken for granted. Of course, you need "to see" what you are doing in order to remain preoccupied with your goal-directed activities, but beyond that there is no good reason (unless, for example, you are a phenomenologist) for you to fixate on the presence of things, other people, and circumstances. The world of know-how conditions us to leave well enough alone.

Of course, many days have their setbacks. The radio alarm doesn't turn on, or a child gets sick with a temperature, or your friend and co-worker is late, or your internet connection is down. Perhaps all of these setbacks occur. Your nerves are shot and grow worse as you stand in a crowded grocery store with checkout lines that are unbelievably long. When you finally make it home and call your parents, the line is busy "for hours!" It has been a frustrating (if not a "horrible") day. You certainly are in no mood "to paint the lousy guestroom."

Such setbacks interrupt the space and time of the world of know-how along with its commonsensical and taken for granted ways of thinking and acting. Be they the result of a sickness, a friend who is late, or a broken technology, these interruptions prompt you to see and relate to things and others differently. The transformation at work here pushes one in the direction of being more observant: What *exactly* is wrong with this radio, this child, this friend? A bedroom, a child's room, and the commute to work take on a sense of urgency. Time flies, goes so slow, and then speeds up again. Moods ebb and flow and change in a flash. The situation can become quite strange and uncanny (*unheimlich*) as places of relative comfort become places of irritation and dismay. A world of know-how being overwhelmed by uncanniness defines a place where it is easy not (*un*) to feel comfortable, secure, and "at home" (*heimlich*). Only a sadomasochist could enjoy putting others and themselves through such an anxious ordeal. When such a situation materializes it is both normal and wise to recall and utilize other habits and routines that you know from past experience may facilitate much needed remedies. Fix the radio or buy a new one, call the doctor, find a "nice" way to express your dissatisfaction with your friend. Damaged and disintegrating worlds of know how call for the thoughts and actions of other domains of know-how to set things right so that one can once again feel at home in the world. Sometimes the situation at hand is simple and easy; other times, however, it can be a living hell.

Such was the case with a community of students, teachers, spouses, and parents from Littleton, Colorado, when, on Tuesday, April 20, 1999, their lives became part of a tragedy known as the "Columbine High School Massacre." At approximately 11:15 that morning, two students—seventeen-year-old Dylan Harris and eighteen-year-old Eric Klebold—entered the school wearing black trench coats and armed with an assault rifle, two sawed-off shotguns, a semi-automatic pistol, and over thirty home-made pipe bombs and grenades. Once in the cafeteria they shouted: "All jocks stand up! We're going to kill every one of you." One witness to the carnage reported that the two boys were laughing, "having the time of their life," as they fired their weapons and set off their bombs. After killing a student athlete, one of the boys was heard to say: "Oh, my God, look at this black kid's brain. Awesome, man!" Before they both committed suicide in the school library at approximately 12:30 P.M., Harris and Klebold had killed twelve students, one teacher, and wounded twenty-one others.[11]

I suspect that in the morning hours that preceded the massacre, students, teachers, spouses, and parents were caught up in the much practiced rituals of know-how: turning off alarm clocks, going to the bathroom, attending to children, eating breakfast, offering loving goodbyes to family members, walking or driving to school, meeting friends, day-dreaming in class or studying hard, gossiping, worrying, laughing, and whenever necessary, dealing with setbacks in the best ways possible. A habitat of habits was alive and well. Then came 11:15 A.M. and the first forty-five minutes of hell that followed. A habitat of habits was literally under fire; worlds of know-how were being destroyed; and new ones came into use in a panic: people screamed and begged for help, ran for their lives, hid under tables, desks and behind doors, prayed, called the police. The news spread quickly. Media coverage was intense. If you were watching television at the time, you, too, could witness some of what was happening at the high school.

How does one cope with such a tragedy? Besides the screaming, begging, running, praying, and news-watching, what must one *know how* to do in order to survive and understand this horrible situation? How would you react to seeing a friend shot, maimed, killed? What was going through the minds of parents and spouses whose loved ones were known to be in the school that day but had not yet been rescued by S.W.A.T. teams? I suspect that as they heard and watched the news, many "religious" and "non-religious" students, teachers, parents, and spouses throughout the country were thinking of their loved ones and murmuring, at least to themselves, such things as "God, forbid!" or "There but for the grace of God go I." Next to the "fight or flight" reaction demonstrated throughout the animal kingdom, one of the most common human reactions to life-threatening situations is to know how to bring God into the situation so that at least some order can be maintained. Indeed, one student was supposedly asked by one of the murderers if she believed in God. "Yes," she said, and then he shot and killed her.[12]

For those who were actually there when it happened or who had some personal tie to the event (e.g., being a parent of a student), the Columbine High School Massacre certainly showed itself to be a heart-breaking and psychologically damaging event. It was an unforgettable tragedy that, as it unfolded, brought about a massive interruption in people's everyday worlds of know-how. Loved ones were dead and their survivors now had to deal with the difficult task of coping with immeasurable loss, of living in a world now void of a source of meaning that had once played a major role in maintaining this world's present and future well-being. The issue that is immediately raised by this situation is thus typically heard as a question of survival: "How am I to go on living without a certain love in my life?" The question expresses heart-felt concern for one's own existence (Being) and its loss of meaning. Such concern lies at the heart of the everyday world of know-how, for this world is built upon the various pragmatic ways that we deal with our personal well-being throughout our lives. An interruption that can shake this world to its very core and possibly even destroy it defines, to say the least, a major existential setback—one that sets us back to the "beginning," to that "primordial" temporal/spatial dimension of existence that, as will be further clarified below, supports all habitats of habits and routines and whose presence is easily taken for granted as these habitats condition us to *their* ways of life and know-how. These ways are human creations; the "beginning" being referred to here, however, is not. As Heidegger continually reminds us, we did not create the fundamental temporal/spatial structure of human being, the way we are "projected" and always "on the way" (*unterwegs*) toward what is not yet, the way we are open to the future. Human being, in other words, did not create what Heidegger, as noted above, describes as the "site," the "clearing," that "place" in existence where Being discloses itself to human beings. An "ontological difference" exists between the two. Taking a closer look at how this difference shows itself in light of some setback will be helpful.

Setbacks in the everyday world of know-how, if only brief and minute, help us realize the place where this difference resides. The world of know-how conditions us to think and speak of this place in terms of common sense measurements and abstractions: seconds, hours, days, weeks, and so on. A setback as overwhelming as the Columbine Massacre, however, takes us beyond this world of "public time." What it thereby gives us to understand is not a set of standards for knowing how to tell and manage time, but rather that upon which these standards take form: the temporality of our Being, the primordial existential process where future, past, and present are interpenetrating and inseparable *ekstases* rather than juxtaposed dimensions defined within an objectified spatiotemporal coordinate. A human being is not a "thing" that merely lives "in" time; it does not exist just "now" and "then" as does a coin in a pocket. Rather, a human being *exists as time*, as a being who is presently living its "having been" that once was its future, and who, at the same time, is presently living out the possibilities that are yet to come. The primordial time of human being is a "unitary phenomenon." The future, past, and present presuppose the ecstatic character of this phenomenon's existence—a character whose beginning is always happening in the actuality of a person's "potentiality-for-Being" and whose ending is commonly understood by such mortal creatures as the occurrence of "death." We are beings who *are open* to our own ultimate end on earth. We are also beings who, as we approach this end, are known to wonder: Where have I come from? Where am I going? How has life gone so far? Have I lived a good life?

Such questions, of course, speak to a larger issue that has been on the minds of human beings ever since they were able to reflect on the awesomeness of their own existence and wonder, "what it means to be." Our prehistoric ancestors most likely pondered the issue when, like us, they were made to feel not totally at home by some setback in their lives (e.g., not being warm enough; suffering from hunger; watching a family member or friend being eaten by a beast). More often than not, the question of Being is raised in moments of disruption, breakdown, crisis—moments wherein our everyday preoccupations in the world of know-how are put on hold and we thereby find ourselves taking more seriously than usual the relationship of life and death and, hence, the question of our Being.

Such moments are well-known for the anxiety they produce—an emotion that signals a significant loss of meaning and stability in our lives. In anxiety we remain open to the uncertainty that is inherent in our temporal existence: that in the face of which we are anxious is not merely the presence of some ontic occurrence raising havoc in our lives, but rather is that primordial condition of existence—the temporal openness of our Being—which makes itself known by way of such an occurrence. This ever-present condition, as Heidegger makes clear, is the true source of anxiety.[13] For example, a person may feel anxious when suddenly stricken by a serious illness, but the experience of this emotion is possible only if the person cares enough about *what is to become* of his or her existence now that it is no longer what it used to be and perhaps may never be again. In anxiety, we stand face to face with the "not yet" of the future and thus with the uncertainty that accompanies the dimension of existence that is always ahead of itself. In anxiety, in other words, we stand face to face with the question of our potentiality-for-Being and how we must put this potential to use if we expect to survive crisis and restore some sense of order (know-how) to our lives. Anxiety attunes us to a place where a call for decision and action is heard.

Let us keep in mind, however, that this place and its call are not human creations. The temporal opening of existence is always already there before any human being can have a say in the matter. Although the Being of this opening shows itself in human being, the two are not one and the same. Being is other than the beings that it sustains and who, in the case of the human, can come to know something of this otherness when the taken-for-granted function of the world of know-how experiences an interruption.

With the Columbine High School Massacre, the otherness of Being was all too apparent. The scene was filled with destruction and death. Anxiety prevailed. The spatial/temporal character of everyday existence was transformed. The moment was terrifying, disorienting, uncanny; people no longer felt at home. From this disturbing environment came a challenging call for thought, action, meaning, and order. Although human beings helped to express this call, its true source was and is more primordial than *their* individual voices. The call originates in the most primordial level of our temporal existence: our openness to the future, the fundamental way we are placed in the world to experience the Being of our lives whenever we have cause to wonder about what it means to be. Setbacks like the Columbine Massacre take us to a place that was there all along, although it was concealed before the setback by habitats (the world of know-how) that were initially constructed as responses to the call heard coming from this place. One might say then that—at this level of space and time—human being is its own evocation and provocation: as it continually happens, our openness to Being calls for the responsiveness of concerned thought and action, for that which enables us, even in the most distressful situations, to take charge of our lives as we assume the responsibility of affirming our freedom through some resolute choice and thereby become personally involved in the creation of meaningful existence. This process is how systems of morality come into being in the first place. The language of morality is the language of responsiveness and responsibility; hence, the essential "challenge-response" logic of moral systems ("Thou shall do this!"; "Thou shall not do that!").

Remember, however, that this particular moral logic is always already operating in the very Being of our temporal existence. Its challenging call is the initial summons for thought, action, meaning, and order. Heidegger associates this summons with the existential "beginnings" of "the call of conscience." This call for responsible thought and action comes to us from a place that we live in everyday but that we did not create. The call of conscience is rooted in something other than the traditional ways of life that constitute and define the "I," the ego, or one's subjectivity. The call of conscience is essentially the call of Being—a call that, for a community in Littleton, Colorado, was and still is difficult not to hear.[14] My discussion of the tragedy faced by this community was offered to prepare readers for a more philosophical discussion of the essential relationship between human being and Being. I need, however, to discuss one more aspect of the Columbine situation before making this move.

Ever since the tragedy happened, the media has kept the public informed about how people involved in the situation have responded to the call of conscience/Being with shock, grief, funerals, memories, moving stories, law suits, and, of course, attempted explanations of why the massacre occurred. The explanation that, at least at the present time, is most "definitive" is this: Harris and Klebold were "outsiders"—two students who were not members of the "in crowd" (with its population of popular, clean-cut kids and athletes) who were known for teasing and bullying people like Harris and Klebold. These two boys, in turn, were known for their alienation and their strange ways of coping with the situation. Indeed, Harris was taking the medication Luvox, which is an antidepressant commonly prescribed for people suffering from Obsessive-Compulsive Disorder (OCD). The boys hung out with each other, played violent video games, listened to German punk rock bands with "messages" of despair, hate, violence, and cruelty, and sometimes greeted each other with a Nazi stiff-armed salute. Harris kept a diary that he filled with "Nazi rhetoric," detailing how he and Klebold had been planning the massacre for the past year. On April 20, Adolph Hitler's birthday, blood would be spilled. The diary also made clear that Harris and his friends were tired of having jocks "putting them down."[15]

Yes, these two boys were strange. How could their parents not have known that something terribly wrong was going on in their children's lives? Accusations of teacher and parental neglect were announced in the media. Moreover, reported the media, being bullied and shamed by one's high school peers was nothing new. The practice could be recalled by many older people who went through the same thing, but who for one reason or another never went so far as to "crack" under the pressure and kill as a result of some childish setbacks in their lives.[16] The *real* bottom line of the massacre was that Harris and Klebold were weak, misguided, and disturbed souls. They could no longer stand their lives; they were incapable of responding to the call of Being in a positive and healthy manner. Bombs had to be ignited and triggers had to be pulled. It was time for revenge; it was time to die.

Harris and Klebold perpetrated the most finalizing act of negative acknowledgment there is. They were murderers, to be sure; and given their suicides, we might also brand them cowards. But if we accept the above explanation as a fair account of why these boys committed their heinous act, then I believe that we also have an obligation to ask a specific question: Would Harris and Klebold have committed their crime if they had received more positive acknowledgment from their peers and others during, say, the last year of their lives? I suspect that this question may make some people feel a bit uneasy and, perhaps, even stimulate outrage because the question allows for the possibility of spreading the blame beyond the killers and on to those innocent folks whose only "crime" was that they just happened to be people who had some role to play in maintaining the "outsider" status of Harris and Klebold. One could certainly argue with my raising of the question by holding on to that bit of cultural common sense that tells us how "insiders" and "outsiders" have always been with us and that such a class distinction should thus be accepted as a fact of life. I, at best, am making a mountain out of a mole hill. Moreover, it must also be admitted that although positive acknowledgment can be a life-giving gift, no "official" law exists that requires us to give it.

Ever since the Columbine Massacre took place, I have wondered what a world would be like if such a law *was* enacted. I suspect that the force of this law would become unbearable. Human beings are not known as creatures who possess the infinite energy it would take to be compassionate every single second of the day. We have not yet evolved—biologically and spiritually—to this level of perfection. Still, however, we are capable of asking a related and relevant question: What would life be like if no one cared enough to acknowledge our existence in a genuine and positive way? As I formulate the answer to the question in this book, I hope to encourage a fantasizing about what it would take to live in a world where positive acknowledgment was the rule of the day. Human beings, of course, would have to be in much better shape given the stamina that would be needed here. And we would also have to sharpen our ability to be keen observers of all that stands before us. Indeed, in the case of Columbine, the problem was not that Harris and Klebold were not *seen* by others—but that not enough (or the right) people took the time to *observe* their situation and the evil that permeated it.

Four months after the Columbine massacre, *The New York Times Magazine* featured a lengthy essay that considered some of the dimensions of such evil and their effect on "The Troubled Life of Boys." In her piece "The Outsiders: How the Picked-on Cope—or Don't," Adrian Nicole LeBlanc shares a host of observations based on her investigation of the New Hampshire regional high school, ConVal, and how, like Columbine, it contains "a brutally enforced teen-age social structure." In describing this structure's "pyramid" nature, LeBlanc writes:

> Boys at the bottom of the pyramid use different strategies to cope—
> turning inward and outward, sometimes in highly destructive ways.
> (There has been a fivefold jump in the homicide and suicide rates of
> boys in the last 40 years, a rise some experts attribute to increasing
> male depression and anger as well as access to guns, among other
> factors.) Most boys live through it, suffer, survive. But the journey
> may be especially deadly now because, as the avalanche of new
> "male identity" literature demonstrates, the old prescriptions for
> behavior no longer hold, and the new ones are ambivalent. Today's
> young males may be feminism's children, but no one is comfortable
> with openhearted or vulnerable boys.

LeBlanc also comments on "the traditional hierarchies" that prevail at the high school:

> ... the popular kids tend to be wealthier and the boys among them
> tend to be jocks. The Gap Girls-Tommy Girls-Polo Girls compose
> the pool of desirable girlfriends, many of whom are athletes as well.
> Below the popular kids, in a shifting order of relative unimportance,
> are the druggies (stoners, deadheads, burnouts, hippies or neo-

hippies), trendies or Valley Girls, preppies, skateboarders and skate-
boarder chicks, nerds and techies, wiggers, rednecks and Goths, better know as freaks. There are troublemakers, losers and floaters—
kids who move from group to group. Real losers are invisible.

To be such "an outcast boy," emphasizes the author, "is to be a 'nonboy,' to be
feminine, to be weak."[17]

LeBlanc is describing an evil that may facilitate an even greater one: cold-
blooded murder. The school's social hierarchy produces a vast amount of negative
acknowledgment. Even the positive acknowledgment that does occur within it—
say, for example, between the members of the jocks or between the members of
the deadheads—carries with it habits and routines that reify the levels of the hierarchy and thereby motivate further negative acknowledgment. I think it is absurd
to excuse the sickness here as something that is "normal" because of its long history. Human beings belong to a species that exalts its own status in the animal
kingdom by offering itself as a show-case of biological and spiritual evolution.[18]
Who, then, in their right mind would want to bolster the effects of this sickness by
accepting and facilitating its presence with a lame excuse?

An environment in which the know-how of positive acknowledgment is
geared to the production of ever more negative acknowledgment marks out a
place of increasing cruelty and brutality—a place wherein it does not pay to spend
much time cultivating a consciousness that is carefully attuned to, and respectful
of, the differences between others and ourselves. There are too many such places
on earth today. For the benefit of all concerned, we need to become more observant of all that stands before us—which is to say, following Heidegger, that we
need to learn how to open ourselves to the call of Being that informs human existence and that thereby warrants the affirmation of heart-felt acknowledgment.

Acknowledging Acknowledgment

Heidegger would have us perform a task that he maintains defines the "highest"
form of action.[19] Indeed, consciousness is an *act* that moves back and forth between seeing the world and observing the world. Acknowledgment heads us in the
direction of observation; hence, it requires us to do what our existence, itself, allows for: be open to the world. Recall that, from Heidegger's phenomenological
perspective, human beings hold a special relationship with Being, for their existence shows itself as the place (the site, clearing, opening) where Being can be
seen, observed with rigor, and acknowledged with care. Acknowledgment requires
that "openhearted" way of being that, as noted above, is sometimes equated, unfortunately, with weakness and femininity. Heidegger's way of making the point,
which was quoted earlier, provides us with a more phenomenologically sensitive
and less chauvinistic/sexist take on the matter: "Acknowledgment lets that toward
which it goes come toward it." The more people remain openhearted as they at-

tune their consciousness to things and others, the better chance acknowledgment has of happening. People who care not to bracket out their prejudices and concomitant stereotypes present themselves as poor candidates for doing what needs to be done when it comes to the practice of acknowledgment.

With the Columbine case, we are reminded of just how hard this task can be. The challenge-response logic that lies at the heart of human existence is most clearly apparent in situations of life and death; for here the issues of survival and personal responsibility are, as they say, "right in your face." Indeed, there are times when the world of know-how and the homey feeling it inspires can suddenly disappear right before one's eyes, leaving one to experience more than ever before what Heidegger terms "the bare 'that it is'" of existence and its way of being open to the future. From this primordial place of space and time comes a call that has a *constructive* ring to it: the future is constantly calling us to acknowledge and make use of our "response-ability" for making thoughtful decisions about how to build and live a meaningful life. Heidegger notes, however, that if we are to remain "authentic" while living the commitment of our decisions, we must be prepared and willing at any moment to question the supposed correctness of what we are thinking and doing as a result of having made these decisions. The constancy of the call demands as much, for it speaks to us of uncertainty and contingency: the future orientation of existence is forever opening us to the possibility of change, of things being otherwise than usual, of how what is yet to come in our lives may require us—for truth's sake—to rethink and revise what we currently hold to be correct about our ongoing commitments, involvements, and interpretive practices.

Notice, then, that along with its constructive nature, the call also has a *deconstructive* ring to it; for it repeatedly calls into question our desire for certainty and stability—a desire that manifests itself whenever we assume the personal responsibility of affirming our freedom through resolute choice in an effort to bring meaning and order to our everyday existence. In short, when listening to the call of conscience/Being, we are told constantly of the importance of being both decisive and open-minded. Owing to the changing circumstances of our lives, what appears to be "right" now may be "wrong" later. Our everyday way of inhabiting the world is always open to questioning, always being challenged by something other than itself (the temporality of Being), something that demands the creation of order if anxiety is not to dominate our lives.

Human being thus shows itself as an opening wherein a primordial and ongoing "struggle" takes place between order (construction) and disorder (deconstruction). The truth of Being has something fundamentally conflicting about it.[20] Setbacks expose us to this conflict; the more disruptive they are the more likely we are to experience the anxiety that arises from the challenge of existence itself, of being called on to own up to one's own existence whereby one must assume the personal responsibility of making decisions and choices that, sooner or later, will have consequences for oneself and others.

Heidegger's assessment of this call was not designed to offer ethical directives for human beings. Phenomenological observation and analysis have the goal of being descriptive, not prescriptive.[21] Heidegger is primarily interested in awakening people from their ontological slumber so that they might become better at *observing* and *acknowledging* the intricacies and essential structure of everyday existence. The phenomenology going on here defines an ontological exercise in the attunement of consciousness. I will now offer a more detailed discussion of what such an exercise entails and how, at least in my opinion, it *does* provide directives for gauging ethical and moral behavior.

The discussion of acknowledgment so far has emphasized certain happenings that define its unfolding nature: the world of know-how; the interruption of this spatial/temporal domain by existential setbacks; coming face-to-face with the question of one's Being; and withstanding the mood of anxiety while observing how it is that one is open to the objective uncertainty of the future. It would seem, then, that for acknowledgment to happen one must learn how to be courageous and steadfast when experiencing the consequences of a most disturbing mood. Heidegger emphasizes this point when he writes about the "*anxiety of conscience*," what it gives us to understand (the temporal unfolding of our Being), what it thereby calls us to do (to think and act in a responsible way), and how in this moment of responsibility one should also experience an "unshakable joy" in being able to take control of one's life.[22] I will be in a better position to say more about this experience of joy after I have clarified the relationship between anxiety and acknowledgment.

Anxiety holds a special place in Heidegger's philosophy, for it is this "mood," more than any other, that brings a person face to face with the question of Being and its concomitant challenge: that of being courageous and resolute. According to Heidegger, "He who is resolute knows no fear; but he understands the possibility of anxiety as the possibility of the very mood which neither inhibits nor bewilders him" but, instead, encourages a clear-headed assessment and praiseworthy response.[23] Caught up in the Columbine situation, one might expect such a person to display the qualities of a "superman" as he or she willingly and heroically risked his or her life to save others. This behavior was reported to have happened during the massacre, as teachers and students tried to protect each other. But is this to suggest, following Heidegger, that all those who allowed anxiety to get the better of them failed the challenge of "authenticity" that was vividly disclosed in the crisis situation?

The way Heidegger treats the issue of anxiety throughout his philosophy makes me think that he would offer a somewhat hard-hearted answer to the question. For my present purposes, however, I need not get caught up in the potential controversy here.[24] Instead, I wish only to emphasize that Heidegger's attraction to anxiety is due in great part to the unsurpassed, disclosing ability of this mood. Anxiety ("Angst"; also translated as "Dread") is unequaled when it comes to clearing the way for acknowledging the truth of Being—or that which is "Other" than a human creation. Heidegger maintains that in the search for truth one must be ever prepared for the experience of this potentially terrifying mood:

> Readiness for dread is to say "Yes!" to the inwardness of things, to fulfill the highest demand which alone touches man to the quick. Man alone of all beings, when addressed by the voice of Being, experiences the marvel of all marvels: that what-is *is*. Therefore the being that is called in its very essence to the truth of Being is always attuned in an essential sense. The clear courage for essential dread guarantees that most mysterious of all possibilities: the experience of Being. For hard by essential dread . . . there dwells awe (*Scheu*). Awe clears and enfolds that region of human being within which man endures, as at home, in the enduring [of Being].[25]

At the heart of human existence lies a challenge, a call, in need of response. In anxiety we are most attuned to this call of Being—a call that speaks of the importance of decisiveness and open-mindedness. The call has both a constructive and deconstructive ring to it: it calls for that which it also calls into question. The call of Being demands courage from those who remain open to it and, in doing so, stand ready to acknowledge how their ways of thinking and acting may not be as authentic and respectful as they could possibly be. Although listening to the call is likely to make us feel uncanny, we should nevertheless realize that this state of not feeling at home is, in fact, the most primordial way in which we dwell on earth and thus are at home in the world. The habits and routines of everyday life condition us to think otherwise, but the fact, sometimes revealed all too clearly by existential crises, nevertheless remains. As William Barrett puts it: "We may chatter about alienation as a cultural or social phenomenon, but all such talk falls short of the deepest dimension in which man is a stranger in his universe. And yet this dimension of strangeness is the peculiar home where he is drawn closest to all that is." Commenting further on this strangeness and its "mystery," Barrett writes:

> Any utopian social arrangement, where what is facilely called "alienation" would cease, would make humankind most truly alienated from its own being. Creatures of a void without knowing it.
>
> Humankind . . . must . . . bear the burden of this mystery. Is it too great, amid our other anxieties, for us to carry? It makes us feel more homeless within the world than any animal can be. Yet is it altogether a burden? Is it not rather a gift too? It is given to us and to no other animal to stand within the mystery. It claims us as its own and we are at home there where no other animal can be. Tonight the stars shine overhead like old and reliable friends. This cosmos is

ours to the degree that we are still able to be enthralled by its stupendous presence.[26]

This last point brings us back to Heidegger's earlier quoted observation regarding how the relationship between anxiety and acknowledgment inspires "awe": human beings are capable of being awestruck by the presencing of what is. Awe defines a state wherein we are open to and are being addressed by something that inspires amazement and wonder; something that, at least for the moment, is beyond total comprehension and that may fill us as much with joy as it does with anxiety. Heidegger spoke of joy in *Being and Time* because with anxiety there comes the opportunity to assume control over one's thoughts and actions and to thereby become "authentic." In his 1929 essay "What Is Metaphyics?" Heidegger also associates awe with a state of mind that has evolved from joy and/or anxiety into a "spell-bound peace" and "the serenity and gentleness of creative longing."[27] Although such a state of mind may appear to be more "religious" than anything else, it is not Heidegger's intention here to transform his phenomenological investigations into a theological project. With its commitment to offering an empirically based description of what is, phenomenology is more scientific than religious in its orientation, and Heidegger's interest in awe and the attunement of consciousness (acknowledgment) that goes with it is directed toward a description of a way of observing the world that is most receptive to the truth of the matter at hand.

Heidegger would certainly point to his own research endeavors as an example of the attunement of consciousness being advocated here. Perhaps a more practical and, hence, better example would be that of the doctor-patient relationship where one finds what Anatole Broyard describes as an "embracing of the patient's condition" that extends beyond a mere biological, chemical, and numerical assessment of the patient's disease and includes a careful consideration of the patient's personhood and overall existential plight. A patient is not just some diseased body lying in some bed. Rather, a patient is a human being whose hopes, beliefs, relationships, and personal needs may also be in a state of distress and disease and who, therefore, is desperate for the sound of caring words and the touch of gentle hands. Broyard wants patients to be seen *and* observed: "Why bother with sick people, why try to save them, if they're not worth acknowledging? When a doctor refuses to acknowledge a patient, he is, in effect, abandoning him to his illness."[28]

Heidegger would have us open ourselves to all that stands before us as Broyard would have physicians open themselves to those they are obligated to serve. In both cases, the encounter is rooted in a heartfelt act of acknowledgment whereby something is both seen and observed with "loving" care. Indeed, love is the emotion known for its capacity of openness and receptivity. Moreover, love is space-binding: the lover feels himself or herself close to the beloved in spite of distance. Acknowledgment is an act whereby we open ourselves to things and to others in order to foster and maintain a close (loving) relationship with them. Setbacks may bring much dis-ease to this relationship. For example: patients can be quite "unattractive" because of what some illness is doing to their bodies and dispositions, or a quarrel between a husband and wife can turn quite nasty. Anxiety can arise in such situations as people are brought face-to-face with uncertainty and the possibility of "worse things to come." Love does not necessarily put an end to anxiety, but it is known to calm down this "dreadful" emotion so that a more peaceful and hopeful environment can take shape; hence, Heidegger's earlier noted notions of "spell-bound peace" and "the serenity and gentleness of creative longing." In *Being and Time*, these notions are described simply as "sober anxiety."[29] As will be discussed below, Heidegger continues to develop the notions in an attempt to describe the attunement of consciousness that promotes acknowledgment and the experience of awe.

He thereby speaks of how acknowledgment and awe involve "sacrifice," "essential thinking," and "releasement," or what he also terms the ability "to let beings be."

Sacrifice, Essential Thinking, and Releasement

Acknowledgment requires sacrifice. What must be sacrificed here, according to Heidegger, is our common tendency to order and understand our surroundings by way of "calculative thought" alone. Such thought fuels the everyday world of know-how; it is willful, practical, and deliberative. As such, notes Heidegger, "its own great usefulness" can only take place as it discloses beings in terms of its own purposive inclinations and everyday activities. "Calculative thought places itself under compulsion to master everything in the logical terms of its procedure."[30] Medical science, for example, is a haven for such thought—as it must be if its practitioners are to use their technical expertise (know-how) to cure a patient's disease. As noted above, however, if physicians intend to treat their patients in a more holistic way, they must supplement such expertise with a competence for caring for the personhood of a given patient. Such competence presupposes the workings of a special type of consciousness/thinking known for its open-minded and receptive ways. We have seen that, following Heidegger, one might speak of this particular attunement of consciousness as the loving mood of sober anxiety. In his later writings, however, Heidegger describes it "simply" as an exercise in "essential thinking."

Essential thinking is nothing more and nothing less than the tie that binds a human being's special relationship to Being. I spoke of this relationship in the second section of this chapter when discussing how human being "*is* essentially" the relationship of "responding to Being." That is, human being is that place/clearing/site/opening in Being where Being can show itself to a consciousness that can see, feel, and hear its presence in the materials of everyday life and that can also think about and articulate an understanding of the perceived event. Human beings are fated to hear the call of Being that discloses itself in everything that is and that thereby "reaches out" to us, "invites" thought, and thus "sets in motion" a process that defines the existential basis of human understanding. Human beings must respond to the call of Being if they are to gain a genuine appreciation not only of whatever it is that concerns them but also of that which makes possible the existence of everything that is and that thereby ought to warrant their utmost respect. "What calls on us to think," writes Heidegger, "needs thinking because what calls us wants itself to be thought about according to its nature. What calls on us to think, demands for itself that it be tended, cared for, husbanded in its own essential nature, by thought."[31] In meeting this demand, whereby we are being true to the essential relationship that we hold with Being, we assume what Heidegger stresses is our highest responsibility and thus ultimate calling: to be "the shepherd of Being" by thinking its truth and bringing it into language.[32] In the next chapter I focus attention on the second part of this responsibility. For now, however, a bit more needs to be said about the responsibility of thinking.

Essential thinking constitutes an act of loving acknowledgment whereby one takes special care to respect the call of Being that discloses itself in the existence ("beingness") of beings, in what and how they are. Expanding on the role played by emotion in this process, Heidegger emphasizes that the call of Being is thus something that needs to be "taken to heart" so that its truth is placed in "safekeeping" and remains "memorable." For Heidegger, taking to heart what the call of Being discloses constitutes an act of "devotion," "a steadfast intimate concentration upon the things that essentially speak to us in every thoughtful meditation."[33] This is how we open ourselves to the call of Being such that, in a moment of "releasement," of "wonder" and "awe," we can experience "the marvel of marvels: that what is is." By way of devotion, which Heidegger also describes as a "'letting be' of what-is," we return "Being's favor" by giving "thankful" thought to what Being first gives us.[34] Heidegger writes:

> When we give thanks we give it for something. We give thanks for something by giving thanks to him whom we have to thank for it. The things for which we owe thanks are not things we have from ourselves. They are given to us. We receive many gifts of many kinds. But the highest and really most lasting gift given to us is always our essential nature [the distinctive relationship we hold with Being], with which we are gifted in such a way that we are what we are only through it. That is why we owe thanks for this endowment, first and unceasingly.[35]

Giving thanks to Being is a matter of the heart, of "taking to heart" what calls on us to think the truth of what is.

Referring to the heart in this way is certainly reminiscent of how the Old Testament speaks to us of "conscience," of that wondrous gift that enables us to be awed by the happenings and mysteries of life and that thereby keeps us in touch with the Lord's call: "I will give them a heart to know me, that I am the Lord" (Jeremiah 24: 7), the One whose Saying—"Let there be . . ."—brought about the original letting-be of what is. As noted earlier, however, in Heidegger's case this Saying and the gift that goes with it come from Being—that which needs beings in order to show itself but also that which is more (other) than everything that is. Might it be the case that this otherness of Being is a sign of God? Heidegger leaves us to answer this question for ourselves. He is doing phenomenology, not theology. And remember, phenomenology is more akin to science than to religion, for like the scientist, the phenomenologist is committed to advancing an empirically based assessment of what is.[36] Yet, one must also remember that, for Heidegger, there remains a crucial difference between scientific thought and phenomenological thought, for in the later a "sacrifice" must be made so that the truth of the matter at hand can show itself beyond the restrictions imposed on it by the ways and means of calculative thought. Heidegger puts it this way:

> In sacrifice there is expressed that hidden *thanking* [essential thinking] which alone does homage to the grace wherewith Being has endowed the nature of man, in order that he may take over in his relationship to Being the guardianship of Being. Original thanking is the echo of Being's favor wherein it clears a space for itself and causes the unique occurrence: That what-is is. This echo is man's answer to the Word of the soundless voice of Being. The speechless answer of his thanking through sacrifice is the source of the human word, which is the prime cause of language as the enunciation of the Word in words.[37]

Despite his being a phenomenologist, Heidegger's discourse here (and throughout his later philosophy) is more reminiscent of the rhetoric of religion than it is the rhetoric of science. A possible explanation for this fact is not hard to figure out: Heidegger is being true to his word and thus speaks to us having already made a necessary sacrifice. He is a self-acclaimed "essential thinker" who is devoted to disclosing the truth of Being and who has thereby entered into a state of "releasement," a "letting go" of ordinary ways of knowing how to calculate and understand all that stands before us. Heidegger thus likens himself to the devoted poet who is forever trying to have language reveal more than it conceals so that he can disclose some truth that remains un-thought and unsaid by those who have yet to learn how their calculative ways of thinking and speaking close them off to the "Saying" of this truth. Like the poet, Heidegger is one who tries to maintain a thoughtful "conversation" with Being—a conversation dedicated to having language become more attuned with the way things are disclosing themselves and thus with the truth of what and how they are. Heidegger maintains that such a conversation is the most responsible way to acknowledge Being, for the "communication" going on here, given its subject matter, is obliged to remain open to that which is itself open (the temporality of Being). What is to come? Who can say for sure? The truth of existence announces itself as an objective uncertainty; Being *is* structured as a challenge, a call, a question, an ongoing process of deconstruction and reconstruction that, in its own silent way, tells of the importance of being open to and awed by the truth.

The world of know-how; the interruptions of setbacks; the deconstructive and reconstructive call of conscience; responsibility; anxiety, joy, love, and awe; essential thinking. We have come a long way with Heidegger in exploring how the attunement of consciousness that allows for acknowledgment is possible. As a phenomenologist, he leads us through an exercise in acknowledging the importance of a life-giving gift that is received with the help of essential thinking. I think it is fair to say that with this gift the world could become a better place. Indeed, what would life be like if no one acknowledged your existence? Acknowledgment is a moral act. Listen, however, to what Heidegger says about the essential thinking that he champions: "Such thinking has no result. It has no effect. It satisfies its essence in that it is. But it is by saying its matter."[38] Thus, the conversation with Being and the sacrifice that goes with it:

> Sacrifice is rooted in the nature of the event through which Being claims man for the truth of Being. Therefore it is that sacrifice brooks no calculation, for calculation always miscalculates sacrifice in terms of the expedient and the inexpedient, no matter whether the aims are set high or low. Such calculation distorts the nature of sacrifice. The search for a purpose dulls the clarity of the awe, the spirit of sacrifice ready prepared for dread, which takes upon itself kinship with the imperishable [Being].[39]

We must learn to think and thank Being, to acknowledge and to be awed by its call. For what purpose? To ask the question is to miss the point for Heidegger; although this is not to say that he fails to realize the necessity of being purposeful. Being, argues Heidegger, speaks its own purpose as it continues to show itself in the existence of beings; we, then, need only learn to listen carefully so as to acknowledge what it has to say about such things as openness, respect, and responsibility. Heidegger credits such listening as being an "ethical" achievement in the most original sense of the term. The basic meaning of *ethos* refers to the "abode" or "dwelling place" that founds our communal relationships with others and wherein a person's virtuous character is developed.[40] To be a good listener, observer, acknowledger is to clear a place in space and time where all things can have a say in what is to become of them. Essential thinking has a purpose and, I submit, it is essentially moral; for with this specific attunement of consciousness we display a commitment for understanding the truth of all that is and for sharing this understanding with others through language. Essential thinking is essential for the receiving and the granting of the life-giving gift of acknowledgment. We need Being and Being needs us. There exists a special relationship between Being and human being. Being calls, and for its sake and ours, we must respond.

Conclusion: The Law of the Beginning

Heidegger's path of thinking returns us to the "beginning," which, for him, remember, is neither God nor the Big Bang, but simply Being—that which we are, but that which is also more than us. Heidegger's lifelong quest was to discover as much about this "otherness" of Being as possible. In a discussion of what he terms "the law of the beginning," wherein he considers the "gift" of Being's openness, Heidegger speaks to the endlessness of his task. What he has to say may sound a bit strange, but if one listens carefully, it is possible to recognize a similarity between what he is talking about and what theologians and scientists admit about God and the Big Bang:

> The beginning does not at first allow itself to emerge as beginning but instead retains in its own inwardness its beginning character. The beginning then first shows itself in the begun, but even there never immediately and as such. Even if the begun appears as the begun, its beginning and ultimately the entire "essence" of the beginning can still remain veiled. Therefore the beginning first unveils itself in what has already come forth from it. As it begins, the beginning leaves behind the proximity of its beginning essence and in that way conceals itself. Therefore an experience of what is at the beginning by no means guarantees the possibility of thinking the beginning itself in its essence. The first beginning is, to be sure, what is decisive for everything; still, it is not the primordial beginning, i.e., the beginning that simultaneously illuminates itself and its essential domain and in that way begins. This beginning of the primordial beginning comes to pass at the end. We know, however, neither the character nor the moment of the ultimate end of history and certainly not its primordial essence.[41]

Being is the beginning: the opening and disclosing of all that is. Heidegger thinks about this event. What he ends up acknowledging is far-reaching and unprecedented in the history of philosophy. Still, however, his thinking is limited to the "begun," to the truth of "what has already come forth" as the existence of beings. The "primordial" beginning, the truth of Being, lies beyond the vantage point—the begun—from which it can be acknowledged, although never completely, as far as we know.

A much earlier version of this "mystery" of Being is found in the teachings of Jewish Mysticism (Kabbalah), which date back to the late Twelfth Century. Kabbalists teach that the common translation of the first line of Genesis ("In the beginning God created the heavens and the earth") is, in fact, a mistranslation, for the actual words in Hebrew can be read another way. Rabbi David Cooper thus tells us that a "kabbalist could say: 'With a beginning, [It] created God (*Elohim*), the heavens and the earth.' That is to say, out of Nothingness the potential to begin was created—Beginningness. Once there was a beginning, God (in a plural form) was created—a God to which the rest of creation could relate. Then the heaven and the earth were created." Cooper then goes on to make the following crucial point: "The implication of this interpretation profoundly affects our entire relationship with God and creation, for it says that all the names we have for God and all the ways in which we relate to God are a few degrees removed from the source of creation that precedes even Nothingness. This is called *Ein Sof*, which is not the name of a thing, but is an ongoing process."[42] "Infinity" is the term commonly associated with the "meaning" of this process. *Ein Sof*, however, is not "restricted" by infinity; rather, it created it. Writes Cooper: "Indeed, we have suddenly run out of words because the idea of 'trans-infinite' is a logical absurdity. What can go beyond infinity? Moreover, what can go beyond the Nothingness that surrounds infinity? This is *Ein Sof*."[43]

I think it is fair to say that this "trans-infinite" happening is what Heidegger is acknowledging when, as noted above, he maintains that "The first beginning is, to be sure, what is decisive for everything; still, it is not the primordial beginning, i.e., the beginning that simultaneously illuminates itself and its essential domain and in that way begins." Of course, this certainly is not to suggest that Heidegger was a closet Kabbalist. Still, the similarities in thinking are striking. Being, *Ein Sof*, the beginning of the beginning, is always other than the begun and thus all that there is in the universe.

And is this not the way scientists also think about the matter? As discussed in chapter two, cosmologists tell us that the universe is an expanding process; it thus follows that the process had a starting point, a beginning that was there "before" the process itself began with a Big Bang. This starting point defines a singularity, a phenomenon of infinite temperature, density, and energy that exists outside of space-time, in a state of "nothingness," the presence of absence. Might the truth of this absence be reduced to some mathematical formulation? "Yes," say many hopeful scientists. "No," say many equally hopeful religious souls. With his response, Heidegger is more on the side of religion than of science; although his phenomenological way of coming to a decision certainly sides more with the empirical motivations of science than it does with the "God-of-the-gaps" thinking of religion. For Heidegger would have us attune our consciousness to what *is* and thereby acknowledge the complex nature and function of Being. At the same time, however, he would also have us pay more careful attention to what scientists too easily take for granted when, in moments of awe, they wonder about the beginnings of the universe and the way it originated in a Big Bang. Heidegger focuses on the relationship that holds between human being and Being itself: a relationship of time, space, place, consciousness, emotion, and responsibility. Scientists would have us look back to what was happening "before the beginning" so that we might be able to capture its essence in equations that reduce it all to numbers. Heidegger, on the other hand, finds his essential directives not in the stars but rather right here on earth: a place in which another place appears and thereby provides an opening for thinking about such matters as God, the Big Bang, and creatures complex enough to ponder how they evolved and where they might be going as their evolution continues.

In this chapter we have concerned ourselves with Heidegger's phenomenological assessment of the matter because, more than religion or science, such an assessment is especially attentive to the existential and ontological workings of the major phenomenon in question here: acknowledgment. With Heidegger, this phenomenon is understood to define the most genuine way of being open to the Being of beings such that we might witness the truth and assume the responsibility of bringing it into language. It is now time to give careful consideration to this responsibility. As we will see, Heidegger still remains helpful here, but only to a point.

Chapter Four

Dwelling Places

Based on what has been said so far about acknowledgment, it should be clear that there is something fundamentally ethical about the phenomenon, its attunement of consciousness, its "essential thinking," its way of being open to the Being of beings. Acknowledgment is an act oriented toward what is other than the person performing the act: it works to clear a "dwelling place" (*ethos*) in space and time where other people and things can be carefully observed and listened to for the purpose of allowing them a say about the truth of their existence. Although its openness may give rise to anxiety, acknowledgment nevertheless maintains a sober outlook out of love for what it is doing for others. By way of acknowledgment, human being maintains a special relationship with Being. Human being is the place where Being shows itself as something that can be understood and expressed. Heidegger thus maintains that "If the name 'ethics,' in keeping with the basic meaning of the word *ethos*, should now say that 'ethics' ponders the abode [or dwelling place] of man, then that thinking which thinks [acknowledges] the truth of Being . . . is in itself the original ethics."[1]

For Heidegger, "ethics" is first and foremost a matter of being true to our fundamental relationship with Being: that is, of making sure that we remain open and receptive to matters that need and thus call for our attention. Heidegger speaks of this original ethics as "the law of Being."[2] The Being of human being *is open to* the future, to what is not yet but that, in all of its uncertainty, is still bound to come our way. Human being is always first on the receiving end of existence, ever in need of being receptive and responsive to the demands of its challenging call. Only by remaining open to the presence of all that stands before us can we answer this call and, in so doing, perhaps *tell* something of its truth. The law of

Being *speaks* of the importance of such ethical behavior. So it is that language has a role to play in enacting this law.

The Language of Being

It is important to realize that Heidegger's understanding of the nature and function of language is first and foremost rooted in ontology. Being calls as it shows itself in beings. Heidegger speaks of this calling/showing of Being as the most genuine "saying of language" (*logos*), a saying that is always already being announced before any given act of expression re-presents it in some symbolic form.[3] With the relationship that holds between Being and human being, there happens the original "bringing-forth" (*poiesis*) of *what is* to our attention. For Heidegger, this means that the dwelling place wherein Being and human being are joined defines a primordial habitat that is first and foremost "poetic": We "dwell poetically" with Being; our temporal and spatial existence is the place where the bringing-forth of all that there is can be witnessed, understood, and, especially with the help of great works of art, displayed.[4]

Great works of art display something of the truth of what is; they thus function to disclose and express something of a more original disclosure. A great work of art functions to call our attention to a more primordial call—that of Being. The whole experience is meant to be quite evocative. Heidegger does not confine this evocation to the realm of "high" or "fine" art. Consider, for example, his description of a bridge that strikes him as being particularly poetic and thus revelatory of the Being of beings.

> The bridge swings over the stream "with ease and power." It does not just connect banks that are already there. The banks emerge as banks only as the bridge crosses the stream. The bridge designedly causes them to lie across from each other. One side is set off against the other by the bridge. Nor do the banks stretch along the stream as indifferent border strips of the dry land. With the banks, the bridge brings to the stream the one and the other expanse of the landscape lying behind them. It brings streams and bank and land into each other's neighborhood. The bridge *gathers* the earth as landscape around the stream. Thus it guides and attends the stream through the meadows. Resting upright in the stream's bed, the bridge-piers bear the swing of the arches that leave the stream's waters to run their course. The waters may wander on quiet and gay, the sky's floods from storm or thaw may shoot past the piers in torrential waves—the bridge is ready for the sky's weather and its fickle nature. Even where the bridge covers the stream, it holds its flow up to the sky by taking it for a moment under the vaulted gateway and then setting it free once more.[5]

Heidegger, whose language here reflects an effort in dwelling poetically, is acknowledging a bridge that he apparently feels was designed and built to acknowledge and thus pay homage to the naturalness of the surrounding environment. The essential purpose of the bridge entails more than being just a mere tool for human travel; it also exists in a way that shows respect for the truth of other matters. The bridge brings "banks" into being that accentuate not only themselves but also a stream and surrounding landscape that give place to the bridge. "The bridge *gathers* the earth as landscape around the stream" and allows its "waters to run their course." Yes, the beauty and truth of nature is a bit spoiled here, but it is also made more evocative because of how the architectural design of some technology dwells poetically with the essential place of the earth.

With Heidegger we are lead to believe that whomever designed and built this technology was, at heart, a poet capable of creating a praiseworthy "work of art" whose instrumental function was carefully integrated with its aesthetic (poetic) function. Heidegger continually tells us throughout his later philosophy how the "work" of the "great poet" grants guidance to those who seek to express the "language of Being" in a most truthful (disclosing) manner: ". . . the responding in which man authentically listens to the appeal [the primordial 'saying'] of language is that which speaks in the element of poetry. The more poetic a poet is—the freer (that is, the more open and ready for the unforeseen) his saying—the greater is the purity with which he submits what he says to an ever more painstaking listening."[6] For Heidegger, then, it is the poet who knows more than most that language "is not a mere tool, one of the many which man possesses; on the contrary, it is only language that affords the very possibility of standing in the openness of the existence. Only where there is language, is there world, i.e., the perpetually altering circuit of decision and production, of action and responsibility, but also of commotion and arbitrariness, of decay and confusion."[7]

Commotion, arbitrariness, decay, confusion. As one who constantly warns about the danger that these states pose to our related abilities to understand the truth and to build communal relationships (dwelling places) on this understanding, Heidegger makes much of the poet's importance for helping to maintain a culture's well-being. For it is the poet, claims Heidegger, who affirms the proper dignity of human being, its most essential and thus authentic calling, by bringing into the language of "mortal speech" a heightened sense of some happening of truth. The poet does this not only as one who has entered into what was referred to in the last chapter as a state of "releasement," a "letting go" of beings so as to allow them to be what they are, but also as one who has developed a sensitivity to the "playful" nature of the "being of language." This playful nature shows itself in how words both reveal and conceal that which they name. The devoted poet is forever trying to have language reveal more than it conceals so that she or he can disclose some truth that remains un-thought and unsaid by those who have yet to learn how their "calculative" ways of thinking and speaking close them off to the "saying" of this truth. The poet is committed to keeping the "conversation" going between human beings and Being. Heidegger thus writes: ". . . poetry is the inaugural naming of being and of the essence of all things—not just any speech, but that particular kind which for the first time brings into the open all that which we then discuss and deal with in everyday language." The poet's conversation with Being, "in which language does truly become actual," forms "the foundation of human existence."[8]

The "greatness" of art—be it architecture, sculpture, painting, linguistic composition, or whatever—lies in its ability to acknowledge and display the truth of its subject matter, the Being of beings (which, as in the case of the bridge noted above, can be quite extensive). Is this to suggest that Heidegger's philosophical investigations of Being are also an ongoing experiment in art, aesthetics, poetry? Listen to the later Heidegger: "It is time to break the habit of overestimating philosophy and of thereby asking too much of it. What is needed in the present world crisis is less philosophy, but more attentiveness in thinking"—that "essential" kind that informs the work of great poets.[9]

Although Heidegger typically retreats to philosophical abstractions (or at least to poetic expression) when he attempts to illustrate the specific ways of such thinking, he nevertheless does identify four criteria that he claims are essential to the "discourse" of poetry and that thereby should be employed when judging the appropriateness or "fittingness" of such discourse. These include "rigor of meditation, carefulness in saying, frugality with words," and the "timeliness" of these words.[10] Such criteria, of course, were first acknowledged and defined by the ancient Greeks and Romans (e.g., Isocrates, Plato, Aristotle, Cicero, Quintilian) as being matters of "rhetorical" competence—that is, of knowing how to organize arguments from the substantive facts and issues of a given case, the emotions of the audience, and the character of the speaker for the purpose of moving ideas to people and people to ideas for the betterment of the citizenry. Heidegger's early lectures on Plato's *Sophist* and Aristotle's *Rhetoric* certainly attest to his understanding of the necessity of this competence.[11] Still, however, as an "essential thinker" taken with the brilliance of such German poets as Friedrich Hölderlin, Stefan George, and Rainer Maria Rilke, Heidegger remains content emphasizing the importance of learning how to dwell poetically over the practical necessity of learning how to dwell rhetorically.

Critics of Heidegger have made much of the inappropriateness of his decision here. Hans-Georg Gadamer—certainly one of Heidegger's most respected students and supporters—puts the matter this way: "What man needs is not just the persistent posing of ultimate questions, but the sense of what is feasible, what is possible, what is correct, here and now. The philosopher, of all people, must, I think, be aware of the tension between what he claims to achieve and the reality in which he finds himself."[12] The philosopher Richard Bernstein is more succinct:

"Our dialogue, and communicative transactions, are not only with Being itself, but with other human beings."[13]

The problem noted here is in great part the result of Heidegger's fanaticism when it comes to stressing the importance of learning how to open oneself to and acknowledge the Being of beings. Still, however, I think it wise not to *underestimate* the importance of such instruction. For the sake of themselves, others, and the environment in general, human beings must learn to dwell poetically; for there is only one earth that can sustain the relationship that human beings hold with Being—a relationship that, as we have seen, is itself an essential dwelling place in need of cultivation and maintenance. Upon these physical and ontological domains are built still other habitats (e.g., factories, skyscrapers, parks, houses) that help us to feel secure, comfortable, and at home in the world. Life is necessarily filled with the practical matters of human dwelling places. Heidegger's thinking about Being and its relationship to poetry lends itself to an assessment of a few of these matters. Those who appropriate this thinking when, for example, writing about "the ethical function of architecture" help to illustrate the applicability of Heidegger's thought—especially how it provides directives for being conscientious and caring when constructing and maintaining some habitat.[14]

For my purposes, however, this use of Heidegger does not go far enough. Although I, too, am interested in how architecture can serve the ethical and moral purpose of helping human beings to dwell poetically on earth, the specific type of architecture of immediate concern here is better known for its "persuasive" character. I speak, of course, of "rhetoric" and the competence it takes to use it effectively in helping people to acknowledge and judge what is good, just, and truthful. As will be discussed in greater detail later on in this chapter, the profession of architecture is not unaware of how its interest in "decoration" aligns it with a common (and at times unflattering) understanding of "rhetoric." But this interest, as typically expressed by architects, does not focus on how the rhetorical competence of people can help bring about "works of art" that transform and give shape to a place and thereby make it into a habitat for developing moral thought and action. This lack of focus, as noted above, is also a feature of Heidegger's philosophy: the topic of rhetorical competence remains more concealed than revealed in his writings. When, however, it comes to assessing the existential function of acknowledgment, the topic necessarily warrants more careful attention. For human beings are creatures who not only dwell poetically, but also rhetorically. Caught up as we are in the midst of the objective uncertainty of our temporal existence, we must hear and respond to the call of Being without ever knowing for sure whether we have finally got it right. *Rhetoric finds a home whenever matters are ambiguous, contestable, and questionable.* "Lacking definitive evidence and being compelled to act are the prerequisites of the rhetorical situation."[15] The call of Being speaks of such matters, and as it does we are reminded of the rhetorical nature of our existence. The rest of this chapter is devoted to a discussion of the type of competence that is needed if this specific nature of ours is to maintain its well-being and strength of character. More, too, will be said about the relationship that may hold between this competence, God, and the Big Bang.

Rhetorically, We Dwell

One of the earliest accounts of the importance of rhetorical competence for establishing and maintaining our social well-being is offered by Isocrates: "Because there has been implanted in us the power to persuade each other and to make clear to each other what we desire, not only have we escaped the life of wild beasts, but we have come together and founded cities and made laws and invented arts; and, generally speaking, there is no institution devised by man which the power of speech has not helped us to establish. For this it is which has laid down laws concerning things just and unjust, and things honorable and base; and if it were not for these ordinances we should not be able to live with one another."[16] As exemplified here, associating rhetorical competence with the creation and preservation of a community's moral ecology is a commonplace of the rhetorical tradition, one that works as a major source of legitimation for teachers of rhetoric. But when "the power to persuade" becomes the all-too-easy target it is made out to be in, for example, Plato's *Gorgias* and *Sophist* and later in Descartes, Locke, Kant, and Hegel, this competence is dissociated from its declared connection with the morality of a community or culture (and more broadly with the human orientation to ideals as guides for behavior).

The rhetorical tradition has had much to say about rhetorical competence in the narrower sense: the civic-minded power to persuade. Conceptualized in terms of the canons of the art of rhetoric, for example, rhetorical competence has been specified as a proficiency in handling the five stages of composing and presenting a speech: *inventio* (invention), *dispositio* (arrangement), *elocutio* (expression), *memoria* (memory), and *pronuntiatio* or *actio* (delivery), as well as an ability to handle the formal divisions of the speech: *exordium* (introduction), *narratio* (narration), *partitio* (division), *confirmatio* (proof), *refutatio* (refutation), and *conclusio* (conclusion). Knowing how to put these elements to use when confronting the contingent demands of a situation may facilitate a person's attempts to be persuasive, but for the ancients, rhetorical competence could also function as an integrative social influence between the self and others.[17]

Beginning with the Sophists, training in rhetorical competence has had as one of its internal goals increasing people's chances of getting an equal hearing for their ideas such that they and their contributions might be recognized and respected as important to the sociopolitical workings of a community.[18] Moreover, as Aristotle would have us understand in expanding on this point, the service provided to the community by its members' rhetorical competence extends beyond mere persuasion to include the development of judgment (*krisis*) and practical

wisdom (*phronesis*). Rhetorical competence lends itself to collaborative deliberation and reflective inquiry (including the self-deliberations of individual members). An audience is not set at a distance in the rhetorical situation. *Rather, it is
acknowledged, engaged, and called into the space of practical concerns.* By facilitating
civic engagement, rhetorical competence helps sustain and enrich the knowledge
of any public, and thus a community's own competence. Through the deliberative
rationality of rhetorical practices, a community can recognize itself and judge
whether to admit the epistemological and moral claims of those who are attempting to influence it.[19] In its very functioning, rhetorical competence gives expression to the communal character of the self's existence and in so doing allows all
concerned to "know together" (Gk. *sun-eidesis*; Lat. *con-scientia*). Maintaining the
health of our communal existence requires nothing less than this moral endeavor,
based as it is on the communicative and rhetorical act of acknowledgment.

Rhetoric and acknowledgment go hand in hand, for as Calvin Schrag reminds us: "The distinctive stamp of rhetorical intentionality is that it reaches out
toward, aims at, is directed to the other as hearer, reader, and audience. This intentionality illustrates not the theoretical reflection of cognitive detachment but
rather the practical engagement of concrete involvement."[20] Indeed, rhetoric
makes its living first and foremost in what, following Heidegger, was described
earlier as the world of know-how. It discovers the materials that are needed for its
work from how people are involved with the everyday concerns and contingencies
of life. The available means of persuasion are found here, and people await the acknowledgment of their particular interests by those who engage them in collaborative deliberation about contestable matters. In this way the know-how of rhetorical competence not only draws from a culture's historically based world of
meaning, it also contributes to the advancement of this intersubjective domain of
understanding. In Heidegger's terms, the know-how of rhetorical competence
must therefore be appreciated as having much to do with "the everydayness of Being with one another," with our "publicness." Heidegger credits Aristotle's rhetoric
with providing "the first systematic hermeneutic" of this communal character of
existence. Moreover, like Aristotle, Heidegger would have us understand how our
everyday way of being with others defines a realm of emotional orientations and
attachments (i.e., moods) that are constantly "attuning" us to situations we are a
part of and that are forever unfolding before our eyes. In offering a gloss of the
Rhetoric, Heidegger writes: "Publicness . . . not only has in general its own way of
having a mood, but needs moods and 'makes' them for itself. It is into such a
mood and out of such a mood that the orator speaks. He must understand the
possibilities of moods in order to rouse them and guide them aright [i.e., in a
right and just manner]."[21]

Such rhetorical competence operates in the immediacy of the present, in the
lived space of the here and now, in the existential and practically oriented world of
know-how. Rhetoric offers an interpretive understanding of this world; it articu-

lates and thus makes explicit something about how people are faring ("dwelling") in their everyday relationships with things and with others and how they might think and act in order to understand better and perhaps improve a particular situation. The effectiveness of rhetoric is dependent on its staying in touch with this emotionally attuned realm of *praxis* and circumspection. For only then can it attend to, with the hope of clarifying and improving, its audience's active relationships with things and with others. In its most elucidating and epiphanic moments, it is not uncommon for rhetoric to assume a poetic nature. Heidegger tells us that "poetry, creative literature, is nothing but the elementary emergence into words, the becoming uncovered, of existence as being in the world [of know-how]. For the others who before it were blind, the world first becomes visible by what is thus spoken."[22] In Heidegger's sense, a poetic interpretation can serve rhetoric well. When used in an appropriate, fitting, and engaging—that is, rhetorically competent—manner, a display of poetic competence may help us improve the ways others are presently seeing, interpreting, and involving themselves with the situations at hand. In short, the practice of rhetorical competence must cultivate in others the practical wisdom that is advanced and sustained by such competence and that no community can afford to be without. The social, political, and moral welfare of our everyday being-with-others, of our publicness, is a major concern of rhetoric.

All of this is to say that the structure of human existence is such that it calls on us to dwell rhetorically. We are creatures who have a special relationship with Being and its way of showing itself, its manner of calling our attention to its presence. We are open to the openness of Being, to a primordial dwelling place where space and time have yet to be reduced to the precise measurements that play a fundamental role in the construction of additional (human-made) dwelling places that help to make us feel at home in the world. Such dwelling places serve our ontological inclination to be social creatures. Human existence is marked with an indelible communal character, a being-with-others who, themselves, are open to the call of Being and who, at least from an ontological standpoint, are free to respond in ways that they deem appropriate. Being calls for this constructive response while at the same time calling it into question. Remember, there always comes uncertainty and contingency with the openness of Being; the call of Being has a deconstructive ring to it. Differences of opinion voiced by others arguing over the "truth" of contested matters remind us of this fact of life. The ontological and social structures of human existence work together to ensure that, at least at the present time in human evolution, we are always in the position of being challenged to dwell both poetically and rhetorically. In meeting this challenge, human beings temper the "struggle for existence" that is rooted in nature's law of "the survival of the fittest" such that the "fittest" now includes "those who are ethically the best."[23]

There are, of course, less noble ways of thinking about rhetoric. In his description of how "publicness" defines a world of common sense and common practice, for instance, Heidegger tends to emphasize its "mass"-like (Plato), "crowd"-like (Kierkegaard), and "herd"-like (Nietzsche) propensity to bring about a mindless conformity in its adherents. That rhetoric can and does play a role in sustaining such publicness is undeniable. With Heidegger, then, it can be said that those who theorize and practice the orator's art are involving themselves with a *techne* whose way of being admits more than a modicum of "inauthenticity."[24] Rhetoric, to be sure, is capable of existing in such a fallen state, but it also admits a competence for acknowledging others such that, when the situation calls for it, they can be roused and guided "in a right and just manner." Heidegger admits as much in his early work and thereby provides ontological support for what philosophers and rhetoricians have admitted for over two thousand years: namely, philosophy is essential for the education of the orator, but it is the "art of eloquence" (*oratio*) practiced by this advocate of the *vita activa* that instructs one on how to equip knowledge of a subject in such a way that it can assume a publicly accessible form and function effectively in the social and political arena.[25] Rhetoric is at work whenever discourse is employed to acknowledge others, to afford them a time and a place to take a stand so that they, too, can have a say in the establishing of truth.

The closest Heidegger comes to recognizing and incorporating this function of rhetoric into his overall philosophy is in his essay "The Origin of the Work of Art," where he notes that "Just as a work cannot be without being created but is essentially in need of creators, so what is created cannot itself come into being without those who preserve it."[26] Heidegger, however, does not characterize the relationship that takes place between the creators and the preservers of the work of art as defining an effort in rhetorical deliberation. Rather, he speaks of the creator of a work of art as being a "poet"—one who has heard and responded to the call of Being by disclosing in some manner the truth of this call. Moreover, Heidegger insists that, like the creator, the preservers must also involve themselves in a poetic act of releasement, "for a work is in actual effect as a work only when we remove ourselves from our commonplace routine and move into what is disclosed by the work, so as to bring our own nature itself to take a stand in the truth of what is."[27] Should the poet—taking a cue from rhetoric—make any attempt to compose his or her creation in such a way that others might stand a better chance of understanding the truth in question? Heidegger does not admit as much. Rather, he presents readers with a theory of *poiesis*, of the bringing-and-showing-forth of truth, that would make rhetoric nothing but a hermeneutic handmaiden to poetry: rhetoric need only concern itself with finding ways of bridging the discursive gap between people and their poets.

I suspect that most rhetoricians might feel a bit uncomfortable with this restrictive view of the orator's art. What about rhetoric's obligation to deal with the contingencies of human existence, to encourage others to do the same, and to thereby help cultivate *phronesis* in our historical situation? Yes, the orator who cares not a whit for learning how to dwell poetically so that he or she can acknowledge the Being (truth) of some matter warrants condemnation as a "sophist" of the worst sort. But what good is a poet who refuses to take the time to create a work of art that can "speak" to an audience, invite their participation in the assessment of the matter at hand, and thereby allow them the opportunity to call into question the artist's ability to "bring-forth" the truth? An exceptionally beautiful house wherein nothing works and whose walls crack and threaten to fall down every time one slams a door hardly qualifies as a safe dwelling place where one can feel at home.

This is not to say that Heidegger would favor building such a house, although the ontological priority he grants to poetry does confuse the issue that concerns me here. To speak of poetry without rhetoric, or rhetoric without poetry, I submit, is to do a disservice to the potential magnificence of these related arts in their making known of truth. Maurice Natanson's study of the rhetoric of Thomas Wolfe and the "epiphanies" or "privileged moments" that this rhetoric makes possible can serve to support this claim.

According to Natanson, an "epiphany is a momentous and instantaneous manifestation of reality; it is a sudden breaking into experience with arterial force, revealing 'that which is' with utter truth and candor. The greatness of an artist may be measured by the epiphanies he gives us, those revelations that turn on vast lights in our consciousness, which in searching out their hidden objects, their shadowed forms, search out in us the gift of understanding."[28] Natanson finds such revelations in Wolfe's rhetoric, in the way he employs language to bring together "meaning and image," "word and reality," so as to inspire "*privileged moments* of consciousness." In such moments, argues Natanson,

> It is not a question of poetic expression or high-flown language; rather it is the victory of language over its object when form fixes content with purity and high purpose. The fixation intended here is the expression of consciousness divorcing from its interest, momentarily, the irrelevancies which bind us to the meanings sedimented in reality. In this sense, [Wolfe's] rhetoric liberates consciousness from a burden of connections and opens it up and out into a world of unlimited truth. It re-teaches us how to *see* what is given us in experience; by its very power and elevation it draws us up to face what hitherto in seeing we have always ignored: rhetoric gives to the privileged moment a privileged status.[29]

Natanson speaks of rhetoric here much like Heidegger speaks of poetry, but still there is a difference. With Natanson we are told of a language that "re-teaches" us how to see (such that we can better observe and acknowledge) whatever it is that now directs our attention, our attunement of consciousness. Those who would teach others about truthful things eventually come to understand that the task at hand, if it is to have any sustained effect, requires a talent for gaining the attention and interest of one's students. Remember Kenneth Burke's words (cited in the introduction): "We interest a man by dealing with his interests" such that in this moment of acknowledgment and identification a dwelling place for collaborative deliberation can take form. Wise teachers know the importance of learning how to dwell poetically. Wiser teachers know the importance of learning how to incorporate rhetoric into the effort. And to do this is to engage oneself in an inventive activity in which a developed sense of "appropriateness" (rhetorical competence) is necessary in order to express oneself in the right way and at the right time.

Rhetorical Invention

Rhetorical competence entails invention: the actual creating of narratives and arguments so as to make them as truthful and effective as possible. The material of this creation finds its source in what is known in the classical rhetorical tradition as *ars topica*, the art of topics. Topics are the "places"—issues, values, commitments, beliefs, likelihoods—that we hold in common with others, that we *dwell in* and *argue over*, and that we use reflectively to find the issues and premises of a specific case. Topics draw from, and then work on, the common sense that informs a given community (*sensus communis*) and that is also taking form as the process of rhetorical invention unfolds and grants acknowledgment to people, things, and circumstances.

When organized into a list of general headings and propositions for making arguments, topics provide a repertoire of responses to practical problems that the thoughtful inquirer can turn to for *re*-sources—sources that can be used again and again on opposite sides of a question as new problems occur. Aristotle's *Rhetoric* I, 3–15, and II, 1–25—in other words, no less than two-thirds of the book—is just such a general inventory, one that Aristotle recognizes can be added to or subtracted from as the scene of its employment changes. More specific inventories or catalogues in principle would include all "how-to" manuals: *The Federalist Papers*, or Benjamin Cardozo's *Nature of the Judicial Process*, or Kierkegaard's *Concluding Unscientific Postscript*, or any number of such texts normally unrecognized as "rhetorics," that is, as collections of topical resources for situated practical thought.[30]

Popular culture's best-known genre of such collections is found in the mall bookstore under the category of "Etiquette." Here, for example, you might come upon John Bridges's book *How to Be a Gentleman: A Contemporary Guide to Common Courtesy*, which teaches such things as "A gentleman never gets so big that he can feel free to say or do things that make others feel small."[31] Such advice is not only *about* a certain way of being rhetorically competent but is also *ex-*

pressed with rhetorical competence. The author is employing the stylistic device or "ornament" of "antithesis" (the juxtaposition of contrasting ideas) to make his point. The effectiveness of this specific device is due in part to the way in which the "logic" of the ornament operates in terms of the "comparative" function of consciousness (e.g., something that is "bigger" is always recognized in conjunction with something that is "smaller"). Moreover, the ornament's effectiveness is also the product of a related ontological feature of human existence, one that has much to do with social and political status and that was examined earlier when discussing Heidegger's phenomenology of *"Dasein"* (or human being). Before they are made out by others to feel "big" or "small," human beings first and foremost share the identity of *being what they are:* creatures whose consciousness of the world provides a "clearing" or "place" where the "truth" of things can reveal itself and be put into language. A fundamental equality marks human existence. One might say, then, that it is in our nature to take offense at being be*littled* by others who think *too much* of themselves. Bridges's advice about the topic of being a gentleman has the ring of truth.

Bridges neither mentions nor reflects on his rhetorical use of antithesis and its ontological underpinnings. He wants only to offer an amusing but sincere book of etiquette, not a philosophically grounded rhetorical manual on the appropriateness of behavior. I have introduced him into the discussion, however, for this very reason. In Greek rhetoric the rhetor aims at finding *to prepon* ("the fitting")—what is right and appropriate for the situation, which in Cicero and Quintilian becomes "propriety" or "decorum," the master principle of rhetoric analogous to ethical *prudentia* or *phronesis* (practical wisdom). Etiquette is motivated by a sense of appropriateness; it defines ways of behaving "properly" in accordance with a set of socially prescribed rules that ought to be followed by a "civilized" society and that inevitably include directives for being rhetorically competent in the presence of others. Rhetorical competence is itself a form of etiquette; hence, the ridicule it has long received from philosophers (beginning with Socrates and Plato) who complain about its preoccupation with techniques for "decorating" discourse in order to appease, entertain, persuade, and manipulate others. What these philosophers typically fail to realize, however, is that within the rhetorical tradition the notion of appropriateness is not simply regarded as a socially and politically informed maneuver that can be used for deceptive and immoral purposes. Rather, appropriateness is also associated with the orderly and harmonious workings of nature. The appropriateness of a well-arranged and fitting piece of discourse can attune an audience to a truthfulness that is not merely the product of human activity. Bridges's use of antithesis is a case in point, even though it appears in an "unscholarly" book produced for the masses, *hoi polloi.*

Hence, one reads in Cicero's treatise on ethics, for example, that "Nature" has endowed "man" with reason, "by which he comprehends the chain of consequences, perceives the causes of things, understands the relation of cause to effect and of effect to cause, draws analogies, . . . connects and associates the present and the future . . . [and thereby] easily surveys the course of his whole life and makes the necessary preparations for its conduct." Moreover, "Nature likewise by the power of reason associates man with man in the common bonds of speech and life." And, continues Cicero, "it is no mean manifestation of Nature and Reason that man is the only animal that has a feeling for order, for propriety, for moderation in word and deed. And so no other animal has a sense of beauty, loveliness, harmony in the visible world; and Nature and Reason, extending the analogy of this from the world of sense to the world of spirit, find that beauty, consistency, order are far more to be maintained in thought and deed."[32] In short, for Cicero and the tradition of "civic republicanism" that evolved from his writings, *ratio* (reason) and *oratio* (the appropriate employment of discourse) are *the* defining attributes of human nature, divine gifts of Providence that link us to the heavens and thereby make it possible for the orator to stand as a "culture-hero": "For if intelligence and reason, by which the human race has some common property with superior beings, are a source of beauty; if men are clearly distinguished from other living creatures because they can use words, how much more excellent than other men is he who, relying on his reason, stands forth with brilliant eloquence?"[33] The "fittest" members of society display the attributes of rhetorical competence.

With Cicero's teachings on appropriateness we learn that the eloquence of rhetoric is not simply something that human beings create as an amusing game. Rather, the use of "ornaments of style" that lend "symmetry" and "brilliance" to discourse and thereby make it more interesting, inviting, and convincing for an audience is rooted in the *logos* of the cosmos that supports our existence—in the "natural eloquence," the harmony and integrity, of "Nature," which "has not brought us into the world to act as if we were created for play or jest, but rather for earnestness and for some more serious and important pursuits."[34] For Cicero, such pursuits are facilitated by humankind's rhetorical competence and include such activities as bringing help to the suppliant, maintaining people's civil rights, and *at the appropriate time* advancing an understanding and appreciation of such existential and spiritual matters as harmony, beauty, and loveliness.

Timeliness (*kairos*), as students of rhetoric are aware, is a vintage rhetorical concept deriving from pre-Socratic drama, philosophy, and oratory, particularly that of Pythagoras, Empedocles, and Gorgias. In Greek drama and literature, *kairos* embraced various meanings: brevity, proportion or moderation (as in Hesiod's "Observe good measure, and proportion [*kairos*] is the best of all things"), what is suited to the moment, the expedient, effective, correct, or appropriate. In early Greek rhetorical theory (e.g., in Gorgias), *kairos* referred to the principle and power (*dunamis*) by which the opportune moment calls forth an intuitive, appropriate response from the perceptive and receptive rhetor (instead of the rhetor's initiating an action after conscious assessment of the situation). It is a power of invention or discovery (*heuresis*) irreducible to mathematical calculation and logic. As such, *kairos* remains beyond the control of the rhetor, coming rather as a gift or even magic (*goetia*).[35] In later rhetorical theory (e.g., in Cicero), however, *kairos* is associated with the orator's active and practical ability to adapt to circumstances and audiences without relying on theoretical rules. *Kairos* thus becomes a concept in rhetorical theory that emphasizes the importance of the orator's being both receptive and responsive to all that stands before him or her. Timeliness, the inventive use of topics and stylistic devices, and acknowledgment go hand in hand. Hence, Cicero's often quoted teaching: "The universal rule in oratory as in life, is to consider propriety. . . ; it is important often in actions as well as in words, in the expression of the face, in gesture and in gait."[36]

Adhering to this rule, the orator's verbal and nonverbal communication take on and display a certain demeanor or character that is fitting and agreeable—appropriate—to an occasion and an audience. It is also designed to help to disclose in a meaningful and compelling (inventive) way what is arguably the truth of some specific subject matter. In his phenomenological assessment of language, Georges Gusdorf associates this entire "artistic" process with what he terms "the ceaseless heroism necessary in pursuing the struggle for style"—a struggle whereby "concern for the right expression is bound up with concern for true reality: accuracy (*justesse*) and integrity (*justice*) are two related virtues."[37] Gusdorf emphasizes, however, that this struggle "is not the privilege of the poet alone" but also confronts each of us in our daily lives. Gusdorf's clarification of this claim is worth noting:

> The writer seems to us testimony to man in his enterprise to impose his mark on the environment. Style expresses the *thread of life*, the movement of a destiny according to its creative meaning. . . . Style establishes man, not simply the style of speaking or writing, but the style of living in general. A person gives himself away in each of his attitudes: one looks after his words as one looks after his clothing. We can look after each of our moments, or else abandon them to a slipshod attitude that indicates a lack of personal discipline, just as do bad manners and poor dress. The struggle for style may here stand as a definition of the whole personality since it is the undertaking of giving an appropriate value to each moment of self-affirmation. Man's presence to himself and the world in his own present raises a constant problem for him. For no solution will put an end to the search, and appropriateness (*justesse*) here is a matter of taste, constantly threatened with falling short or going too far: it isn't far from simplicity to studied elegance and affectation, from refinement to coyness or preciousness. The gift of proper expression is the privilege of certain beings who intuitively know the balance-point and show, in the face of the most unexpected difficulty, that

they are equal to the circumstances. . . . Each of us, even the most
simple of mortals, is charged with finding the expression to fit his
situation. Each of us is charged with realizing himself in a language,
a personal echo of the language of all which represents his contribution to the human world. The struggle for style is the struggle for
consciousness (*la vie spirituelle*).[38]

For Gusdorf, as for the rhetorician influenced by the teachings of those like
Cicero, style is something that possesses much existential and ontological weight.
It shows itself in one's very being, in the way a person lives and communicates
with others. Indeed, the struggle for style is the everyday struggle to be seen, observed, listened to, acknowledged: to find a place to dwell in the company and
comfort of one's family, friends, colleagues, and even strangers who might help, or
be helped by, you. By way of style, we open and present ourselves and our ideas
and beliefs to others. Style is a "showing-forth" (*epideixis*) of a human being's particular way of being, an epideictic display of who we are—or at least of who we
would like to be. Caught up in the ebb and flow of social existence, each of us "is
charged with finding the expression to fit his [or her] situation." As we engage in
this task we offer a focal point for the attunement of consciousness, for the attentiveness of others who might be caring enough to take the time to get to know
who we truly are and what we truly think about some matter. For those like the
"great artist" who are "bound up with concern for true reality," writes Gusdorf,

> the effort never ceases; at the slightest relaxation, the new form de-
> generates into a formula. There comes a moment when the power is
> lost, when style seems an empty imitation of itself, a whole jumble
> of conditioned responses in which the person is the victim rather
> than the master. The great artist avoids imitating even himself. He
> continually undertakes the task of remaining vigilantly aware of the
> world and words, a task forever unfinished because the world changes
> and is renewed, and living man with it.[39]

Thus, the ever-present issue of appropriateness, of discerning what is right and fitting to do and to say given the situation, the audience at hand, and one's desire to
reveal what is believed to be the truth of something in need of acknowledgment.

By now it should be clear that acknowledgment is a moral action that in its
most positive mode is dedicated to making time and space for the disclosing of
truth. Appropriateness helps to facilitate this action by lending itself to the rhetorical task of creating dwelling places wherein people can collaborate about and
know together matters of importance. Human beings are gifted with the potential
for developing the capacity to perform such an artistic and moral feat. To the extent that one believes that what we are talking about here is a "divine" gift, then *the
exemplar of rhetorical appropriateness is readily at hand*. We can "read" the mo-

ment of creation in rhetorical terms: "In the beginning was the Word, and the Word was with God, and the Word was God" (John 1:1). The ultimate moment of creation, when the arrangement, coherence, and integrity—in short, the style—of all that there is was brought into being, is appropriateness par excellence.[40] There is no greater right thing, right time, and right way; there is no holier answer to the supreme metaphysical question: Why is there something rather than nothing? With the Word, the revelation of truth, darkness became light and out of nothingness came something of immense complexity and beauty. The "rhetoric of religion" has long argued the point. The "rhetoric of science" has long responded with caution: Getting at the truth of *what is* need not inspire metaphysical gymnastics; let us begin with the Big Bang and then move on empirically and mathematically from there. I will have more to say about this argument in the last section of this chapter. Now, however, as a way of further advancing an understanding of the relationship between acknowledgment and appropriateness, I want to take a closer look at rhetoric's capacity for "showing forth" (*epideixis*) the truth of its subject matter.

Epideictic Rhetoric

In his lectures on rhetoric and how this art contributes to the creation and the preservation of a culture's interpretive understanding and domains of meaning, the nineteenth-century classicist and philosopher Friedrich Nietzsche made much of how the metaphorical structure of language, with all its tropes and figures, forever stands between anyone who would use language to tell the truth of things and the truth of things themselves:

> There is obviously no unrhetorical "naturalness" of language to which one could appeal; language itself is the result of purely rhetorical arts [and their inventional use of topics and ornaments of style]. The power to discover and to make operative that which works and impresses, with respect to each thing, a power which Aristotle calls rhetoric, is, at the same, the essence of language; the latter is based just as little as rhetoric is upon that which is true, upon the essence of things.

Nietzsche thus insists that

> Language does not desire to instruct, but to convey to others a subjective impulse and its acceptance. Man, who forms language, does not perceive things or events, but *impulses:* he does not communicate sensations, but merely copies of sensations. The sensation, evoked through a nerve impulse, does not take in the thing itself: This sensation is presented externally through an image. . . . The full

essence of things will never be grasped. Our utterances by no means wait until our perception and experience have provided us with a many-sided, somehow respectable knowledge of things; they result immediately when the impulse is perceived. Instead of the thing, the sensation takes in only a *sign*.[41]

For Nietzsche, then, language creates "fictions," not "truths."

In the hands of such philosophers, historians, and literary theorists as Jacques Derrida, Michel Foucault, and Paul de Man, Nietzsche's teachings on the relationship between rhetoric, language, and truth help form the basis of the twentieth-century program of "postmodern" criticism. Commonly known as "deconstructionism," this criticism in its most extreme form appeals to the "true" fictional character of language in order to promote an endless questioning of any authoritative grounds for meaning and truth. Against what is arguably most important in the rhetorical tradition—establishing a dwelling place where collaborative deliberation may help to set, at least for a while, such grounds—deconstructionists threaten to reduce "rhetoric" to an unstable figurality in which topics and proofs are subordinated to, and finally subsumed by, unauthorized and unstable tropes and figures. I take exception to this rather simplistic understanding of rhetoric; although as I clarify below my reasons for doing so, it should also become clear how I find deconstructive criticism to be important for the study of acknowledgment.

The problem I have with deconstructionism's extreme understanding of rhetoric is epitomized in the work of Paul de Man. He reads Nietzsche as saying that rhetoric is first and foremost a system of tropes and figures, rather than a practical art concerned with the cultivation of good judgment (*krisis*) and practical wisdom (*phronesis*).[42] Not only do I find this reading of Nietzsche to be questionable, but I also find it to be blind to an understanding of rhetoric that goes back to the ancient Greeks and that has been examined and employed by such notable literary and rhetorical critics as Kenneth Burke. Throughout his many writings, Burke makes clear that the range of rhetorical materials generated by *topoi* defines a continuum—a holding-in-tension—of topics commonly received as places for arguments ("providing evidence"), and tropes and other techniques used as means of disclosure (the symbolic display of "worldly" phenomena). *Dispositio* and *narratio*, for example, were for the ancients not merely artificial embellishments, much less (merely or exclusively) unstable pitfalls for authors and audiences, but rather substantive resources in league, if not always on a level, with arguments for making one's case.[43] Regarding that genre of rhetoric most steeped in these techniques of showing (of *narratio*)—namely "epideictic"—Quintilian has said: "Indeed I am not sure that this is not the most important department of rhetoric in actual practice."[44] I would put it more directly: When it comes to getting at the truth of things and involving others in the process, epideictic discourse *is* rhetoric's most important department.

With this claim I grant epideictic rhetoric an ontological depth that remains unobserved by the classicist E. M. Cope, who would have us understand epideictic rhetoric in this way: "It is the ... demonstrative, showy, ostentatious, declamatory kind: so called because speeches of this sort are composed for 'show' or 'exhibition,' *epideixis*, and their [primary] object is to display the orator's powers, and to amuse an audience ... who are therefore *theoroi* rather than *kritai*, like spectators at a theatre ... [who have no] serious interest or real issue at stake."[45] Nietzsche also thinks of epideictic rhetoric in this way, and de Man offers no correction. But a correction is needed, for epideictic rhetoric is not simply a tool for amusement. Hence, the suggestion offered and developed by the rhetorical theorist and critic Lawrence Rosenfield, who makes the following three claims about the phenomenon:

> First, we need to look at epideictic in conjunction with notions of luminosity which the pre-Socrates knew as the stimulus for mental activity; epideictic discourse is unique among public address types [i.e., deliberative and forensic rhetoric] in that it *lets be what lies before us* so that we may *acknowledge* the radiance that is present to us. Second, epideictic's effort to acknowledge Being's radiance enables the listener who approaches what *is* in *a spirit of appreciative attention* to join with the speaker in *taking reality to heart*. Third, there is a distinctive form of understanding evoked in epideictic celebration, and this mental participation differs from inferences and judgments more common to public community in *giving thought to what we witness*, and such *thoughtful beholding in commemoration constitutes memorializing.*[46] (emphasis added)

I emphasize Rosenfield's three claims here in order to make a point that is quite obvious when examining his entire essay and its endnotes: He speaks of epideictic discourse much as Heidegger speaks of poetry. Recall that, for Heidegger, *poiesis* is a "bringing-forth" of truth by way of "essential thinking." And this is how Rosenfield would have us understand the genuine function of epideictic rhetoric: a "beholding" and a "showing forth" of what *is*. According to Rosenfield, we "submit to the spell of the epideictic speaker in the sense that we heed him out of respect for his authority, for his capacity to behold, attend to, and dwell appreciatively in the midst of the reality that is ordinarily closed off to us in the rush of our daily lives."[47] The spell of the epideictic speaker, in other words, is exactly like that of Heidegger's "great poets." In fact, drawing inspiration and direction from Heidegger, Rosenfield goes so far as to suggest that, unlike in deliberative and forensic rhetoric, "in epideictic the auditor is purely a beholder," which is to say that he or she is no different from Heidegger's "preservers" of great works of art. Rosenfield insists that

Epideictic neither teaches nor admonishes—it functions only to provoke thought, to envelope its participants in reminders of excellence and therefore to rescue it in memory. . . . Yet if epideictic discourse is rare it is only because its necessary constituents—openness of mind, felt reverence for reality, enthusiasm for life, the ability to congeal significant experiences in memorable language—are also rare.[48]

I have no problem with Rosenfield's drawing inspiration and direction from one who never acknowledged the greatness of epideictic discourse *per se*.[49] However, what is bothersome about his dependence on Heidegger is that, when all is said and done, Rosenfield offers no explanation for why we should not just think of the epideictic speaker as a poet rather than a rhetor, or, conversely, why the poet should not be thought of as an epideictic speaker or great orator. Such an explanation is also lacking in Heidegger, although, as discussed earlier, he never places the practically oriented thought of the orator on the same grand level as the essential thinking of the poet.

Rhetoricians who, for one reason or another, are not comfortable with Heideggerian ontology may find Rosenfield's thoughts on epideictic discourse as yet another instance of a colleague bowing down to philosophy and thereby admitting rhetoric's lower-class status. I, however, do not think so unkindly of his arguments and suggestions. Like Rosenfield, I wish to claim that it is a mistake to restrict one's understanding of the "showing-forth" function of epideictic rhetoric to a manipulative exercise of amusement and persuasion whereby a coming to know of what *is*, is afforded inappropriate respect. Moreover, I want to propose that *epideixis is poiesis* but with a bit of a twist: one that helps to make sure that the acknowledgment that must take place in the work of the rhetor/poet is robust enough in its consideration of both its subject matter *and* its audience. Heidegger and Rosenfield leave readers with the impression that the best thing the audience can do is to follow the lead of the artist ("authority"), learn to let beings be, and thereby become witnesses to the truth. For, indeed, the great artist is there to answer the call of Being rather than worry about how best to arrange a persuasive argument. I submit, however, that the process is much more involved than that.

Consider this: Rosenfield's artist is one who would raise the confessional nature of acknowledgment beyond the banality of everyday existence and toward the truth of Being—someone like Aleksandr Solzhenitsyn, the Nobel laureate and author of *The Gulag Archipelago*. This survivor of Soviet atrocities, argues Rosenfield, is a perfect example of his noble epideictic speaker; hence, we are told that because "he willingly bore witness to the entire degradation of the Soviet concentration camps, because he gazed unflinchingly at a monstrosity that the rest of mankind chose to look away from, Solzhenitsyn's commemoration testifies to our capacity for life, truth, and human dignity even as it disparages the venality of those responsible for the evil."[50]

Solzhenitsyn did not just *see* certain circumstances, he *observed* them, *acknowledged* their presence in great detail, and confessed and shared his assessments of them in an awarding-winning book. But the award was given not merely because this author spoke about the truth of these circumstances, but also because he knew how to present his experiences in a well-told, captivating, emotionally moving, and persuasive narrative or "showing" (*narratio*) that is not easily forgotten. Epideictic discourse is offered not only with the truth in mind but also by way of a talent for acknowledging others whom the artist desires to instruct as she or he gains and maintains their interests.[51] The talent is that of the rhetorician who can disclose the truth such that it can be understood and taken to heart by others who have yet to form a genuine appreciation of the matters at hand. This is what epideictic rhetoric is all about: a desire for truth; a willingness to open oneself to what *is;* the courage to confess, to admit publicly one's worldview; and the skill to present this confession in an appropriate and thus fitting manner to others who wait for their interests to be acknowledged by artists who seek their undivided attention and their acceptance of an *argument in the making.* Like Heidegger, Rosenfield has little to say about the intricacies of this skill, for epideictic rhetoric, at least as he sees it, unfolds first and foremost as a disclosing of truth rather than as a carefully composed argument (with such things as tropes, figures, examples, stories, and stated and unstated definitions of terms). I, on the other hand, take issue with such a perception. Epideictic rhetoric necessarily involves the ways and means of argumentation, for even the most simple and well-accepted definition has a history steeped in argument.[52]

Solzhenitsyn is an epideictic speaker, although for more reasons than those recognized by Rosenfield. The difference between his view and the one being advocated here is worth emphasizing, especially because not all efforts in epideictic rhetoric are as "clear-cut" and thus as easy to recognize as Solzhenitsyn's. For who but a sociopath, someone who could care less about evil and the sufferings of others, would deny the worth of what this Russian author has to say? A more complicated rhetorical situation would be one where the rhetoric of "good reasons" ultimately fails because what will count as good and what will count as reasons are the very issues at stake. For example, what do we say to someone who denies basic freedoms to women or children or homosexuals or other races? How does a religious believer speak to an unbeliever and vice versa? Is there any common ground on which those who advocate the morality of physician-assisted suicide might converse with defenders of the right to life? Thinking about such questions, Ludwig Wittgenstein once remarked: "Where two principles really do meet which cannot be reconciled with one another, then each man declares the other a fool and a heretic. . . . I would 'combat' the other man—but wouldn't I give him reasons? Certainly, but how far do they go? At the end of reasons comes *persuasion.*"[53]

Although Wittgenstein does not elaborate on this point, a provocative but unfortunately neglected essay by the philosopher Raphael Demos entitled "On Persuasion" provides what I take to be a fair-minded assessment of the matter that is not inconsistent with a Wittgensteinian philosophy of language. Demos argues both that divergent theories or world-views may equally explain the "facts" and that "to explain the facts is not enough; a theory must be true."[54] Yet, such truth is not an easy matter of superior arguments, because the very ideas of argument and reason are contested. For Demos, the superiority of one theory or world-view over another resides instead in the "cumulative force of minute considerations"; ultimately "it is a conflict between patterns. Persuasion is not a mechanical process, but a living growth in which elements are gradually assimilated, and ultimately modify those very tissues which assimilate them."[55] Persuasion, then, is a matter of our "acknowledging" the pattern of accumulated particulars—coming to an experience of this pattern beyond mere intellectual understandings—and this realization is achieved by "evocation":

> Often the reason why so much discussion among individuals is futile is that what one person realizes vividly, the other does not. Evocation is the process by which vividness is conveyed; it is the presentation of a viewpoint in such a manner that it becomes real for the public. It is said that argument is the way by which an individual experience is made common property; in fact, an argument has much less persuasive force than the vivid evocation of an experience. The enumeration of all the relevant points in favor of a theory and against its opposite can never be completed; far more effective is it to state a viewpoint in all its concreteness and in all its significant implications, and then stop; the arguments become relevant only after this stage has been completed.[56]

Rosenfield, I suspect, would agree: the process of evocation is a showing-forth (*epideixis*) of what is, and it is this process that warrants priority over argument. Demos, however, is suggesting more than that. He makes two points that are especially important for my purposes: first, that one realizes something vividly, and second that *what* one realizes is a "pattern" or "whole" within which everything else makes sense. Wittgenstein puts it this way: "When we first begin to believe anything, what we *believe* is not a single proposition, it is a whole system of propositions. (Light dawns gradually over the whole.)"; "it is not single axioms that strike me as obvious, it is a system in which consequences and premises give one another *mutual* support."[57] Charles Taylor refers to such patterns as our moral "frameworks," whose supports are our "hypergoods," that is, those "strong evaluations" or intuitions of goods that we believe deserve admiration and adherence beyond our own desires and wishes—in short, that belong to human beings *as* humans. For Taylor, as for Wittgenstein and Demos, adherence to these frameworks is a matter of practical reason, and also consists in the vivid realization of some whole, but with this addition: that there be an "epistemic gain" in converting from A to B. This transition (or persuasion) for Taylor is grounded in (inter)personal confession and story: "Practical reasoning . . . is a reasoning in transitions. It aims to establish, not that some position is correct absolutely, but rather that some position is superior to some other." Moreover, notes Taylor,

> This form of argument has its source in biographical narrative. We are convinced that a certain view is superior because we have *lived a transition* which we understand as error-reducing and hence as epistemic gain. I see that I was confused about the relation of resentment and love, or I see that there is a depth to love that I was insensitive to before. But this doesn't mean that we don't and can't argue. Our conviction that we have grown morally can be challenged by another. It may, after all, be illusion. And then we argue; and arguing here is contesting between interpretations of what I have been living.[58]

I trust that my exception to Rosenfield's *argument* regarding epideictic rhetoric is now clear: Yes, the process of evocation is a showing-forth of what *is*, but this process is not without the influence of persuasion if its goal is to have others take an interest in, understand, and accept what is being disclosed by some artist—be he or she a speaker, writer, or any other type of creative soul whose work of art clears a place in time and space for people to acknowledge and know-together what is arguably the truth of some matter. Indeed, epideictic discourse is inevitably open to argument, for the dwelling place it seeks to establish must be situated within the flow of another (ontological) process that is forever opening us up to the objective uncertainty of the future. Remember, the structure of human existence is such that it not only calls us to construct a world of understanding and meaning, but it also calls into question the truth of what we have constructed. No mortal "authority" remains unchallenged by this constructive and deconstructive call for resoluteness and open-mindedness. This call speaks to who we are as creatures that are fated to dwell on earth both poetically and rhetorically. It is a moral vocation, one of learning to "let beings be" and, in turn, of trying to know together (by way of discussion, argument, and persuasion) the truth of all that stands before us. It is a vocation that requires ethical and rhetorical fitness.

The Moral Vocation

Derrida offers the following description of this vocation while defending Heidegger's ontology against the critique of another one of his teachers, Emmanuel Levinas (a phenomenologist and Talmudic scholar whom I will have more to say about shortly):

> It conditions the respect for the other as what it is: other. Without this acknowledgment, which is not a knowledge, or let us say without this "letting-be" of an existent (Other) as something existing outside me in the essence of what it is (first in its alterity [or "otherness"]), no ethics would be possible. . . . To let the other be in its existence and essence as other means that what gains access to thought, or (and) what thought gains access to, is that which is essence and that which is existence; and that which is the Being which they both presuppose. Without this, no letting-be would be possible, and first of all, the letting be of respect and of the ethical commandment addressing itself to freedom. Violence would reign to such a degree that it would no longer even be able to appear and be named.[59]

We are saved from an all-encompassing violence by our ability to attune our consciousness toward things and others so that they can be acknowledged and respected for what, who, and how they are. In once again employing Derrida to help make a point that is essential to the current project, I at the same time reintroduce a philosopher and literary theorist whose program of deconstructive criticism is something I promised to return to before completing this chapter. Now is the time to fulfill that promise. With what I have to say about deconstruction, I continue to make an argument for the social, political, and moral importance of rhetorical competence. I will thus have more to say about such related topics as space, time, place, emotion, *topoi*, and the disclosive and persuasive functions of epideictic discourse. The discussion of all of these matters will eventually lead, once again, to a consideration of how acknowledgment, God, and the Big Bang are possibly related. This time, however, my stretch of the imagination will be aided by a fuller understanding of how the rhetorical competence of human beings allows them the honorable opportunity of being what I term "home-makers"—creatures who are wise enough to construct those special places where "the heart" is supposed to be. This activity is rooted in what was referred to above as the moral vocation of human being, a calling that has both a deconstructive and reconstructive ring to it.

Deconstruction. Derrida's above description of this vocation echoes Heidegger's assessment of the fundamental relationship that holds between Being and human being (*Dasein*): we are those beings who exist in such a way that we make a place for Being to show and call attention to itself. This showing and call (for essential thought) defines the "ethical commandment" upon which all moral systems are based. The commandment calls for a respecting of the Being of beings, for a letting-be of what gives and shows itself to and for thought and that thus is "other" than the consciousness that perceives it. Derrida aligns deconstruction with one way of answering this call. He writes: ". . . deconstruction is, in itself, a positive response to an alterity which necessarily calls, summons or motivates it. Deconstruction is therefore vocation—a response to a call."[60]

Moreover, Derrida would have us understand that deconstruction offers itself to others as a way of helping them to realize that "every culture needs an element of self-interrogation and of distance from itself, if it is to transform itself" and thereby become something different, something other and perhaps "better" than what it presently is under the "official political codes of governing reality."[61] Deconstruction, in other words, is especially attuned to that deconstructive dimension of the moral vocation of human being that shows forth in the temporal openness of this being's existence and that continually calls into question the truthfulness of whatever human beings create in order to make their lives meaningful. Deconstruction does something of what existence tells it to do: it is a critical activity; it *"intervenes"* in meaning systems in order to call attention to the potential pitfalls that accompany our strict adherence to these systems and that are too often taken for granted and forgotten when "all is well" with the system's functioning. Derrida thus emphasizes that the vocation and evocation of his way of doing criticism are one and the same: like existence itself, deconstruction operates to interrupt and "destabilize" whatever it is that directs its attention.[62] Recall that Heidegger associates this interruption with the call of conscience (Being) and the experience of anxiety that this call brings about. Might it therefore be said that deconstruction defines an effort to create the discomforting emotion of anxiety in others? It would seem so. Deconstruction is a vocation whose evocation is a provocation designed to make us feel uncanny, *unheimlich*, "not at home" with our meaningful surroundings. Deconstruction instigates "setbacks" in our lives. And this act of rhetorical intervention is done out of respect for the "otherness" of the other.

Heidegger, as we have seen, traced this otherness back to Being itself, to that which shows itself in our very existence, although it is not a human creation. With Derrida, on the other hand, otherness is more a matter of what he terms "the play of *différance*." This play, according to Derrida, defines the basic rhetorical economy of language that, as indicated earlier, attracted Nietzsche's attention. It is the way in which language functions not only as a semiotic system of differences, of arbitrary and conventionalized signifier/signified relationships and oppositions, but also as a "temporizing" (or "deferring") movement of significations whereby any given semiotic system of meaning, as it takes form, always enters into an "intertextual" relationship with some *other* system that it is currently transforming.[63]

For Derrida, a person's "self" is always situated in and comes to "know" itself through this play of *différance*. The self of an existing individual, he therefore maintains, can never be unto itself. For, caught up in the play and rhetorical texture of *différance*, the self perpetually finds itself carrying some "trace" of the "other than self," some trace of past systems of meaning that, whether recognized or not, are there with the self as its constant co-authors who speak, for example, of how the self should see itself as being "good" or "bad," "superior" or "inferior," in the valued center of society or on its margins. Societies are known for placing meanings/selves on the margins in order to secure the well-being of the status quo. In American society, some classic examples of the "other" would be people whose "meaning" is "known" in light of their being female, physically disabled, Jewish, old, non-white, gay, or any combination of these characteristics, and who thereby have most likely come to know the pain and suffering of being marginalized, of having to live a life of "social death" with its lack of positive acknowledgment.

In its most socially and politically relevant form, deconstructive criticism is dedicated to initiating a process of deliberation that can rectify conditions of social death by encouraging people to rethink their "truthful" conceptions of reality so that what these conceptions end up placing on the margins of society might receive more positive acknowledgment. Such criticism is advanced not only by those who dwell in the "ivory towers" of academe, but can also be found in the ongoing national debate over the justifiability and social acceptability of euthanasia and physician-assisted suicide. The controversial narrative entitled "It's Over, Debbie," which was written by an anonymous physician and published in the *Journal of the American Medical Association*, is one important example.[64]

The narrative presents a first-person account of how the author "supposedly" engaged in the illegal practice of active euthanasia. Yet, when one pays particular attention to what this narrative is doing—*how* it means, not just *what* it means—the author's confession can be read as a well-designed rhetorical and deconstructive experiment in "uncertainty" and "ambiguity," an experiment that denies itself and its readers a sense of closure. For example, Debbie is reported to have said, "let's get this over with" when the physician was about to "sedate" her. What is not clear, however, is whether Debbie's statement was a request from a competent patient to be put to sleep "for good." With its uncertainty and ambiguity, the story opens up a space for deliberation and calls for a response, for the production of other texts that can perhaps educate people about matters that inform and motivate the euthanasia debate, matters that remain unclear in a story whose "truth" might in fact be a "fiction." The physician's narrative is thus designed to get readers involved in the rhetorical process of public moral argument—answering the many questions raised by the narrative's uncertainty and ambiguity is left up to us. Although this way of acknowledging and displaying "respect" toward others proved to be quite threatening and anxiety-provoking for the medical establishment, it also proved to be quite successful in generating response from the general public. This success is evidenced in the many responses that the text inspired from people both inside and outside the medical establishment, people who voiced passionate arguments for the "right to die" or for the "right to life" and who read the story as supporting their *particular* and *opposing* stances on the issue.

The deconstructive rhetoric found in "It's Over, Debbie" works primarily as a rhetorical intervention into the discourse of others. As noted above, deconstruction commits this act in order to destabilize this discourse, its reified meanings, and thus its purported "truth" claims. Truth is put up for grabs when deconstruction enters the scene and creates anxiety with its interruptive discourse. The interruption is intended to have us recall the uncertainty and contingency of human existence. Deconstruction is a disclosing and a showing-forth of a more primordial evocation and epideictic display of what *is* (and *is not*). With the rhetoric of deconstruction, we learn of a "saying" that is always "other" than what is "said" about it in the rhetoric of any symbolic system (including that of the deconstructive critic).

This last way of putting the matter is significant for, perhaps as you already realize, the formulation implies that the primordial saying of human existence (the call of conscience/Being/Otherness) may be properly understood as the most original epideictic event there is to be empirically experienced and observed. And this being the case, it can also be said that with this event we are given the purest instance of epideictic rhetoric that there is: what Levinas terms "rhetoric without eloquence."[65] Levinas puts the matter this way because, although he acknowledges that rhetorical *praxis* is by its very nature *other-oriented*, he also holds a very narrow understanding of "eloquence." He equates the term with the selfish use of language to manipulate and exploit our interlocutor or audience. Eloquence, claims Levinas, inhibits our ability to hear the one true "discourse," which never goes away: the "saying" of existence and its "otherness"—a saying that, for human beings, is most pronounced in the evocative presence (the "face") of another's being. Not the otherness of Being, but rather the otherness of other people is what is most important for Levinas. This "human" dimension of alterity stands as an ever-present rhetorical interruption that calls the self into question as it speaks first and foremost of the goodness of life and how it ought to be respected. "Where art Thou?" "Here I am!"[66] This interruptive transaction gives motivation to the activity of the deconstructive critic, to his or her use of discourse to open a space for deliberation, to the clearing of a place in any formalized language game or system of meaning such that those who are marginalized by the customary rules of the game might be granted the opportunity of becoming a more major and recognizable player. As worked out by Levinas and Derrida, deconstruction answers a call for acknowledgment that comes especially from those who are in need of help and who are seeking a more humane dwelling place to live. Deconstruction is a way of breaking ground so that such a dwelling place might be built.

Yet, what typically is missing in the discourses of deconstructive critics is a well-developed plan of *reconstruction* that would show exactly how people who are being marginalized and experiencing social death could improve their lot. Of course, such a plan, as Derrida readily admits, would be "incommensurate" with "the call" that inspires the moral vocation of deconstructive criticism.[67] The other calls, "Where art thou?" and the deconstructionist responds, "Here I am!" But he shows up without a positive plan of action; hence, the potential danger of allowing deconstructionism to be on the scene for too long. It is a devoted witness to evil happenings, admit its critics, but that in and of itself is not enough to prevent other evildoers from filling the gap left open by those who, when all is said and done, leave us only with self-interrogating words: Are you being just in all that you say and do?[68]

Reconstruction. Constructing a dwelling place that the self and the other can gladly call home presupposes some past event of groundbreaking. But what good does it do to initiate such a deconstructive activity if nobody is willing and able to take the next reconstructive step and become a home-maker? Remember: the call of Being/conscience/the Other functions in both a deconstructive *and* reconstructive way. Existing and surviving in the everyday world not only requires a rhetorical competence for calling into question the thought and actions of people whose power intentionally or unintentionally promotes social death. The well-being of human being also requires a rhetorical competence for inventing and creating from the materials (topics) at hand domains of meaning that can provide a sense of order for those in dire need of such dwelling places. I have already discussed this second, but equally important, dimension of rhetorical competence in some detail. A few additional comments about it, however, will be helpful in order to further prepare the reader for the case studies that are offered in the remaining chapters of the book.

As we direct our rhetorical competence from doing deconstructive things (ground-breaking) to doing reconstructive things, we accept the responsibility of becoming *home-makers*, builders of those special places where "the heart" is supposed to be. The rhetorically competent speaker or writer is a linguistic architect whose symbolic constructions both create and invite others into a place where they can dwell and feel at home while thinking about and discussing the truth of some matter that the rhetor/architect has already attempted to disclose and show forth in a specific way with his or her work of art. Such a work of art thus assumes an epideictic function. With architecture in mind, we might also speak of the work as an "edifying" discourse (to edify, Latin: *aedificare*: *aedes*, "dwelling" + *ficare*, "to make" or "to build") whose communal character (*ethos*) takes form as the artist uses materials (tropes, figures, topics, arguments, narratives, emotions) to attract our attention, maintain our interest, and encourage us to judge the work as being praiseworthy and persuasive.

Maintaining a bias that is steeped in Platonic philosophy, the edificatory nature of a work of art may be degraded as being mere "decoration" that is added on to the work for aesthetic purposes. This standpoint is the basis of the bifurcation between rhetoric and science, where one is seen as essentially "stylistic ornamentation and embellishment" while the other is considered "rational" discourse on the supposed "truth" of reality. As already discussed, however, an artist's "style" is not necessarily antithetical to the disclosing of truth. Take, for example, the passionate, colorful, and mesmerizing moods and style of Vincent Van Gogh. His artistic disclosures re-present the "truth" of things in a way that transcends the representational power of some "straightforward" equation offering an "empirical" account of the physics at work, for instance, in the being of a sunflower. Of course, Van Gogh's *Sunflowers* are not "the thing itself," but those famous brush stokes and color combinations that compose the painting are more than a mere decorative technique. Rather, they make up his style and his way of expressing himself, of being evocative, epideictic, edifying, and truthful about a thing of beauty, which, with the space and time he gives it, may help viewers to see such beauty as never before. The content of Van Gogh's painting is simple enough to see and recognize, but it is the form that discloses the sunflowers and that allows them to come "alive" so that they can be observed and acknowledged for what they are.

Or let us think once again about an example that was introduced in chapter 1: Lincoln's Gettysburg Address. In this masterpiece of rhetorical competence, which "remade America" as it set forth what historian Garry Wills describes as a "revolution" in thought and speech, we witness a work of art whose distinctive and appropriate use of grammar, syntax, signs, tempo, topics, tropes, figures, emotion, narrative, and argument creates a dwelling place of eulogized time and space, an opening in the midst of immense loss and suffering. With this opening there is still hope to be found as we acknowledge the devotion and courage not of individuals dressed in blue or gray but of those "brave men, living and dead, who struggled here" and who would have us realize "that the nation shall, under God, have a new birth of freedom, and that the government of the people, by the people, and for the people, shall not perish from the earth."[69] The form and content of Lincoln's Address are inextricably bound together in a rhetorical disclosure of Being and conscience that calls for assistance in building a common *ethos*—dwelling place, character, ethic—for the nation. The Gettysburg Address is rationally designed and decorated in order to have us acknowledge and know together something of the truth of being-with-and-for-others, of feeling at home in their company, and of treating them in a just and moral way. To dwell with Lincoln at Gettysburg is to learn how important it is to have a heart that is open to the world and, hence, to the experience of wonder and awe that shows itself in acts of commitment, courage, and sacrifice.

Of course, the lesson here is an old one. King David, for example, spoke of it in the twenty-third Psalm when he acknowledged his confidence in the grace of God while he walked "through the valley of the shadow of death": ". . . Surely goodness and mercy shall follow me all the days of my life, and I will dwell in the house of the Lord forever." Lincoln, too, would have his audience dwell "under God." There is something "spiritual" about his Address. With his epideictic/edifying discourse, Lincoln not only acknowledges others, but also his and their Creator: *the* maker/builder/architect of the universe, whose "house" is meant to be our home, the place that came into being with the initial speaking of the Word, the first and greatest act of *epideixis* (showing-forth) "known" to humankind. Acknowledging, at least for the sake of argument, that this Word was designed to be emotional, instructive, and persuasive, might it also be said that "In the beginning was the Word" and it was rhetorical?

I trust that with all that has been said so far about the goodness of rhetorical competence, the reader will not accuse me of being disrespectful in raising this question. God the rhetorician, the linguistic architect, whose first act of acknowledgment ("Let there be!") granted us a place to dwell in the company of others who, like God, need the life-giving gift of acknowledgment. "Where art thou?" "Here I am!" This all-important exchange takes place throughout the Old and New Testament. It also takes place in everyday life. What would life be like if no one cared enough to acknowledge your existence? For someone like Levinas, the "secret of [God's] semantics" is found in the face of the other, in a presence that is a living memory of this question's importance and where it ought to lead us. We are called out of ourselves by the other who is in need of assistance. As Levinas puts it, " [the other] requires me. The face looks at me, calls out to me. It claims me. What does it ask for? Not to leave it alone. An answer: Here I am."[70] With the otherness (alterity) of the other comes a responsibility that is always before us and that no human being can totally meet, for there are too many others in need of help. The exigency, in its totality, transcends our finite grasp. Look for yourself! What are you to do? Perhaps you might pray for guidance and assistance. Levinas asks: "Is not the face of one's fellow man the original locus in which transcendence calls an authority with a silent voice in which God comes to the mind?"[71] And what exactly is the object of this event of consciousness? One typically begins answering this question, notes Levinas, "by accepting his Word in the name of the social authority of religion." But how, asks Levinas, are we "to be sure that the Word thus accepted is indeed that spoken by God? The original experience must be sought."[72]

Conclusion: At Home in the Universe

We are back to where we started in chapter 2: the original experience, the "beginning"—known by religious souls in a holy way, by scientists in an explosive and mathematical way, and by phenomenologists in an ontological way. Thus the many references so far to God, the Big Bang, and Being. I have suggested that Western religion and philosophy offer ways of understanding how rhetoric has a fundamental role to play in the "beginning" that calls for acknowledgment. But what about science? Might any of its practitioners be willing to admit that rhetorical competence, or at least its primordial ingredients, existed within the singularity whose explosion can still be heard radiating through the universe? This singularity and all the materials that came from it certainly qualify as instances of Being, things whose presence (otherness) caught the attention of at least one species who evolved from the Big Bang and who can hear and respond to its call, to its showing-forth or epideictic (rhetorical) display of truth. Looking at matters in this way, it seems fair to say that when the Big Bang happened so did rhetoric. It just took a while for it to be acknowledged.

I suspect, however, that such reasoning will most likely be less than satisfying to scientists who, despite the many arguments they offer for how the calling of human beings entails a "responsibility" for continuing "the great intellectual endeavor of finding the final laws of nature," might still rightly point out that what has been said about acknowledgment and rhetoric so far does not necessarily presuppose the presence of some "mind-stuff" and whatever intelligence it might possess. Divine intervention? As noted in chapter 2, this retreat to "the God-of-the-gaps" is considered a cop-out by the hardcore scientist who, like the Nobel Prize–winning physicist Steven Weinberg, maintains that "the only way that any sort of science can proceed is to assume that there is not divine intervention and to see how far one can get with this assumption."[73]

Weinberg does not believe that science will find an interested God in the final laws of nature, for all "our experience throughout the history of science has tended in the opposite direction, toward a chilling impersonality in the laws of nature."[74] Moreover, writes Weinberg, "Remembrance of the Holocaust leaves me unsympathetic to attempts to justify the ways of God to man. If there is a God that has special plans for humans, then He has taken very great pains to hide His concern for us. To me it would seem impolite if not impious to bother such a God with our prayers."[75]

Weinberg speaks of a God whose rhetorical competence is, at best, headed in the direction of negative acknowledgment of the worst kind: unconcern, social death, and, at times, total annihilation. Weinberg admits that he does not believe in such a God, for *any* notion of "God" is but a "metaphor" for the "mystery" that is found in nature, a mystery that science continues to expose and rationally explain. "Today for real mystery one has to look to cosmology and elementary particle physics. For those who see no conflict between science and religion, the retreat of religion from the ground occupied by science is nearly complete."[76] What has yet to be conquered by science is most likely to inspire "an almost irresistible temptation" to believe in a Creator intent on making us feel at "home" in the universe. For Weinberg, however, there is "honor" to be found in resisting this temptation, which he acknowledges "is only a thin substitute for the consolations of religion," but "is not entirely without satisfactions of its own."[77] These satisfactions include the sheer "excitement" and "enjoyment" of doing science, making "aesthetic judgments" about the "beauty" of some theory (its "simplicity" and "inevitability"), and the satisfaction that comes with scientific progress and how it can help "to preserve a sane world." Expanding on this last point, Weinberg writes: "It is not the certainty of scientific knowledge that fits it for this role, but its *uncertainty*. Seeing scientists change their minds again and again about matters that can be studied directly in laboratory experiments, how can one take seriously the claims of religious tradition and sacred writings to certain knowledge about matters beyond human experience?"[78]

We are discussing whether the scientist who refrains from considering how a caring God and the Big Bang's beginning are related might still grant rhetoric a role in this original experience. Given his assessment of God's status, Weinberg has no reason to attend to the issue. Yet, he still leaves an opening for further consideration of the matter when (1) he speaks of the importance of scientists' changing their minds in the face of that major catalyst of science *and* rhetoric: uncertainty; and (2) when he admits how aesthetic judgments play a role in science.

Weinberg fails to recognize the relationship that exists between uncertainty and rhetoric. Perhaps, like his fellow physicist David Bohm, he believes that it is not rhetoric but "dialogue" that enables the scientist to engage in rational collaborative deliberation with his or her colleagues. Writes Bohm:

> Conviction and persuasion are not called for in a dialogue. The word "convince" means to win, and the word "persuade" is similar. It's based on the same root as are "suave" and "sweet." People sometimes try to persuade by sweet talk or to convince by strong talk. Both come to the same thing, though, and neither of them is relevant. There's no point in being persuaded or convinced. That's not really coherent or rational. If something is right, you don't need to be persuaded. If somebody has to persuade you, then there is probably some doubt about it.[79]

Bohm, in short, is denying that rhetoric (certainly depicted in a narrow-minded and uninformed way) has a role to play in scientific dialogue. I, however, must disagree, especially in light of the literature on the "rhetoric of science," which makes it clear how scientific dialogue constitutes a rhetorical process that presupposes a history of both great and small minds being persuaded and convinced by arguments unfolding in the face of uncertainty.[80]

Science acknowledges and respects both uncertainty and the dialogue that it calls for; therefore it should also acknowledge itself as being, at least in part, a rhetorical enterprise. Of course, such a confession doesn't necessarily mean that rhetoric had a role to play in the Big Bang. But the confession continues to keep the matter open. Consider, for example, what the physicist and Nobel Prize recipient Richard Feynman has to say about the scientist's acknowledgment of uncertainty: "Every scientific law, every scientific principle, every statement of the results of an observation is some kind of a summary which leaves out details, because nothing can be stated precisely." Feynman thus maintains that

> All scientific knowledge is uncertain. This experience with doubt and uncertainty is important. I believe that it is of very great value, and one that extends beyond science. I believe that to solve any problem that has never been solved before, you have to leave the door to the unknown ajar. You have to permit the possibility that you do not have it exactly right. Otherwise, if you have made up your mind already, you might not solve it. . . . Scientists are used to this. We know that it is consistent to be able to live and not know. Some people say, "How can you *live* without knowing?" I do not know what they mean. I always live without knowledge. That is easy. How you get to know is what I want to know.[81]

Feynman goes on to stress how this "freedom to doubt" allows science to thrive and how he feels a responsibility as a "citizen-scientist" to "proclaim the value of this freedom and to teach that doubt is not to be feared, but that it is to be welcomed as the possibility of a new potential for human beings. If you know that you are not sure, you have a chance to improve the situation. I want to demand this freedom for future generations."[82]

What Feynman is arguing for is nothing more and nothing less than what comes with the temporality of human existence and its openness to the future: the ethical responsibility of answering the call of Being/conscience, a call which challenges people to affirm their freedom of choice. Indeed, argues Feynman, "openness of possibility is an opportunity. Doubt and discussion are essential to progress."[83] As a way of justifying the moral urgency of their art, rhetoricians have been making the same argument for over two thousand years. Feynman's continuation of his argument is worth noting:

> Why do we grapple with problems? We are only in the beginning. We have plenty of time to solve the problems. The only way that we will make a mistake is that in the impetuous youth of humanity we will decide we know the answer. This is it. No one else can think of anything else. And we will jam. We will confine man to the limited imagination of today's human beings.
>
> We are not smart. We are dumb. We are ignorant. We must maintain an open channel.[84]

Given all that has been said in this chapter, I trust it is clear that to maintain an open channel is to remain true to the openness and objective uncertainty of our temporal existence. Human temporality has a deconstructive and reconstructive ring to it, which necessarily calls on the rhetorical competence of human beings, or what Feynman, in a rhetorically delightful moment, describes as "atoms with curiosity" who look at themselves, wonder why they wonder, and thereby help to promote the evolution of moral consciousness.[85]

So was rhetoric at work in the Big Bang's beginning, when the potential for *everything* that *is* actually came into being in an awesome, epideictic display of truth? I continue to ask the question because I am interested in the history of acknowledgment, the story of a life-giving phenomenon whose rhetorical functioning warrants careful consideration. Western religion and philosophy have helped clarify this belief. It would be nice to have science on my side, too, given its influential presence in the world today. That many (if not most?) scientists are reluctant to offer this support, even as they argue for the importance of acknowledging uncertainty, should perhaps give us pause for thought. Is not science supposed to be consistently open to possibility? Of course it is; hence, its constant questioning of its findings. Science is a process of construction and deconstruction; it follows the lead of existence. Scientists can do this without having a taste for theology, philosophy, or rhetorical theory. Yes, there are rhetorically competent and incompetent arguments to be found throughout the history of science, but such arguments are conditioned to give way to mathematics and its precise way of disclosing truth. What's rhetorical about $2 + 2 = 4$, or $E = MC^2$? Something of the nature of the Big Bang can be measured; something of the nature of its singularity can be understood by investigating black holes and where they lead.

Of course, no one yet knows (or ever will know) for sure how it all ends, for, according to the calculations of science, there is no way for a human being or any of its technological creations to travel toward the singularity of a black hole without being smashed to bits before even coming close to what lies at the "bottom" or the "beginning" of this cosmic pit. With its ultimate respect for uncertainty, science can say with great certainty that we will never know *all there is to know* about the truth of the Big Bang and what came before it. Uncertainty will always keep us guessing, measuring, arguing, philosophizing, and perhaps even praying to One who, at any moment, we are told, is willing to do what no one else may care to do: acknowledge our existence. Why is it this way? Was there an "ingredient" for uncertainty in the singularity that, as Feynman puts it, "belched" the Big Bang?[86] Was that part of the "plan": to make sure that beings would eventually evolve who were complex enough to wonder about and thus acknowledge their beginnings and thereby engage in behavior that is crucial to their well-being? If so, then we "atoms with curiosity" were fated to become rhetorical beings (at least for the moment).

But wait a minute! What plan? The temporal call of Being, which, remember, is not a human creation, is known to encourage human beings to think of their beginnings in terms of some grand design. Hence, these beings' belief in God, that first "rhetor" whose awesome Word, gift, act of acknowledgment transformed space and time, cleared a dwelling place for things to exist and to live, and thereby made it possible for human beings to have a home in the universe and to share with others the life-giving gift that these beings were given in the beginning. Could this beginning be without a plan? Science is right: Who can say for sure?

Yet, as science rightly raises this question, it at the same time speaks to us of aesthetic matters: the "structure," "order," "harmony," and "beauty" that marks the life of the cosmos. "The Universe we live in is beautiful," writes physicist Lee Smolin in articulating his theory of "cosmological natural selection," and "it is so at least partly for the same reason a beautiful landscape or a beautiful city is, because a multitude of phenomena are taking place on a vast array of scales. . . . Indeed, in our universe we not only find structure on a variety of scales, *we find structure on every scale we have so far explored*"—from quarks, electrons, and neutrinos to the spiral wave of the whole galaxy.[87] Smolin thus maintains that "perhaps for the first time in human history, we know enough to imagine how a universe like ours might have come to be without the infinite intelligence and foresight of a god. For is it not conceivable that the universe is as we find it to be because it made itself; because the order, structure and beauty we see reflected at every scale [and re-presented in "elegant" mathematical equations] are the manifestations of a continual process of self-organization, of self-tuning, that has acted over very long periods of time?"[88]

From a rhetorical standpoint, Smolin is, of course, speaking about a process that exhibits "appropriateness" and "style." Although he opts for the elegance and beauty of mathematics over rhetorical invention when it comes to revealing the true workings of the process, he nevertheless is a wonderful writer whose prose is as clear as it is compelling and pleasing to the ear. Listen, for example, to the way he concludes his argument for a self-organizing, godless universe:

> The world will always be here, and it will always be different, more varied, more interesting, more alive, but still always the world in all its complexity and incompleteness. There is nothing behind it, no absolute or platonic world to transcend to. All there is of Nature is what is around us. All there is of Being is relations among real, sensible things. All we have of natural law is a world that has made itself. All we may expect of human law is what we can negotiate among ourselves, and what we take as our responsibility. All we may gain of knowledge must be drawn from what we can see with our own eyes and what others tell us they have seen with their eyes. All we may expect of justice is compassion. All we may look up to as judges are each other. All that is possible of utopia is what we make with our own hands. Pray let it be enough.[89]

Smolin writes with rhetorical competence. There is a symmetry and rhythm to his sentence structure that is appealing. It would be fair to say that his style is *appropriate* to his topic. Moreover, what he asks of human beings—negotiation, responsibility, compassionate and wise judgment—certainly presupposes an appreciation for the need to develop rhetorical competence. Such a need, according to Smolin, is an evolutionary outcome of "processes of self-organization" that lend order to chaos and that are not grounded in some ultimate or final principle.[90] We are all we have to help others and ourselves as we raise the question "Where art thou?" and offer a response: "Here I am!" "Pray that it be enough." We would be wise to structure our prayers in a rhetorically appropriate way so as to make them more effective. At the present time in its evolution, Nature requires nothing less. It is a matter of being fit. We *are* creatures who appreciate and are moved by the right, fitting, and timely use of words.

Although Smolin ends his book on a high rhetorical note, I feel confident in saying that it is not his intention to suggest that there was something fundamentally rhetorical about the Big Bang. Still, if it were not for the appropriateness—the harmony and beauty—of the universe, he would have nothing to talk about in a rhetorically appropriate way. For someone like Steven Weinberg, however, who does "dream" of constructing a "final theory," the nature of this appropriateness demands further inquiry:

> It is when we study truly fundamental problems that we expect to find beautiful answers. We believe that, if we ask why the world is the way it is and then ask why that answer is the way it is, at the end of this chain of explanations we shall find a few simple principles of compelling beauty. We think this in part because our historical experience teaches us that as we look beneath the surface of things, we find more and more beauty. Plato and the neo-Platonists taught that the beauty we see in nature is a reflection of the beauty of the ultimate, the *nous*. For us, too, the beauty of present theories is an anticipation, a premonition, of the beauty of the final theory. And in any case, we would not accept any theory as final unless it were beautiful.[91]

Weinberg grants the appropriateness of beauty a transcendental status; it is something "that is built into the structure of the universe at a very deep level." As already noted above, Weinberg does not credit God with this accomplishment, for that would be foolish for a scientist to do. Discovering the beauty and truth of the ultimate laws of nature does not require divine guidance. Human intelligence, commitment, state-of-the-art technology, and mathematics are enough. These things have long served and will continue to serve in that "demystification of the heavens" that has lead those like Weinberg to believe that beyond the order, symmetry, harmony, and beauty—a.k.a. appropriateness—of the cosmos there is "nothing." Or as Weinberg also likes to put it: "the more the universe seems comprehensible the more it seems pointless"—which is not to say "that science teaches us that the universe is pointless, but rather that the universe itself suggests no point."[92] As a way of countering the charges of cynicism that he realizes are bound to be evoked by this claim, Weinberg says this:

> But if there is no solace in the fruits of our research, there is at least some consolation in the research itself. Men and women are not content to comfort themselves with tales of gods and giants, or to confine their thoughts to the daily affairs of life; they also build telescopes and satellites and accelerators, and sit at their desks for endless hours working out the meaning of the data they gather. The effort to understand the universe is one of the very few things that lifts human life a little above the level of farce, and gives it some of the grace of tragedy.[93]

In the Judeo-Christian tradition, the "lift" that comes with the "grace of tragedy" marks an epiphanous moment whereby one's suffering becomes instructive for a better life (be it one's own or another's) and thereby enables a person to remain open to, acknowledge, and share an understanding of the loving-kindness of God. The moment is "most appropriate" because it is one in which "the true beauty" of human being is displayed—a beauty whose distinguished purpose is to cultivate "the good" here on earth.[94] The "grace of tragedy" is but an oxymoron when dissociated from this purpose. An oxymoron is a rhetorical figure (Gk. "a witty, paradoxical saying") employed for effect, for stimulating the attunement of consciousness when making a point. Weinberg's point is that, with the universe in mind, it is pointedly foolish to grant it more than it is worth. There is a beauty, an appropriateness, to the universe that can be acknowledged by scientists and other interested folk who, in turn, can think well of themselves because they can engage in this act. Beyond this, things like rhetorical competence and God don't really matter, unless one chooses to use his or her rhetorical competence to call into question those who think otherwise.

Like Weinberg, the physicist Brian Greene is committed to the view that his profession's calling is to acknowledge the appropriateness, or what he calls the "elegance," of the universe without appealing to "the God-of-the-gaps." Greene is one of the world's leading "string theorists." String theory advances the cosmological dreams of those who seek a final theory, a "theory of everything (T.O.E.)." According to Greene, who speaks of such a theory in a more optimistic way than Weinberg does,

> The discovery of the T.O.E.—the ultimate explanation of the universe at its most microscopic level, a theory that does not rely on any deeper explanation—would provide the firmest foundation on which to *build* our understanding of the world. Its discovery would

mark a beginning, not an end. The ultimate theory would provide an unshakable pillar of coherence forever assuring us that the universe is a comprehensible place.[95]

And with the mathematical findings supporting string theory, such a pillar is taking form, for the theory declares

> that the "stuff" of all matter and all forces is the *same*. Each elementary particle is composed of a single string—that is, each particle *is* a string—and all strings are absolutely identical. Differences between the particles arise because their respective strings undergo different resonant vibrational patterns. What appear to be different elementary particles are actually different "notes" on a fundamental string. The universe—being composed of an enormous number of these strings—is akin to a cosmic symphony.[96]

Introduced by the Big Bang, this symphony gives substance, form, and function to life and brings into being the "symmetries of nature." By this construct "physicists mean that nature treats every moment in time and every location in space identically—symmetrically—by ensuring that the same fundamental laws are in operation. Much in the same manner that they affect art and music, such symmetries are deeply satisfying; they highlight an order and a coherence in the workings of nature"—which is rightly called "beautiful."[97] The complexity and beauty of this symphony and its symmetries are astonishing—and more: "In fact," writes Greene, "the mathematics of string theory is so complicated that, to date, no one even knows the exact equations of the theory. Instead, physicists know only approximations to these equations, and even the approximate equations are so complicated that they as yet have been only partially solved."[98] The evolution of human intelligence has a way to go before it can come to terms with and understand what "essentially" keeps the cosmos in tune and allows it to play on into the future. Greene and his colleagues must therefore admit that their specific measures of the appropriateness of the cosmos, at the very least, may be somewhat off the mark and thus inappropriate. Still, Greene is encouraged by a host of ongoing scientific findings and speaks of string theory as leading the scientific community in the direction of "unified-theory paradise."[99] Here would be the ultimate and thus most appropriate dwelling place for comprehending what it *really* means to speak of what *is* right, fitting, and timely—the essence of appropriateness, or what Stephen Hawking once described as "the mind of God."[100] Perhaps, then, it would be appropriate to credit string theory with discovering the "holiest" rhetoric that there is.

Because the presence of rhetoric presupposes a motivating intention on the part of some orator or "intelligent designer," I doubt Greene and his fellow physicists would spend much time considering this suggestion. It is too metaphysical for their tastes. But as long as science continues its search to discover the fundamental principle that grants order, beauty, harmony, symmetry—in short, appropriateness—to the evolving universe, the suggestion must remain a possibility.[101] As noted earlier when we discussed certain views of Richard Feynman, the ethic of science requires as much: an openness to and an acknowledgment of the presence of what *is* and the uncertainty that is concomitant with this presence.

Science and religion agree: the original experience, the initial happening, must be sought and its truth acknowledged. The *call* to do this may have nothing to do with God or the Big Bang, but as phenomenological research helps to make clear, it certainly is "coded" into the ontological structure of human existence, with its different dimensions of alterity or otherness. The universe has evolved to the point where the question can be asked by one of its species that "knows" of its "own importance": What would life be like if nobody cared enough to acknowledge your existence, to say "Here I am!" when you called out "Where art thou?" and thus to offer you a place in his or her life where, if only for the moment, you might dwell together in a caring way? As noted in chapter one, with this added living space comes the opportunity for a new beginning, a second chance, whereby one might improve his or her lot in life. Acknowledgment is a gift worth sharing, time and again, for the good of humankind—those creatures who more often than not need to feel at home in their dwelling places. Science and religion accept the burden of trying to fulfill this need with their respective teachings about where we came from, how we got here, and what we have to look forward to in the future. These teachings are empty if they are not about some matter and manner of appropriateness rooted in nature. Science and religion are committed to finding the most appropriate ways of disclosing and "showing forth" this most fundamental phenomenon. It is, like it or not, a rhetorical task, an epideictic adventure. The goal is to help us understand our place in the universe, or what both science and religion sometimes refer to as our "home." In the next chapter, I focus more closely on the existential reality of this commonly used metaphor. What exactly is being referred to when, at a certain moment in time and space, one admits that he or she feels at home—be it in the universe or in any smaller and more localized habitat? Addressing this question enables us to take another step toward understanding the scope and function of acknowledgment.

Chapter Five

Home

"Please, make yourself at home!" These are generous words for house guests to hear, for they welcome people into a habitat that, at least as it is commonly defined, is supposed to be a place of security, convenience, cordiality, relaxation, happiness, and love; a place that encourages the development of personal relationships and strong family ties; a place where one need not worry about "being oneself"; in short, a place of genuine care and comfort.[1] A house that is authentically a home is an abode or dwelling place whose inhabitants ought to know that, no matter how bad things become, here still exists a haven of shelter and forgiveness. Indeed, if people really mean what they say with the words "Please, make yourself at home," then those who receive this invitation are right to expect that their hosts will go out of their way to accommodate their guests' needs and behaviors. The invitation need no longer even be uttered with close friends and family, for such people are already expected to know that their presence is welcomed and will be accommodated with open arms—even when company is not expected and the house is a wreck. Once it becomes an open and standing invitation to certain others, "Please, make yourself at home" is meant as an unconditional form of positive acknowledgment: *"Mi casa es su casa!"*

Of course, this generous acknowledgment is easier to give when guests are willing to abide by an unspoken rule of decorum that I suspect is more often than not at work in the homeowner's mind when he or she utters the invitation. Stated in its most straightforward form, the rule is this: don't be a pig, a slob, a nuisance, a freeloader, a "guest" whose presence is more of a source of worry, anger, frustration, and repugnance than a source of comfort. Unless they are masochistic, homeowners do not invite their guests to "make themselves at home" in such a way that the homeowners will become miserable in their company. One's home is far too special a place for that to happen. I say this with more in mind about the matter than what has been noted so far.

According to Agnes Heller, "integral to the average everyday life is awareness of a fixed point in space, a firm position from which we 'proceed' (whether every day or over larger periods of time) and to which we return in due course. This firm position is what we call 'home.'"[2] Indeed, one's home is both a place of origin *and* a destination that is longed for after a busy day, a weary journey, or even an enjoyable vacation. It is satisfying to be able to say and *really* mean that "it's good to be back home."

The meaning of this saying is rooted in the nature of human being: specifically, how we exist as *animalia metaphysica*, creatures who, in having to deal with the uncertainty of our temporal existence and the anxiety that such uncertainty inspires, have also developed a passionate longing for some degree of meaning, order, and completeness in our lives. This metaphysical urge is at work, for example, when religious souls pray to God, when scientists formulate mathematical equations in an attempt to identify the ultimate laws of the universe, and when philosophers address the ontological question of what it means to be a human being. Such endeavors display what William Earle describes as "a nostalgia for something final and absolute."[3] This description is especially appropriate considering that the feeling identified here—"nostalgia," from the Greek *nostos:* to return home—speaks of that state of being wherein one is "homesick." Such sickness threatens the well-being of *animalia metaphysica*.

I thus believe that Gaston Bachelard, in his phenomenological study of how people experience intimate places, is right to insist that the house become home "is one of the greatest powers of integration for the thoughts, memories and dreams of mankind. . . . Without it, man would be a dispersed being. It maintains him through the storms of the heavens and through those of life."[4] Moreover, as Bachelard notes, "the house we were born in has engraved within us the hierarchy of the various functions of inhabiting [a place]. We are the diagram of the functions of inhabiting that particular house, and all the other houses are but variations on a fundamental [and metaphysical] theme. The word habit is too worn a word to express this passionate liaison of our bodies, which do not forget, with an unforgettable house."[5] The relationship that holds between the two observations that Bachelard makes here is significant: A home offers an alternative to a nomadic existence, grants us shelter from the elements, and provides a refuge wherein we can feel more comfortable when learning how to cope with the difficulties of everyday life.[6] To be sure, the home is an educational environment, a place where we learn to crawl, walk, talk, eat, play, converse, be good and bad, and to care for others who are busy caring for us as they teach their loved ones all kinds of things. As one inhabits a home, it, in turn, begins and continues to inhabit oneself. Hence, for example, the possibility of becoming upset with a guest's table manners and wondering if he or she "was raised in a pig sty." Our bodies are home to our home's ways of being a social, political, moral, and, like it or not, unforgettable environment.

Sigmund Freud refers to the female body as the "former home of all human beings."[7] The issue of one's well-being certainly begins in this home. Although I have never met a person who can recall what it was like to be nurtured in the womb, there is substantial popular literature that details how the female owners of this home remember all the "labor" that it took to care for and give birth to their babies. Homes are worth remembering for the lives and dreams that they help make possible.

With life, however, comes death. As the saying goes: "As soon as you are born you are old enough to die." Before the twentieth century, when hospitals acquired enough scientific and technological know how to assume the responsibility of "personal and loving care," home was the place where people went to die, where they could be cared for in the deathbeds of their rooms by members of their family who came together in the home to love and make peace with someone who, as it might be said, was about "to return home to their Maker."[8] Even in death we can still have a home—both in heaven *and* here on earth. Of these two homes, heaven, of course, is the more "spiritual" place to rest in peace. On earth, however, the metaphysical inclination is still needed, for those who have passed away are dependent on accommodations made by the living. Pericles' funeral oration on the Athenian dead in the first year of the Peloponnesian war provides a classic piece of epideictic rhetoric that both refers to and performs this early task. The Greek General insists that his fellow soldiers, in sacrificing their lives to defend their homeland, have

> won praises that never grow old, the most splendid of sepulchers— not the sepulcher in which their bodies are laid, but where their glory remains eternal in men's minds, always there on the right occasion to stir others to speech or to action. For famous men have the whole earth as their memorial: it is not only the inscriptions on their graves in their own country that mark them out; no, in foreign lands also, not in any visible form but in people's hearts, their memory abides and grows.[9]

By way of our minds and hearts we provide accommodations that enable the dearly departed *to come back to life*, to be there with us and to guide us as we carry on their teachings. Here on earth, our lived bodies offer a home for the dead. Pericles' speech is designed to bring this point home to an audience whose members, he believes, need not only "commiseration" but also "comfort."[10] Home is *the* metaphysical symbol for this longed-for state of being, and Pericles' epideictic rhetoric creates a narrative structure whose *ethos* (dwelling place) caters to this human desire. As he offers unqualified praise for his fallen comrades, Pericles constructs a home where personal relationships and strong family ties can be acknowledged and where people can know-together something of their goodness.

My move to Pericles is strategic of course, for it brings back into play a central concern of this book: how rhetoric, functioning as a tool of acknowledgment, transforms time and space in order to provide a dwelling place (a home) for people to gain some understanding of truth and to cultivate moral thought and action. This task lies at the heart of the rhetorical tradition and its teachings on the ethics of rhetorical competence. The effectiveness of such competence presupposes on the part of the orator an appreciation of a certain fact of life associated with the ontological and metaphysical nature of human being: The more people feel at home with another's arguments and world-views, the more they are likely to remain open to what the other has to say. Such openness, on the part of both orator and audience, allows for genuine acknowledgment to take place. It may be possible to employ rhetoric simply as a means of manipulation and deceit, but it also offers itself as a tool for collaborative deliberation whereby people are encouraged to take an active role in discovering and remaining open to all that needs to be observed in a given situation if disputable matters are to be resolved in a reasonable and truthful manner.

In his discussion of the rhetorical competence that must be at work here, Quintilian makes much of a topic that, as noted above, is related to the significance of one's home: memory. According to Quintilian, "it is memory which has brought oratory to its present position of glory. For it provides the orator not merely with the order of his thoughts, but even of his words, nor is its power limited to stringing merely a few words together; its capacity for endurance is inexhaustible, and even in the longest pleadings the patience of the audience flags long before the memory of the speaker."[11] Quintilian then notes: "This fact may even be advanced as an argument that there must be some art of memory and that the natural gift can be helped by reason, since training enables us to do things which we cannot do before we have had any training or practice."[12] A good memory is a prerequisite of rhetorical competence for, at the very least, it enables an orator to remain coherent and consistent in advancing a position, and coherency and consistency are two things that help an audience to begin feeling comfortable (at home) with what they are hearing. Quintilian suggests that perhaps the best way for the orator to cultivate the art of memory is to learn to associate topics and lines of argument with "localities": "For when we return to a place after considerable absence, we not merely recognize the place itself, but remember things that we did there, and recall the persons whom we met and even the unuttered thoughts which passed through our minds when we were there before."[13] The specific locality that Quintilian recommends as a model for the arrangement of rhetoric is "a spacious house divided into a number of rooms": "The first thought is placed, as it were, in the forecourt; the second, let us say, in the living-room; the remainder are placed in due order all around the *impluvium* and entrusted not merely to bedrooms and parlours, but even to the care of statues and the like. This done, as soon as the memory of the facts requires to be revived, all these places are visited in turn and the various deposits are demanded from their custodians, as the sight of each recalls the respective details."[14]

Although Quintilian has nothing to say about the ontological and metaphysical significance of his chosen mnemonic device, he nevertheless ends up associating rhetorical competence with a locality that, as mentioned above, is one of the greatest powers of integration for our thoughts, memories, and dreams. The rhetorical and ethical achievement of acknowledgment defines an activity of *home-making* that is aided by thinking about a place called home—a place filled with rooms, decorative and symbolic furnishings (e.g., statues), loved ones, and the memories associated with such sources of comfort.

Throughout the remaining chapters of this book I will be discussing various additional matters that contribute to the character of the relationship being emphasized here between acknowledgment, rhetoric, and the home. In the present chapter, however, I want to continue establishing some common ground for understanding the three related topics. I do this with the help of Robert Frost's poem, "The Death of the Hired Man"—a poem that, as will be detailed below, works rhetorically to call the meaning of home into question and, in so doing, invites readers to ponder what a home ought to be and how it should make one feel. As my reading of the poem unfolds, I will have occasion to refer to architectural design theory—as well as to reintroduce the topics of religion and science—for the purpose of providing a more complete picture of what it means to make people feel at home.

A Rhetoric of Home

Mary sat musing on the lamp-flame at the table,
Waiting for Warren. When she heard his step,
She ran on tiptoe down the darkened passage
To meet him in the doorway with the news
And put him on his guard. "Silas is back."
She pushed him outward with her through the door
And shut it after her. "Be kind," she said.
She took the market things from Warren's arms
And set them on the porch, then drew him down
To sit beside her on the wooden steps.

So begins Frost's poem "The Death of the Hired Man."[15] The remaining one hundred fifty-five lines detail a conversation between Mary and her husband, Warren, in which they talk about how he, especially, should acknowledge the presence of his on-again-off-again hired man, Silas. In the course of this conversation we learn more about who Silas is, how he is thought of by Mary and Warren, and why he is back "home." When the topic of home comes up, Mary and Warren dispute its meaning. This dispute, along with the initial interruption of their daily lives by Silas's presence, sounds for Mary and Warren what was described in chapter 3 as the call of conscience. The rhetoric they employ in responding to this call constitutes their conversation. Frost's poem, in other words, is essentially about the related topics of acknowledgment, home, and rhetoric.

But why, then, the emphasis on "death" in the title? Recalling how the meaning of home can entail a consideration of death provides a clue. I make use of this clue in due time.[16]

"Silas is back," Mary says, and adds to this fact a request: "Be kind." This request certainly raises the issue of acknowledgment. Warren's reply is somewhat defensive: "When was I ever anything but kind to him? But I'll not have the fellow back . . . I told him so last haying, didn't I? If he left then, I said, that ended it. What good is he? Who else will harbor him/ At his age for the little he can do?" As Warren continues with his reply, we learn that Silas is not dependable: "Off he goes always when I need him most. He thinks he ought to earn a little pay/ Enough at least to buy tobacco with, [s]o he won't have to beg and be beholden." Warren admits that he cannot afford to pay Silas a fixed wage, although he wishes this were possible so that Silas could begin "bettering himself." But Warren doubts that Silas honestly desires this goal, for the man is a drifter with no authentic ties to anyone: he leaves "In haying time, when any help is scarce. In winter he comes back to us. I'm done."

Warren's acknowledgment of Silas (who he has yet to see directly) is limited by the "rationality" of a pragmatic and utilitarian outlook that farmers, for their own well-being, are wise to maintain. Such rationality is the *modus operandi* of what Heidegger terms "calculative thought." Recall that such thought "places itself under compulsion to master everything in the logical terms of its procedure."[17] Medical science, for example, employs calculative thought in its high-tech "war" against disease. The downside of this type of thinking shows itself, however, when the personhood of patients is lost in the rush to treat them only "by the numbers" (the numerical data made possible by technological instruments). The rationality of calculative thought encourages a reductionistic view of people. Silas is thus seen by Warren as being first and foremost a commodity, a tool whose thrifty purchase provides a means to an end. Silas is a hired hand, a worker, a cog in a wheel that is failing and is thus is no longer dependable. "What good is he?" The question speaks of a law of nature: survival of the fittest.

Mary, however, acknowledges Silas more as a person than as an instrument. She protects him from Warren's cold-hearted remarks: "Sh! not so loud: he'll hear you." And having actually been with him since he returned, her reaction speaks more directly to the matter at hand: "He's worn out. He's asleep beside the stove.

When I came up from Bowe's I found him here,/ Huddled against the barn door fast asleep,/ A miserable sight, and frightening, too—I wasn't looking for him— and he's changed. Wait till you see." She goes on to explain how she "gave him tea and tried to make him smoke. I tried to make him talk about his travels. Nothing would do: he just kept nodding off."

Warren, however, is more interested in knowing whether Silas "said he'd come to ditch the meadow for me." Mary reacts to her husband's uncaring query with disappointment and scorn: "Warren!" Pressed again to answer his question, Mary responds: "Of course he did. What would you have him say? Surely you wouldn't grudge the poor old man/ Some humble way to save his self-respect. He added, if you really care to know,/ He meant to clear the upper pasture, too." But then, immediately, she becomes more existential again: "Warren, I wish you could have heard the way/ He jumbled everything. I stopped to look/ Two or three times—he made me feel so queer—/ To see if he was talking in his sleep. He ran on Harold Wilson—you remember—/ The boy you had in haying four years since," and was always arguing with Silas when they worked together pitching and stacking hay. "After so many years he still keeps finding/ Good arguments he sees he might have used. I sympathize. I know just how it feels to/ Think of the right thing to say too late." Mary has a sense for the importance of appropriateness.

Continuing to report on what Silas had to say, Mary recounts his reaction to learning that the boy finished school and was now teaching college. Silas "thinks young Wilson is a likely lad, though daft/ On education." The boy cares more for Latin than he does about "how to find water with a hazel prong." Silas wishes he had "another chance/ To teach him how to build a load of hay." Warren interrupts to admit that, indeed, "that's Silas' one accomplishment": he is well-skilled in the know-how of haying. Mary once again steers the conversation back toward Silas's personhood: "He thinks if he could teach him that, he'd be/ Some good perhaps to someone in the world. He hates to see a boy the fool of books. Poor Silas, so concerned with other folk,/ And nothing to look backward to with pride,/ And nothing to look forward to with hope,/ So now and never any different."

Mary is shocked and depressed by Silas's presence. Warren, on the other hand, seems more bothered than anything else by how this presence has brought about an unexpected and unwanted interruption to the routines of his day. Recall that such an interruption can sound a call of conscience. Silas's presence raises a question to his witnesses: "Where art thou?" By way of their conversation, Mary and Warren are establishing premises on which to answer "Here I am!" Having only past memories of Silas the worker and his wife's words to go on, Warren is not unsettled enough to answer the call by going beyond the calculative workings of his instrumental outlook. He thereby sentences Silas to a life of social death, of having to continue to maintain a lower class status and live on the margins of society. Haying is what Silas is good for, nothing else. Owing to the deficiency of positive acknowledgment at work here, it makes sense to speak of "the death of the hired man." Silas is worthless, until he can show his talent for working with hay. In a world that demands industrious behavior, a talented man whose talents are rapidly declining may be better off dead.

Picking up where she left off, and with her husband's restricted sense of the situation in mind, Mary discloses a somewhat different impression: "Warren . . . he has come home to die: You needn't be afraid he'll leave you this time." Warren gently mocks his wife: "Home . . . Yes, what else but home?" Mary's reply adds force to the call of conscience already at work in the situation: "It all depends on what you mean by home. Of course he's nothing to us, any more/ Than was the hound that came a stranger to us/ Out of the woods, worn out upon the trail." Perhaps bothered by the suggestiveness of this analogy, Warren counters it with a rather callous definition of the topic: "Home is the place where, when you have to go there,/ They have to take you in." And Mary, again, takes her husband to task: "I should have called it/ Something that you somehow haven't to deserve."

Mary and Warren disagree about the meaning of a place called home, a topic that, like Silas, suddenly becomes an issue, an interruption, in their everyday lives. Warren's definition of home lacks any sense of heartfelt emotion. Mary's definition, although not as clearly expressed as her husband's, certainly goes further. For home is not merely a place where people, whether they like it or not, are obliged to take you in. Home, when all is said and done, is where one goes to die so that he or she might pass away in the company of others who genuinely care about what is happening and who are there to offer comfort at a time of great need. As discussed earlier, humankind's mortal coil is more often than not a source of anxiety, that "uncanny" (*unheimlich*) feeling that arises when things like our bodies or cherished meanings break down and that makes it so difficult for us to feel "at home" (*heimlich*) with our life and where it seems to be going. Coming face to face with death is worse when one is all alone, without anyone who seems to care. Silas lives a nomadic existence; he is homeless. But he has returned to a place where things might be different, at least if Mary has her way.

Mary's sense of home does not totally preclude Warren's take on the matter, but it does call the rigidity and narrowness of his view into question. Silas's presence registers a call of conscience, and now the same can be said of Mary's words. Warren remains quiet for a moment, pondering Mary's last statement regarding how home is "something you somehow haven't to deserve." When he responds he seems to be a bit more open to the association between home and people who care: "Silas has better claim on us you think/ Than does his brother? Thirteen little miles/ As the road winds would bring him to his door. Silas has walked that far no doubt today. Why doesn't he go there? His brother's rich . . . ." Mary agrees that Silas's brother "ought to help" and she declares that she will "see to that if there is need." She also insists that Warren "have some pity on Silas. Do you think/ If he had any pride in claiming kin/ Or anything he looked for from his brother,/ He'd keep so still about him all this time?" Warren wonders out loud "what's between them." Mary is quick to answer: "Silas is what he is—we wouldn't mind Him—/ But just the kind that kinsfolk can't abide. He never did a thing so bad. He don't know why he isn't quite as good/ As anybody. Worthless though he is,/ He won't be made ashamed to please his brother." Warren's response is telling of a heart acquiring more feeling: "*I can't think Si ever hurt anyone.*"

Warren is becoming more open to the situation, and Mary takes advantage of this opening with a shrewd yet sincere rhetorical move: "No, but he hurt my heart the way he lay/ And rolled his old head on that sharp-edged chair-back. He wouldn't let me put him on the lounge. You must go in and see what you can do. I made the bed up for him there tonight. You'll be surprised at him—how much he's broken. His working days are done; I'm sure of it." Warren is still a bit skeptical: "I'd not be in a hurry to say that." Mary maintains that her judgment was not hurried. "Go, look, see for yourself."

The moment is now at hand for Warren to acknowledge, not just think about, Silas's condition. What would life be like if no one acknowledged your existence? The question, I think it is fair to say, has been on Mary's mind throughout the conversation with her husband. So much so, in fact, that, as Warren enters their home, Mary expresses yet another caution in an attempt to guarantee Silas's self-respect and to make the man feel at home: "But, Warren, please remember how it is: He's come to help you ditch the meadow. He has a plan. You mustn't laugh at him. He may not speak of it, and then he may." When Warren returned— "too soon, it seemed to [Mary]"—he "Slipped to her side, caught up her hand and waited." Mary questioned her husband: "Warren?" "'Dead,' was all he answered."

We can only wonder whether Silas felt at home when he died. Mary tried her best to attend to this task of conscience. "Where art thou?" "Here I am!" Warren's response to the call took too long to be of any good. An ideological outlook got in the way. The rhetoric informing this outlook appears throughout the conversation and is especially noticeable in contrast with Mary's rhetoric. Warren sees Silas first and foremost in terms of his "use" value. As a farmer whose work is demanding and perhaps not especially profitable, Warren is not "wrong" to make such an evaluation. In light of the situation at hand, however, the evaluation proves inappropriate given its consequence of promoting the marginalization and isolation— the social death—of a man who apparently does not want to be alone when he dies. No, Silas has come *home* to die. He is in desperate need of someone whose appreciation of fitness is not limited to physical strength but also entails a good amount of ethical and moral sensitivity. Warren's understanding of home lacks the feeling that is necessary to accommodate a hired man's last request. The premises of his argument are not supportive of another type of premises that are called to mind when admitting that "home is where the heart is." The habitat built on Warren's rhetoric is less of a home than a house, less of a place of hospitality and comfort than a place where they "have to take you in" whether they like it or not.

In her work *Geography of Home*, interior designer Akiko Busch speaks of the essential connection between the rhetorical art of "arranging words" and the architectural art of "designing places":

> Both of these are about finding the logical order of things, about assembling these aggregates of experience in a way that makes sense. A room, like a page, offers us the space to do this. Sometimes that sense of order comes with the way words are arranged on the page. Other times it may come with the way objects have been assembled in a room. Both are ways of finding those arrangements with which we can live. . . . Another word for that is fit [or appropriateness]. And this is the way I try to define design, as having to do with how things fit—how things fit the hand, how furniture fits the body, how people fit in buildings, and how buildings fit the landscape. . . . And if we think of design as being about fit, we consider not only the physical dimensions, but the moral and social ones as well.[18]

Silas no longer fits into Warren's way of being at home on the farm, a scheduled existence that is arranged and designed to accomplish a hard but good day's work. Mary presumably plays an essential role in this place: cooking, cleaning, and helping with any number of additional chores, perhaps including fieldwork. She offers no complaints about her way of being at home on the farm, although, of course, her outlook on the matter exceeds Warren's with respect to its capacity for positive acknowledgment of someone like Silas. Taking a closer look at this capacity as it is presented in Frost's poem can help to advance our understanding of the relationship between acknowledgment, rhetoric, and home.

Mary's acknowledgment of Silas is the result of a call of conscience that is heard as soon as his sickly presence interrupts her day. "Where art thou?" The moment was "frightening." Silas was a "miserable sight." Mary didn't recognize him at first, for she "wasn't looking for him." This person who, until that moment, was recognized and appreciated in a calculative way for the most part—as a hired man who was good at haying. But now Silas was not "himself," and Mary could not help but know that there was something terribly wrong. Such knowledge presupposes the attunement of consciousness whereby acknowledgment can begin taking form as one's taken for granted ways of seeing the world assume a more observant function, one that, to repeat Heidegger's description of the process, "lets that toward which it goes come toward it."

Faced with Silas's unsettling (deconstructive) presence, Mary perceived something other than a hired man, something more moving and fragile, something that had to be "dragged" into the house so that he could be attended to and cared for as he continued to lose and regain consciousness.

This response to the call of conscience was, of course, the decent thing to do. Warren, one hopes, would have done the same thing if he had been the first to be awed by Silas's presence. But would he have remained open to the ongoing call of this being? Would he have continued to sacrifice his calculative understanding of a hired man so that, in a moment of "releasement," of "'letting be' of what-is," he could "take to heart," hear the truth of, and remember all that Silas was trying to say? In short, was Warren capable of dwelling poetically with this suffering soul?

Mary certainly was. She engaged in the moral act of listening carefully to Silas's speech as he mentioned ditching the meadow and clearing the upper pasture, and as he "ran on" about the youth Wilson. Indeed, Mary was attentive as Silas noted that he had continued to think of "good arguments" that he could have used with this college boy, how he wished he had another chance "to teach him how to build a load of hay," and how, if he taught the boy that, "he'd be/ Some good perhaps to someone in the world." Listening to these thoughts and observing their source, Mary understood that Silas was in need of special comfort, for he had come home to die. In his highly praised work on the historical relationship between comfort and home, Witold Rybczynski writes: "We must discover for ourselves the mystery of comfort, for without it, our dwellings will indeed be machines instead of homes."[19] Machines play an important role in farm life. The same can be said of homes. Hard work without any expectation of eventual comfort defines a hellish life. The man who was dying in her home deserved more than that, for his life, even as he now faced Mary, was lacking so much: "Poor Silas, so concerned for other folk,/And nothing to look backward to with pride,/And nothing to look forward to with hope,/So now and never any different."

Mary is never more poetic than when she utters these sad words. She had opened herself to Silas's presence, listened closely to his speech, took it to heart, and then spoke her memory of a man who she sympathized with as he tried to find good and timely arguments to validate his life. Mary's words acknowledge the goodness of a person whose life was overwhelmed with failure. But there was still time, perhaps, to make Silas feel at home—a feeling that, at least for Mary, "you somehow haven't to deserve." Although no justification for this belief is offered, Mary does suggest, in talking about Silas's brother, that the feeling is not totally dependent on the actions of one's kinsfolk. Such folk, even if they were in someway hurt by a family member, still "ought to help" in caring for the needs of their kin. This suggestion encourages a sympathetic response from Warren ("I can't think Si ever hurt anyone")—one that certainly provides an opening for Mary's next remark: "No but he hurt my heart the way he lay/And rolled his old head on that sharp-edged chair-back."

Earlier I characterized this remark as being a shrewd yet sincere rhetorical move. This assessment assumes that Mary, who, like Silas, knows "just how it feels/To think of the right thing to say too late," was being intentionally strategic with her speech. Yet, even if the intention was not at work on a conscious level, the

remark still indicates a noticeable degree of rhetorical competence in that it is especially "appropriate," right and fitting, for the conversational moment. Mary is
attempting to construct a "good argument" on Silas's behalf, an argument that will
inspire proper judgment and action on Warren's part. The argument is for sympathy, compassion, and mercy; for an attunement of consciousness that can acknowledge Silas's being and *all* that goes with it. Such acknowledgment is fostered
by a remark that would have Warren identify with Silas by way of his wife. Mary is
"hurting," and this admission further personalizes the situation for Warren. As
Kenneth Burke would put it, there now exists a "consubstantiality"—a common
bond of understanding—between the three characters.[20] Owing to Mary's persis-
tence, she and her husband are on their way to knowing together what they ought
to do about Silas's condition and his immediate needs. Although Warren's calculating way of seeing Silas still makes him a bit skeptical, he is nevertheless moved
to action.

Abraham Heschel tells us that a human being is that creature who

> insists not only on being satisfied but also on being able to satisfy,
> on *being a need* not only on *having needs*. Personal needs come and
> go, but one anxiety remains: *Am I needed?* There is no man who has
> not been moved by that anxiety. . . . The only way to avoid despair is
> *to be a need* rather than an end. *Happiness*, in fact, may be defined as
> the *certainty of being needed.*[21]

Silas needed to be needed as a respected hired man who, given his present condition, also needed a place to feel comfortable, a place called "home." Warren, presumably, was now in the position to attend to these needs. Mary had already begun the process by caring for and listening to Silas and by speaking to her
husband in a way that functioned rhetorically to open a space in time where Warren could reconsider both his meaning of home and his assessment of one who
had come home to die. Warren's eventual acknowledgment of the matters at hand
presupposes the occurrence of such an existential transformation of everyday life.
The transformation took place as Silas's presence sounded a call of conscience and
as Mary's response to this call enhanced its importance and urgency for her husband. "Where art thou?" A "Here I am!" is sounded as Warren walks into his
home.

But the question still remains: Did Silas feel at home when he died? Walter
Jost maintains that with Warren's "last respectful pronouncement" ("Dead"),
Frost and his characters mark "the outermost bound of effective rhetoric and
speech," that "appropriate time and place to quit all rhetoric, leave off talk, recognize what talk can never fully say."[22] Although I am much indebted to Jost's reading of Frost, I think his position here must be amended a bit, especially if the full

potential of Frost's poem for adding to an understanding of the relationship between acknowledgment, home, and rhetoric is to be actualized.

In one sense, death puts an end to rhetoric, for as they say: "dead men tell no tales." In another sense, however, death calls for rhetoric that can speak on behalf of those who have passed away and that can thereby attend to what was discussed earlier as a human being's metaphysical need for completeness. We are *animalia metaphysica*, creatures who have a nostalgia, a "homesickness," for something final and absolute. Recall, too, how such sickness haunts us when we imagine our own deaths and funerals and people not showing up to pay their respects. To repeat a point made in the introduction: Even when we have passed to the most out-of-the-way place there is, we still crave the goodness of positive acknowledgment— the way it brings us to mind and keeps us alive. We want to be remembered for our accomplishments; we want to live on in the bodies, the hearts and minds, of others. The epideictic rhetoric of the funeral oration or eulogy grew out of this metaphysical need. Remember the above example of Pericles and the "comfort" he offered to those who lost loved ones and friends in the Peloponnesian War.

Although Mary and Warren's conversation about Silas occurs before either of them knows that he has died, we might still read Frost's poem as a eulogy in the making. For as the conversation unfolds, a showing-forth of Silas's character is displayed in both the good and the bad that is said about him. Frost's arrangement of this conversation is rhetorically designed in such a way that readers are lead to believe that, despite his flaws, Silas is still someone who is "so concerned for other folk" and who thereby warrants positive acknowledgment from them. Was Silas told this by Mary as she answered his call of conscience? He certainly did not hear it from Warren, whose response to his wife's call of conscience came too late. Was Silas suffering physically as well as ontologically from a serious bout of homesickness?

Frost's poem is about a dying man who is in need of acknowledgment, a home, and kind words (appropriate rhetoric). It is also about people being called into question by each others' presence and current ways of being. This call is rooted in the temporal and challenging structure of existence The challenge is there because we are not immortal, but rather finite beings driven by a metaphysical urge to find meaning and order in our lives, to reconstruct what is called into question by our being-towards-death. Frost's poem is a case study in this deconstructive/reconstructive process. Mary and Warren are called on to be what I have termed "home-makers": people challenged with the architectural and rhetorical task of creating a dwelling place that, at least for the moment, can provide comfort for themselves and others. The conversation in "The Death of a Hired Man" is offered as an edifying discourse on that place where the heart (conscience) is suppose to be. By ending the conversation in the way that he does, however, Frost closes on a deconstructive note. Uncertainty prevails: Did Silas feel at home when he died? And what about Mary and Warren? How did they feel as they sat hand in hand on the front porch steps when all was said and done?

From the traditional standpoint of architectural design, the front porch of a house serves an important social function—one meant to add a "homey" quality to the habitat. A front porch invites people to sit and stay awhile, to gossip and share news, to relax and feel comfortable; it is a visitor's introduction to what remains to be seen inside the home.[23] Throughout their conversation, Mary's behavior is more consistent than Warren's with respect to this "opening" function of the front porch. Mary is open to Silas's presence, to his needs for acknowledgment, comfort, compassionate rhetoric, and a home. Was just being inside Mary's home enough for Silas to overcome his homesickness? Besides the porch and the darkened passageway that leads to a room with a stove (the kitchen?)—the same room where Silas died sitting in a chair with a "sharp-edged" back—the reader knows nothing about how the rest of the house was further arranged to make it feel homey. No, Frost's poem is focused primarily on the rhetorical architecture of the conversation, which comes into being and is advanced by the ways that the call of conscience is sounded and answered. Influenced more by Mary than by Warren, this architecture creates a "poetic" dwelling place that allows for an openness to the environment, a "letting-be" of what is, and a respectful appreciation of *its* way of "showing-forth" its nature. In this place, Silas can be acknowledged as someone who is more than the hired man that Warren has habitually calculated him to be.

This way of describing the workings of Frost's poem admits, of course, a specific philosophical orientation, for it is phrased in the rhetoric of phenomenology whereby a certain interpretive understanding is given to such related phenomena as acknowledgment, being, dwelling, the call of conscience, ethics, and death. Phenomenology, especially from a Heideggerian perspective, understands this last phenomenon as being the most deconstructive happening there is. The finitude of *animalia metaphysica*, our "Being-unto-death," is the ground upon which our nostalgia (homesickness) for order and completeness arises. Death, therefore, also calls on the reconstructive capabilities of human beings. With Frost's poem in mind, we thus have good reason to wonder if Mary and Warren's conversation simply came to an end with Warren's last pronouncement ("Dead") of Silas's condition. Certainly, what Jost terms the "rhetorical drift" of the conversation is not headed back toward Warren's calculative and cold-hearted way of thinking about Silas and the meaning of home ("the place where, when you have to go there/They have to take you in").[24] No, Mary is the lead rhetorical architect here, and she is constructing a dwelling place meant to be more comforting than that. Listening to her speak, one is hard-pressed not to recall the adage: "Home is where the heart is." Home defines a place where conscience is cultivated. We do not emerge from our first home, the womb, already knowing for sure what is right and wrong. Conscience needs instruction in order to evolve toward all that is good. Mary instructs Warren. Who, however, instructed her? Where do her sympathetic and merciful ways of being come from? Why does she acknowledge Silas and home differently than her husband does?

In light of the phenomenological reading of Frost's poem that has been offered so far, I trust that it makes sense to think of this difference as having something to do with the tension that exists between the calculative rationality of scientific thought and the more religious outlook of metaphysical thought. As discussed earlier, religion gives the most well-known and hopeful directives for responding to the call of conscience that is embedded in our temporal existence and that speaks to us of such things as personal responsibility and death. Science "knows" this end-point of being in strictly physiological terms: the cessation of activity in the central nervous system, especially as indicated by a flat electroencephalogram for a predetermined length of time (i.e., "brain death"). Religion, on the other hand, sees death as the beginning of an after-life in "heaven," the most sacred of all homes. In its strict allegiance to "empirical" reality, science forbids itself such a metaphysical move, although, as seen in the words of Stuart Kauffman, it sometimes allows "God" a role in filling the gaps of its evolutionary (and hopeful) outlook:

> We cannot know the true consequences of our own best actions. All we players can do is be locally wise, not globally wise. All we can do, all anyone can do, is hitch up our pants, put on our galoshes, and get on with it the best we can. Only God has the wisdom to understand the final law, the throws of the quantum dice. Only God can foretell the future. We, myopic after 3.45 billion years of design, cannot.... We enter a new millennium. It is best to do so with gentle reverence for the ever-changing and unpredictable places in the sun that we craft ever anew for one another. We are all at home in the universe, poised to sanctify by our best, brief, only stay.[25]

Science has much to tell us about the universe. However, I have yet to find one of its practitioners taking the time to clarify what he or she means by "home." Instead, as seen in Kauffman, it is a term that, at best, sounds as if it has something to do with the greatest home-maker that can be imagined: "God." More often than not, the scientist introduces the term for purely rhetorical purposes; that is, as a way of making us feel comfortable with "the scale and fabric of the universe that is our home."[26] Science uses the word "home" as a soothing metaphor for something whose truth extends far beyond our conceptual reach, something that speaks of the deficiency of the metaphor in grasping this truth and all that goes with it. Still, however, there is that profession—architecture—that is best known for appropriating the findings and technological directives of science for the purpose of designing and building houses and other habitats. Hence, the birth of "modern" architecture and the belief, as Le Corbusier puts it, that "The house is a machine for living in."[27]

Coming from one of the most influential architects of the twentieth century, this definition is, in great part, the result of the scientific and technological accomplishments of the industrial revolution. According to Le Corbusier, modern architecture should concern itself with the construction of places that are "in tune with a universe whose laws we obey, recognize, and respect."[28] Le Corbusier also puts it this way:

> Every modern man has the mechanical sense. The feeling for mechanics exists and is justified by our daily activities. This feeling in regard to machinery is one of respect, gratitude and esteem.
>
> Machinery includes economy as an essential factor leading to minute selection. There is a moral sentiment in the feeling for mechanics.
>
> The man who is intelligent, cold and calm has grown wings to himself.
>
> Men—intelligent, cold and calm—are needed to build the house and to lay out the town.[29]

And when speaking about the house he has in mind, Le Corbusier writes: "There is no shame in living in a house without a pointed roof, with walls as smooth as sheet iron, with windows like those of factories. And one can be proud of having a house as serviceable as a typewriter."[30]

This is not to say, however, that Le Corbusier does not have "a heart" when it comes to designing and building houses; for he certainly makes clear in his writings that "Architecture is the art above all others which achieves a state of platonic grandeur, mathematical order, speculation, the perception of harmony which lies in emotional relationships. This is the *aim* of architecture."[31] Indeed, says Le Corbusier, we must take the notion of "architectural emotion" seriously: "The purpose of construction is TO MAKE THINGS HOLD TOGETHER; of architecture TO MOVE US."[32] Architecture achieves this end when "certain harmonies" happen within its work—harmonies that ring true with the laws of the universe that speak to us of the values of efficiency, economy, utility, and practicality. Warren ran his farm with these values in mind; hence, his predominant way of calculating Silas's worth in an "intelligent, cold and calm" manner. But did he feel guilty when he was too late to comfort Silas? Do you think he and Mary might have talked about their feelings afterword?

Although Mary's livelihood was also dependent on the above-noted values, she, of course, was more than "intelligent, cold and calm" when dealing with the situation at hand. Her rhetoric admitted as much: Silas needed more comfort than a machine could offer. He needed a home, not just a house, where he could live out the remainder of his days and die in peace. It hurt Mary's heart to think that Silas was without such a special place to be. Conscience called: "Where art thou?" It was time to say "Here I am!" to one who was "so concerned for other folk"; it was time to open one's heart and not be callous in the face of misery. The Bible speaks of callousness—"stubbornness of heart," "hardness of heart"—as being the root of sin.[33] The prophets reproach Israel for this sin and the lack of sensibility and acknowledgment that result from it. "He sees many things but does not observe them; His ears are open, but he does not hear. . . . You have never heard, you have never known. From of old your ear has not been opened."[34]

The rhetoric of the Judeo-Christian tradition is rooted in the moral requirement of acknowledgment, whereby one must learn to both see and observe what is. Thus the story of Jacob, who wakes up in the desert after having his great dream about a ladder reaching to heaven with angels going up and down it, and who then is awestruck by the realization that "Surely God was in this place and I did not know it" (at least until now). Jacob's epiphany comes about as he observes and acknowledges a place that has always been in view, but could not be truly seen without enhanced insight. In the Rabbinic tradition, the Hebrew word for what Jacob acknowledges—a "place," makom—is also a name for God. This place is the "house of God" that invites humankind to enter into a conversation about what it really means to make oneself at home.[35] Raising the stone that was his pillow from a horizontal to a vertical position, Jacob creates an altar for this place of places. According to Karsten Harries, "This simple alter, a celebratory representation of the supporting stone, as well as a representation of the dream ladder, becomes the archetype of the church and perhaps of sacred architecture: building as a response to the genius loci, to the divinity dwelling in that place."[36] Indeed, acknowledgment transforms space and time and thereby opens a place where people can commune and know together what it takes to live in peace and harmony with all that is.

I cannot imagine Mary and Warren having nothing more to say about someone who deserved more acknowledgment then he received while he was still alive. These are country-folk. Sure, they value the utility of calculative thought, but the environment in which they dwell is also known to be a source of another mindset—one that is conditioned by the country environment to appreciate what James Kunstler describes as "rural charm." Such charm is rooted in

> the opportunity to live in connection with the rich patterns of other organisms, namely plants and animals, and their interactions with natural patterns like the seasons or the cycles of day and night. These patterns include the processes of birth and decay, and they excite our senses in ways that their artificial replacements do not. A hike through meadows and woods in real farm country in May is exhilarating because of the extravaganza of patterns of emerging life operating in concert; the buds unfurling on the trees, the trilliums

blooming, the insects buzzing in the air, the birds singing as they build their nests, the little wild mammals scurrying about, the perfumes and tantalizing stinks of the cow pastures and the sloughs. We feel more alive in places like this. We are literally drawn into sensual participation with these patterns, charmed by the living activities of creatures and organisms with whom we share a kinship.[37]

Kunstler does not have religion in mind when making this point. Rather, abiding by a cosmological and evolutionary point of view, he maintains that such rural charm is itself rooted in the "self-correcting mechanisms of the teleologic process that we call nature, or *the ever-unfolding universe.*" Moreover, he claims that "we are hard-wired to appreciate [its] patterns. It is part of the neurological pattern of our own nature to be excited by them."[38] There is a beauty, a charm, and an appropriateness to the universe that can make us feel good if only we remain open to it. Mary observed something good in Silas. She spoke of this to Warren. Her rhetoric was moving. It certainly would be appropriate if Warren broke the silence so as to continue a conversation about a dearly departed soul. The ever-unfolding universe calls for such a response. Perhaps God does, too.

Did Silas die in peace? Did he feel at home as he passed away—alone—while sitting in an uncomfortable chair? How did Warren feel when he arrived too late? How did Mary feel as Warren held her hand? There is still a rhetorical situation going on when Frost ends his poem—a situation that continues to sound a call of conscience that calls into question the thoughts and actions of two characters who remain in close proximity to death and thus to that feature of life known for being a primary source of sadness, dread, and anxiety. Frost leaves it up to his readers to deal with the situation at hand.

Along with Mary and Warren, we must take on the role of being home-makers. The rhetorical competence needed to perform this task has long been institutionalized, for example, in humankind's burial rituals, with their various strategies for helping the living talk about and cope with their loss. Such rituals provide ready-made dwelling places where people are given the space and time to know together something about life and death. Such togetherness is known to bring comfort to those who have lost loved ones and whose lives are now lonelier. Loneliness is a state that cries out "Where art thou?" The sadness, dread, and anxiety that oftentimes accompany this state are not impossible to deal with, as long as there are others who are willing to comfort us with their helpful presence and speech: "Here I am!" Such a heartfelt response provides the most natural and genuine medication that humankind has for dealing with the horrible disease of being all alone.

Silas is dead and Mary and Warren sit hand in hand. I have been trying to imagine what these two characters are bound to say at this moment in their situation. Frost forces the issue in the way that he has rhetorically constructed his poem.

He sounds a call of conscience; he invites us to join his characters and him in the moral vocation of being a good home-maker. Levinas defines the interpersonal and communicative bond that is necessarily a feature of this vocation as being an essential ingredient for the creation and evolution of *any* institutionalized religion, for all religions require the "caress" that this bond provides in bringing people together so that they can do for others what they would have others do for them: acknowledge their presence.[39] There is something "religious" going on between Mary and Warren as they talk about Silas and as they silently sit together hand in hand. "The Death of a Hired Man" closes with home-makers bonded in a simple caress. Perhaps Frost figured that this ending was good enough as he thought about Mary's and Warren's ongoing conversation. For a caress can say and do a lot when it comes to the performance of acknowledgment.

Chapter Six

The Caress

I think it is fair to say that the "meaning" of "The Death of the Hired Man" is affected by the way the poem ends. Holding another's hand in a time of distress is reassuring and comforting. With such a simple caress, we can acknowledge someone non-verbally while still "saying" a lot: Here I am! You are not alone! Let me help! We can deal with things together!

Maybe if he had acted sooner, Warren could have held Silas's hand as this caring and needful soul passed away. Maybe Silas would have then felt more at home. But at least Warren was there for Mary, and she was there for him. They had each other to hold on to in the presence of death and while experiencing the heart-sickness of grief. Such sickness is not conducive to people feeling at home with their selves, others, and the immediate environment. A caress, however, can help to encourage this feeling of comfort as it transforms space and time by opening the lonely and suffering individual to another, whose touch is meant to bring about a more comfortable dwelling place for this individual. Acknowledgment and the caress go hand and hand; they work together to accomplish the ethical task of home-making. When one is sick and thus in need of comfort, the home is a good place to be.[1]

The caress is not only an act that Frost refers to; it is also something that he performs with his discourse. The performance admits rhetorical competence: a story is told in a certain way so that it may "touch" us and arouse our interest in and concern for matters deemed important by at least one other person whose calling demands the talent of having a way with words. Those who identify with and "love" Frost's poetry are caught up in the caress that it offers with its rhetorical way of being there for others, of opening us to its subject matter and opening its subject matter to us. Acknowledgment is made possible by such opening acts and the places they bring into being—places where people and things can dwell together poetically and rhetorically for the benefit of all concerned; places that speak an invitation: "Please, make yourself at home."

In this chapter I advance my discussion of acknowledgment by taking a closer look at the ontological, metaphysical, and rhetorical workings of the caress that promotes the development of this life-giving gift. The discussion unfolds primarily in light of the phenomenological investigations of Emmanuel Levinas who, in extending Heidegger's assessment of the meaning and truth of Being, provides what I take to be the most far-ranging exploration of how human existence is, itself, structured as a caress. I follow this discussion with a case study in chapter 7 that dramatizes how the rhetorical workings of the caress manifest themselves in the everyday world of practical concern. Frost, we have seen, offers some direction regarding the matter with his "The Death of the Hired Man." The artifact I employ to move us further along in this direction is the award-winning film *Ordinary People* (based on the novel of the same name by Judith Guest). Concerning myself once again with an artistic "re-presentation" of the topic in question will allow me to address directly an ambiguity in Levinas's assessment of the moral function of rhetoric, especially as this function is appropriated by artists who seek to instruct others about some truth in an entertaining way.

The Ontological, Metaphysical, and Rhetorical Nature of the Caress

Human beings are subjected to a caress before they know of its existence. In its most amoral form, this caress is the embrace of space, which we *feel* as gravity. Space, writes Brian Greene, "is the medium by which the gravitational force is communicated."[2] In its most original form as an act of loving-kindness, the caress takes place in our "first home" as the physiology of the womb undergoes the necessary transformations to accommodate the biological event and progress of conception. The process here, of course, entails the touching of two beings: the developing fetus and the body of an expectant mother who has the option to help safeguard her health and the health of her child by exercising good prenatal care. Such care is an exemplar of a self answering the call of a defenseless and thus vulnerable other: "Where art thou?" "Here I am!"[3]

A home is a place for a caress to happen. A caress is something that can help us feel at home. This feeling may arise with something as simple as a gentle pat, a kind word, or a warm smile from another. Such acts are a source of nourishment for a self who may feel alone and isolated in the company of others. But acknowledgment requires more than the mere presence of people who, for whatever reason, are too busy to initiate a caress and the comfort it has to offer.

We are brought to life by a caress that is rooted in millions of years of biological evolution and that most people continue to crave throughout their lives.
We are creatures whose well-being requires acknowledgment from those who
would have us return the favor. Indeed, we are social beings—born from others
and, right from the start, in need of family, friends, and even strangers who are
willing to open themselves to and acknowledge our presence, be it joyful or desperate. "The social relation itself," writes Levinas, "is not just another relation, one
among so many others that can be produced in being, but is its ultimate event."[4]
This event shows itself in our everyday ways of being with others at home, work,
and play. For Levinas, the "goodness" of the event is made possible by the way
human existence is fundamentally structured as a caress or what he also terms a
"being-for" others. This primordial and moral way of being, maintains Levinas, is
something that is always already at work in human existence and, hence, "chooses
us" before we decide to exercise our will and respond to others in any given situation. Human being has a dimension to it that exists on "the hither side of freedom
and non-freedom"—a life-giving dimension that is first and foremost not a human creation and that, for Levinas, must therefore "have the meaning of a 'goodness despite itself,' a goodness always older than . . . [any human] choice. Its value,
that is, its excellence or goodness, the goodness of goodness, is alone able to coun-
terbalance . . . [whatever] violence . . . [may come about with] the choice."[5]
    Levinas's phenomenological assessment of the caress that lies at the heart of
human existence and that shows itself in the caring nature of social relationships
unfolds throughout his entire corpus. The assessment, to say the least, is involved,
complex, and at times a bit "mysterious," especially when Levinas employs certain
metaphors and analogies or allows his discourse to assume a hyperbolic bent in
order to reveal "the thing itself," whose truth lies beyond the limited and habitual
conceptual capacity of everyday language-use. With such rhetorical maneuvers,
which are a mainstay of his Judaic heritage, Levinas stretches his reader's mind so
that he or she might realize, among other things, how human being is informed
by a moral impulse that shows something of itself in the "otherness" or "alterity"
of others, but whose actual source is, as he puts it, "otherwise than being." Levinas
is always on the move from ontology to metaphysics—a move that, as will be detailed below, promotes the view that "ethics" has priority over any other mode of
philosophical analysis. This view and Levinas's understanding of the caress go
hand in hand.
    Although I do not intend to burden the reader with an in-depth analysis of
all of the intricate, complex, and mysterious moves that constitute Levinas's understanding of the ethics of the caress, my discussion and critical assessment of
this understanding will require me to pay special attention to certain related topics
that cannot be overlooked when coming to terms with what Levinas has to say
about the matter. These topics include Being, the love of life, and the alterity or
otherness of existence. I introduce and explain these topics as I return now to

Levinas's interest in the "social relation" and discuss why he would have us recognize that the "everyday life" of this relation "is a preoccupation with salvation."[6]

Being's Caress

In everyday life, writes Levinas, "we are surrounded by beings and things with which we maintain relationships. Through sight, touch, sympathy and cooperative work, we are with others. All these relationships are transitive: I touch an object, I see the other. But I *am* not the other." Levinas is stating the obvious here in order to make a point that typically only comes to mind when "the continual play of our relations with the world is interrupted" by events that call into question the taken-for-granted ways that we relate to things and to others: "It is . . . the being in me, the fact that I exist, my *existing*, that constitutes the absolutely intransitive element [of everyday life], something without intentionality or relationship. One can exchange everything between beings except existing. In this sense, to be is to be isolated by existing."[7] Such a state of isolation, according to Levinas, defines the most primordial and painful form of solitude or loneliness that can be suffered by human beings. "Solitude is the very unity of the existent, the fact that there is something in existing starting from which existence occurs. The subject is alone because it is one [with its being] . . . it cannot detach itself from itself" and remain alive to be what it is.[8]

An example of someone who is likely to experience the pain and suffering of being would be a person whose well-being has been interrupted by a serious and incapacitating illness. This illness, among other things, undercuts the person's mastery of existence; breeds despair, helplessness, and a feeling of abandonment; and thereby directs the person to question life's meaning, purpose, and ultimate worth. In such a state of suffering, writes Levinas, "there is an absence of all refuge. It is the fact of being directly exposed to being. It is made up of the impossibility of fleeing or retreating. The whole acuity of suffering lies in this impossibility of retreat. It is the fact of being backed up against life and being."[9] Silas was so situated when Mary first found him.

When Levinas speaks of how everyday life is a preoccupation with salvation, he has in mind all those habits of thought and action that we employ to maintain the intersubjective realm of our social relationships—a realm of common sense and common practice that provides us with some degree of protection and distraction from the pain and suffering that accompanies being. A case in point is doing what is "right and decent" in order to help ease the pain and suffering of one who is ill. Such ways of salvation are also evident in Annie Dillard's conversation with the little boy that she recounts in "A Hill Far Away" that was discussed in chapter 1. Recall, for example, how the boy keeps asking questions of Dillard in order to prolong her company and thereby postpone his being alone once again. Common courtesy demands that she respond. With her own salvation in mind, however, Dillard eventually ends the conversation. Perhaps the boy, still seeking salvation, will now return to playing with the family dogs. After all, play is a common form of salvation that helps keep even the loneliest soul from the pain and suffering of "dying from boredom"—that way of being where life becomes a "drag," or what Levinas describes as a state of "weariness."

Levinas emphasizes that this particular existential state is especially revealing of an essential attribute of Being, for "There exists a weariness which is a weariness of everything and everyone, and above all a weariness of oneself." Levinas goes on to explain: The original source of weariness

> is not a particular form of our life—our surroundings, because they are dull and ordinary, our circle of friends, because they are vulgar and cruel; [rather,] the weariness concerns existence itself. Instead of forgetting itself in the essential levity of a smile, where existence is effected innocently, where it floats in its fullness as though weightless and where, gratuitous and graceful, its expansion is like a vanishing, in weariness existence is like the reminder of a commitment to exist, with all the seriousness and harshness of an unrevokable contract. One has to do something, one has to aspire after and undertake. . . . [T]he obligation of this contract remains incumbent on us like an inevitable "one must." It animates the need to act and to undertake, makes that necessity poignant. Weariness is the impossible refusal of this ultimate obligation.[10]

Whenever we are weary—due to boredom, labor, heartbreak, or some other form of hardship—we learn something fundamental about what it means *to be*. Being, writes Levinas, holds us in the caress of a "suffocating embrace" that is always challenging us to overcome its inherent pain and suffering by way of action—the very thing whose constant performance sooner or later incites fatigue and weariness and thereby leads us back to a suffocating embrace.[11] The logic here appears senseless, if not sadistic. In order to hold off the abject weariness of existence, we must do things that are prone to make us tired and weary over time. It is the "myth of Sisyphus," *for real*. Commenting on the "numbness of fatigue" that can be produced with this ongoing endeavor, Levinas notes:

> The numbness of fatigue is a telling characteristic. It is an impossibility of following through, a constant and increasing lag between being and what it remains attached to, like a hand little by little letting slip what it is trying to hold on to, letting go even while it tightens its grip. Fatigue is not just the cause of this letting go, it is the slackening itself. It is so inasmuch as it does not occur simply in a hand that is letting slip the weight it finds tiring to lift, but in one that is holding on to what it is letting slip, even when it has let it

drop but remains taut with the effort. For there is fatigue only in effort and labor.[12]

Being demands action; we must take up the burden of existence in order to temper its suffocating embrace. The fatigue here can be so overwhelming that giving up the endeavor may seem to be the only sensible option at times; hence, the related arguments for the "rationality" of suicide and voluntary euthanasia.[13] With the Columbine High School Massacre that was discussed in chapter 3, we also see how horrible acts of vengeance can come into play when dealing with fatigue. When our existence becomes a living hell due to the pain and suffering of Being, one can end up believing that there is nothing life-giving about the solitude of Being; it is simply a matter of the survival of the fittest in the struggle to exist. For Levinas, however, this belief could not be further from the truth.

Love of Life

Although he admits that the solitude of Being brings about fatigue, pain, and suffering, Levinas also maintains that this "solitude is necessary in order for there to be a freedom of beginning, the existent's mastery over existing—that is, in brief, in order for there to be an existent. Solitude is thus not only a despair and an abandonment, but also a virility, a pride and a sovereignty."[14] Human beings can take control of themselves and, even in the face of horrifying circumstances, display courage and responsibility. For Levinas, this "heroic" capacity indicates that along with the solitude, fatigue, pain, suffering, and weariness of being, there also comes "the love of life"—a love that is, in fact, presupposed by the darker side of being. Here is how Levinas puts it:

> At the origin there is a being gratified, a citizen of paradise. The "emptiness" felt implies that the need which becomes aware of it abides already in the midst of an enjoyment—be it that of the air one breathes. It anticipates the joy of satisfaction, which is *better* than ataraxy. Far from putting the sensible life in question, pain takes place within its horizon and refers to the joy of living. Already and henceforth life is loved. . . . Every opposition to life takes refuge in life and refers to its values. This is the *love of life*, a pre-established harmony with what is yet to come to us. . . . The love of life . . . loves the happiness of being. Life loved is the very enjoyment of life, contentment—already appreciated in the refusal I bear against it, where contentment is refused in the name of contentment itself [as seen in those people who are content only when their lives are so busy that there is little or no time to relax and enjoy life].[15]

The love of life that stirs in our being, or what Levinas terms "the primordial positivity of enjoyment," is what allows us to find some value in pain and suffering. Commenting further on how the workings of this enjoyment figure in the life of a person, Levinas writes:

> In its opposition to being [that is, suffering, pain], the I seeks refuge in being itself [that is, in the gift of life and the "goodness" that accompanies it]. Suicide is tragic, for death does not bring a resolution to all the problems to which birth gave rise, and is powerless to humiliate the values of the earth—whence Macbeth's final cry in confronting death, defeat because the universe is not destroyed at the same time as his life. Suffering at the same time despairs for being riveted to being—and loves the being to which it is riveted. It knows the impossibility of quitting life: what tragedy! what comedy[!] . . . The *taedium vitae* is steeped in the love of the life it rejects; despair does not break with the ideal of joy.[16]

The religious correlate of what Levinas is saying here is found in God's creative Word—"Let there be!"—and in God's subsequent command to "choose life" over death (Deuteronomy 30:19). Science's take on the matter eliminates metaphysics in order to stick to the "facts": In the beginning was a singularity, then a Big Bang and an expanding universe in which life arose and evolved into creatures (i.e., human beings) whose biochemistry registers the love of life in such physiological mechanisms as the autonomic nervous system (with its way, for example, of keeping us breathing) and the immune system (which, of course, stands guard against microscopic organisms that are hostile to the body's well-being).[17]

Although Levinas shows little interest in emphasizing what science can tell us about a human being's love of life, as a phenomenologist he, too, would have us stick to the facts in order to understand the matter better and, as will become ever more evident in what follows, to appreciate its "religious" implications. Remember, for Levinas, everyday life is a preoccupation with "salvation," of making use of our love of life in order to deal with the pain and suffering of Being's suffocating embrace. With Being's caress there also comes an impulse *to act* and thereby to move beyond whatever distressing circumstances are at hand. Levinas associates this ontological impulse with what he describes as "the Desire for the new": "That the New and Renewal are peaks of human life, that one can define the human by the desire for the new and by the capacity of renewal—is perhaps a basic truth, but a truth [nonetheless]."[18] Desire is our love of life in action: "At the very moment when the world seems to break up we still take it seriously and still perform reasonable acts and undertakings; the condemned man still drinks his glass of rum," trying at least to enjoy the moment and, especially if he knows himself to be innocent, perhaps hoping that before the sentence is carried out a reprieve will be given.[19]

A classic literary depiction of this situation is offered by Dostoevsky as he has one of the central characters in *The Idiot* share the story of a man whose confrontation with death is based on an actual experience of the author:

> This man had once been led out with the others to the scaffold and a sentence of death was read over him. . . . Twenty minutes later a reprieve was read to them, and they were condemned to another punishment instead. Yet the interval between those two sentences, twenty minutes or at least a quarter of an hour, he passed in the fullest conviction that he would die in a few minutes. . . . The priest went to each in turn with a cross. He had only five minutes more to live. He told me that those five minutes seemed to him an infinite time, a vast wealth. . . . But he said that nothing was so dreadful at the time as the continual thought, "What if I were not to die! What if I could go back to life—what eternity! And it would all be mine! I would turn every minute into an age; I would lose nothing, I would count every minute as it passed, I would not waste one!" He said that this idea turned to such fury at last that he longed to be shot quickly.[20]

The teaching here, as noted by William Barrett, emphasizes that "in the face of death, life has an absolute value. The meaning of death is precisely its revelation of this value."[21]

Levinas maintains this view of death throughout his writings, for he believes, as indicated above, that "Every opposition to life takes refuge in life and refers to its values. This is the *love of life*, a pre-established harmony with what is yet to come to us." With this last sentence, Levinas supplies an important directive for understanding what I take to be the most important topic of his philosophy—one that is identified as he continues his phenomenological inquiry into the related topics of the caress, the pain and joy of Being, life, desire and action, and the ways of salvation of everyday existence. The "pre-established harmony with what is yet to come to us" is fundamentally a matter of the temporality of human existence and the *otherness* or *alterity* that is consubstantial with it.

Otherness

Continuing his description of the relationship that holds between death and the love of life, Levinas emphasizes that "What is important about the approach of death is that at a certain moment we are no longer *able to be able*"; that is, no longer capable of acting in order to maintain some mastery over existence. Death "marks the end of the subject's virility and heroism"; it "is the impossibility of having a project." Levinas stresses that the approach of death "indicates that we are in relation with something that is absolutely other, something bearing alterity not as a provisional determination we can assimilate through enjoyment, but as something whose very existence is made of alterity."[22] Our love of life happens in the face of otherness. Levinas thereby maintains that "existence is pluralist. Here the plural is not a multiplicity of existents; it appears in existing itself. A plurality insinuates itself into the very existing of the existent." A common way of expressing this existential reality is to say that "death is a part of life." Levinas, on the other hand, makes the point in a way that is more precise in its treatment of alterity: "In death the existing of the existent is alienated. To be sure, the other [l'Autre] that is announced [in the approach of death] does not possess this existing as the subject possesses it; its hold over my existing is mysterious. It is not unknown but unknowable, refractory to all light."[23]

In acknowledging the mystery of the otherness of death, we remain open to the possibility that the "whole truth" of death is not merely reducible to the moment when the body's physiological functions abruptly come to an end. Rather, from a phenomenological point of view, death is a happening of otherness that approaches from out of "what is yet to come to us"; it shows itself in the "intentionality" of human temporality and thus in the unfolding of the future. Things such as clocks and calendars are the result of our ability to make something out of this intentionality. But the intentionality that is presupposed by such devices is not, itself, a human creation. Besides the otherness of death that insinuates itself into our existence, there is also the otherness of temporality that is always already happening before we reconfigure its workings and that, in a manner of speaking, sets the stage on which the otherness of death makes its appearance.

Temporality and Transcendence: The anxiety that we experience upon coming face to face with the otherness of death defines a state of being that is grounded in another mode of otherness: one whose nature is "transcendence," the continual process of going beyond what is the case now. This process gives direction to the desire for the new and the love of life that this desire, with its capacity for renewal, acts out with the hope of making our circumstances better than they happen to be at the present time. Death would be meaningless if not for the love of life that stirs in our being (the transcending temporality of human existence), opens us to the ongoing future, and thereby grants us the possibility of having hope even as the pain of Being becomes ever more insufferable and perhaps even makes us believe that we would be better off dead. With hope, there not only comes the possibility of better days ahead but also of a time and place that lies beyond death and that is cared for by a loving God. Indeed, transcendence and the hope that it makes possible can encourage us to believe in a realm ("heaven") that is not of this world and that holds the promise of pardon and, hence, of a new beginning. Using this utopian belief as an orientation to the future, to what is yet to come to us, we might agree with Levinas that "the true object of hope is the Messiah, or salvation."[24]

Recall that Levinas uses this last term to identify the fundamental preoccupation of everyday life whereby we are caught up in the struggle of forming and maintaining relationships with things and with others in order to deal with and overcome the pain and suffering of Being. We exist in the suffocating embrace of Being's caress. But with this caress there also comes the capacity of the love of life—a capacity that informs both our physiology and our everyday concerns and actions, especially as they function to promote our salvation from the pain and suffering of Being. With all of this in mind, we might wonder whether Levinas's use of the term "salvation" in this existential context is a rhetorical maneuver designed to portray his philosophy as an approach to the mysterious and awe-inspiring presence of God's absolute alterity. I believe it is, although Levinas would have his readers understand that he has "no ambition to be a preacher"; rather, his primary philosophical interest is to "understand the word 'God' as a significant word."[25]

The Word "God": God comes to mind as human beings struggle with their finitude while immersed in a process that is more than a human creation and that, with this dimension of otherness at work, speaks of something that is not simply finite but rather has something "in-finite" about it. Owing to their cognitive capacity, human beings can ponder how their finitude is marked by an infinite process of transcendence, or what Levinas terms "the futuration of the future" and they can thereby grant meaning to something whose dynamic way of being in process poses a challenge to human beings to assume the responsibility for their actions. According to Levinas, this "imperative signification of the future" certainly lends itself to being understood as "an order that would be the word of God or, still more exactly, the very coming of God to the idea and its insertion into a vocabulary—whence comes the 'recognizing' and naming of God in every possible Revelation." This is not to say, however, that Levinas would have us understand the "futuration of the future" as being a *proof* of God's existence; rather, as he emphasizes, this process, and the mystery it discloses as it moves on continuously, can at best be conceptualized as "'the fall of God into meaning.' This is the singular intrigue of the duration of time . . . up to Saint Augustine himself—time as the to-God [*a-Dieu*] of theology!"[26]

Levinas is interested in a Mystery that shows something of itself in the transcending temporality of human existence and thus in a process that is other than, and more than, a human construction. Commenting on the otherness that marks existence and what it means for human being, Rabbi Abraham Heschel notes:

> If man is not more than human, then he is less than human. Man is but a short, critical stage between the animal and the spiritual. His state is one of constant wavering, of soaring or descending. Undevi-

ating humanity is nonexistent. The emancipated man is yet to emerge.

Man is more than what he is to himself. In his reason he may be limited, in his will he may be wicked, yet he stands in a relation to God which he may betray but not sever and which constitutes the essential meaning of his life. He is the knot in which heaven and earth are interlaced.[27]

Although this way of putting the matter may be far too religious for some readers to accept, it still speaks of something that, as Levinas observes, lies at the heart of human existence and that makes it possible for any individual self to have a life. Human beings must necessarily dwell in the presence of otherness. "Being is produced as multiple and as split into same [the self] and other; this is its ultimate structure."[28] Existence is pluralist. There is no self without the otherness of death and the transcending temporality of our being that simultaneously holds us in its caress and points beyond itself to infinity, or what Levinas also describes as that which is "otherwise than being."[29] Levinas uses this description as a guiding metaphor for thinking about the absolute alterity of God, the wholly Other. But again, this description and the thinking it is meant to encourage are not intended as a scheme for proving God's existence. Rather, the otherness that can be termed "God" is always more than words can convey. Rabbi David Cooper's discussion of this point is worth noting:

> What is God? In a way, there is no God. Our perception of God usually leads to a misunderstanding that seriously undermines our spiritual development.
>
> God is not what we think It is. God is not a thing, a being, a noun. It does not exist, as existence is defined, for It takes up no space and is not bound by time. Jewish mystics [Kabbalists] often refer to It as *Ein Sof*, which means Endlessness.
>
> *Ein Sof* should never be conceptualized in any way. It should not be called Creator, Almighty, Father, Mother, Infinite, the One, Brahma, Buddhamind, Allah, *Adonoy, Elohim, El*, or *Shaddai*; and It should never, never be called He. It is none of these names, and It has no gender.[30]

Cooper's discussion of *Ein Sof*, you may recall, was first introduced in chapter 3 when considering Heidegger's notion of "the law of Being" and its application to what came "before" the Big Bang: the mystery of Nothingness. *Ein Sof* is not restricted by the infinity that is thought to describe this mystery; rather It created the endlessness of the mystery. *Ein Sof* is trans-infinite, it is the source and ongoing process of creation. Cooper emphasizes that the struggle "to know" what the truth of this process is, "is the key to all Kabbalah and the lifeblood of all Jewish practice." Moreover, he notes that the "secret teaching in developing this [knowing] relationship with the Unknowable is hidden in the mystical foundation of the nature of relationship itself."[31]

In any relationship there necessarily exists the phenomenon of otherness: of something that is other than something else being joined in some way to this something else. Death and transcending temporality make up the otherness of existence that joins one's "self" together with God. Søren Kierkegaard provides what many consider to be the most influential "existentialist" analysis of the entire matter with his investigations of and speculations about the experience of "selfhood."[32] Levinas, on the other hand, would have us pay closer attention not to ourselves but rather to the presence of others in our lives in order to come to terms with the nature of relationship itself in a most genuine way. For with this presence we witness a "face" of otherness (alterity) whose "expression" converts the caress of Being into a "saying" that, more so than death and temporality, speaks to us of the source and "sacredness" of the "good."

The Presence of the Other. Levinas's specific term for the presence of the other (and the self, who is also an other to other selves) is the "face," or what he defines as "the expressive in the Other (and the whole human body is in this sense more or less face)."[33] Elsewhere he writes: "A face has a meaning not by virtue of the relationships in which it is found, but out of itself; that is what expression is. A face is the presentation of an entity as an entity, its personal presentation, . . . the existence of a substance, a thing in itself"; "A face is the very identity of a being. There he manifests himself out of himself, and not on the basis of concepts."[34]

This way of speaking about the face reflects a phenomenological orientation toward the matter. Levinas is thus attending to something that comes *before* what someone like the sociologist Erving Goffman means by face. Without ever acknowledging that he is doing so, Goffman identifies and studies a sense of face that rhetorical theorists have long known as a person's "good character" or *ethos*: "Face is an image of self delineated in terms of approved social attributes—albeit an image that others may share, as when a person makes a good showing for his profession or religion by making a good showing for himself." Goffman thus emphasizes a notion of face that goes no further than the "face-work" or learned behavior of "self-regulating participants in social encounters."[35]

For Levinas, however, the face of the other in its simple "nakedness," its mere presence before it subscribes to the socially circumscribed rituals of self-presentation, is its own good showing—a showing that is good first and foremost because it discloses something of the miracle and mystery of life. Understood from the standpoint of phenomenology, such a disclosure constitutes a primordial discourse or "saying" (*logos*) that offers itself for understanding. The saying of the face is a showing-forth of a most fundamental truth, or what Levinas describes as an "epiphany" that reveals the "vulnerability" of the human body. Levinas listens carefully to this saying that comes with the presence of the other's being, with his or her face. "In the approach of a face the flesh becomes word, the caress a saying." "Face and discourse are tied," writes Levinas. "The face speaks . . . it is in this [primordial signification] that it renders possible and begins all discourse" that we eventually express in oral and written form.[36] The saying power of language thus originates with our coming face-to-face with the otherness of others, and before these others ever open their mouths or write a single word.

Recall that in my discussion of Heidegger in chapter 3, I connected this saying power of language to his assessment of how the disclosing or "showing-forth" of a human being's temporal existence admits a "call of conscience" that summons a person to assume the ethical responsibility of affirming his or her freedom though resolute choice, as well as to "know together" with others. Heidegger associated this epideictic event with the revelatory function of poetry. I, on the other hand, suggested that the event must also be understood as the happening of a primordial rhetorical interruption that, primarily by way of anxiety and joy, calls us to think and act for the benefit of ourselves and others, to dwell with and for others, and thus to become rhetorically competent home-makers. The moral vocation of human being is heard in the discourse of the purest instance of epideictic rhetoric that there is: the call of conscience of our temporal existence.

With Levinas's phenomenology of the epiphany of the face, he, too, allows this "primordial event of communication" to be associated not only with the call of conscience but also with rhetoric—albeit a rhetoric that, as briefly noted above, is void of eloquence. I will expand on this matter shortly. For now, however, it is enough to alert the reader to this rhetorical move on Levinas's part. More needs to be said about the "good showing" of the face and its ethics before the matter of rhetoric can be further addressed.

Moral Consciousness: The "otherness" of the face marks a fundamental difference characterizing everyday existence—a difference that distinguishes one's self from others and that thereby serves as a catalyst for inspiring moral consciousness. Alterity, the otherness of others, is what, in a moment of "interruption," calls the self's attention away from its preoccupation with its personal business and toward the source of the interruption. The scientist, engineer, and philosopher R. Buckminster Fuller has a wonderful way of speaking of the significance of this event:

> Life's original event/And the game of life's /Order of play/Are involuntarily initiated/And inherently subject to modification/By the a priori mystery/Within which consciousness first formulates/And from which enveloping and permeating mystery/Consciousness never completely separates/But which it often ignores/Then forgets altogether/Or deliberately disdains/And consciousness begins/As an awareness of otherness/Which otherness awareness requires

time/And all statements by consciousness/Are in the comparative terms/Of prior observations of consciousness/ ("It's warmer, it's quicker, it's bigger/Than the other or others")/Minimal consciousness evokes time/As a nonsimultaneous sequence of experiences/Consciousness dawns/With the second experience/This is why consciousness/Identified the basic increment of time/As being a second/Not until the second experience/Did time and consciousness/Combine as human life/*Time, relativity, and consciousness*/Are always and only coexistent functions/Of an a priori Universe/Which, beginning with the twoness of secondness/Is inherently plural.[37]

Levinas would not disagree. Consciousness begins with an awareness of otherness and thus with "the inevitable orientation of being 'starting from oneself' toward 'the Other.'"[38] For Levinas, the importance of this movement toward the other cannot be overemphasized, for this movement is the basis of the birth of one's subjectivity and moral character: "I am defined as a subjectivity, as a particular person, as an 'I,' precisely because I am exposed to the other. It is my inescapable and incontrovertible answerability to the other that makes me an individual 'I.' . . . I can never escape the fact that the other has demanded a response from me before I affirm my freedom not to respond to his demand."[39] With this demand comes the ethical responsibility of thinking and acting with others in mind. The other is a source of interruption, a calling into question of consciousness that raises the issue of accountability—"Are you being just in all that you say and do?"—and thereby summons the moral capacity of human being to action. "This is certainly not a philosopher's invention," writes Levinas, "but the first given of moral consciousness, which could be defined as the consciousness of the privilege the other has relative to me. Justice well ordered begins with the other."[40]

Compassionate and conscientious souls presumably raise the question of justice as often as they can. The question interrupts, slows down, and perhaps brings the taken-for-granted routines and rituals that make up one's rule-governed everyday social encounters to a halt. And although the question directs one's concern toward the self and its possible improvement, it is raised initially because of what Levinas describes as "one's fear for the Other," a fear for how one's personal freedom can place a serious burden on others. Elaborating on this point, Levinas writes: "My being-in-the-world or my 'place in the sun' [Pascal] . . . have these not also been the usurpation of spaces belonging to the other man whom I have already oppressed or starved, or driven out into a third world; are they not acts of repulsing, excluding, exiling, stripping, killing?" Indeed, says Levinas, as social creatures whose communal well-being is dependent on others, we are obligated to feel a "fear for all the violence and murder [our] existing might generate, in spite of its conscious and intentional innocence."[41] We can pay this debt only by listening and responding to the other's call for acknowledgment, respect, companionship, help, and perhaps love. As finite beings, however, we can never pay the debt in full; for as soon as we choose to respond to the call of the other, a sacrifice must be made that increases the overall debt. What is sacrificed are the obligations to which we *also* have to respond, in the same way, in the same instance, to all the others whose calls beg for acknowledgment. Still, something of the debt must be paid. Imagine what life would be like if nobody acknowledged your existence. Or, if you will, imagine being Silas without Mary: a poor, unfit, and dying creature about whom nobody seems to care.

In appropriating Levinas's philosophy as I am doing here, it is crucial to be clear about the nature of this debt of acknowledgment. With the presence and saying of the face there comes a call—"Where art thou?"—in need of a response: "Here I am!" The debt that takes form here is not grounded in what Levinas terms the "inter-personal commerce" of everyday social interaction. Rather, the debt originates in the more ontological realm of what Levinas describes as the "inter-human," which "lies in a non-indifference of one to another, in a responsibility of one for another. The inter-human is prior to the reciprocity of this responsibility, which inscribes itself in impersonal laws, and becomes superimposed on the pure altruism of this responsibility inscribed in the ethical position of the self as self." Moreover, writes Levinas, the "inter-human lies also in the recourse that people have to one another for help, before the marvelous alterity of the Other has been banalized or dimmed in a simple exchange of courtesies which become established in an 'inter-personal commerce' of customs." The inter-human, in other words, defines a primordial dimension of existence where, as Levinas describes it, "intersubjective space is initially asymmetrical": the self's most original way of "being-with" others is a "being-for" others, out of which any particular act of moral acknowledgment is borne.[42] The social workings of community are made possible by an altruistic and thus moral impulse that lies at the heart of human being. Human existence is structured in a way that has the self move toward the other before the self can even raise the related issues of reciprocity and moral responsibility. Morality originates and evolves in a movement of being-for others (which is exactly what others are doing when they are responsible enough to acknowledge and assist *other* selves).[43] Levinas's phenomenological inquiry of existence thereby concludes that ethics, not ontology, is "first philosophy" and that rhetoric, as will be discussed below, has a significant role to play in this philosophy. In developing this last point, I will at the same time suggest how Levinas's philosophy is itself a case study in the rhetorical workings of the caress.

Ethics and Rhetoric

"When I speak of first philosophy," writes Levinas, "I am referring to a philosophy of dialogue that cannot not be an ethics. Even the philosophy that questions the meaning of being [ontology] does so on the basis of the encounter with the other."[44] As detailed above, Levinas's understanding of this encounter entails a consideration of otherness or alterity and its manifestation in death, temporality and transcendence, our thinking of the mystery of infinity (or what can be *named* "God"), and the presence of other people. Human being is permeated with and surrounded by otherness, which holds us in its caress, exists as *the* source of existential interruptions of everyday life, and speaks to us by way of the pain and suffering of Being, the love of life, a temporality that allows for hope and pardon, and the presence of other selves whose pain and suffering call for acknowledgment and help and who, in turn, may return the favor whenever the need arises. "Where art thou?" "Here I am!" The self's most fundamental relationship with the other takes form in response to a call for acknowledgment, in a dialogue of and about ethical responsibility, a dialogue that begins in what Levinas terms "the proximity of the other."

> The proximity of the other is the face's meaning, and it means from the very start in a way that goes beyond those plastic forms which forever try to cover the face like a mask of their presence to perception. But always the face shows through these forms. Prior to any particular expression and beneath all particular expressions, which cover over and protect with an immediately adopted face or countenance, there is the nakedness and destitution of the expression as such, that is to say extreme exposure, defenselessness, vulnerability itself. . . . The Other becomes my neighbor [in the most fraternal and moral sense of the term] precisely through the way the face summons me, calls for me, begs for me [with its interrupting presence], and in so doing recalls my responsibility, and calls me into question.[45]

Levinas speaks to us of an existential bond—the "fraternity with the neighbor"—whose caress is prior to every chosen bond and is presupposed by such heartfelt emotions as "pity, compassion, [and] pardon." In this primordial state of proximity, "the contact in which I approach the neighbor is not a manifestation or a knowledge, but the ethical event of communication which is presupposed by every transmission of messages, which establishes the universality in which words and propositions will be stated."[46] The face speaks, and the essence of its discourse is ethical, for the saying going on here calls the self out of selfishness and toward the responsibility and goodness of being-for others. We are creatures, claims Levinas, that exist in a constant caress with others, a caress that holds us "hostage" to their needs and that thereby defines a state of having been "chosen without assuming the choice," where responsibility for the other is always placed before the self's freedom, and thus where the issue of justice is forever being raised in and through an ongoing dialogue between the self and others.

Levinas writes of a dialogue, an ethical event of communication, that speaks before he does, that comes to him from outside his self, and whose truth, permeated as it is by alterity, always exceeds whatever can be said about it. Levinas is forever trying to say something truthful about this event. The face speaks; its saying is a nonverbal expression of otherness, a silent but all-important call for acknowledgment: "Where art thou?" Levinas writes: "One could call this situation religion, the situation where outside of all dogmas, all speculation about the divine or— God forbid—about the sacred and its violences, one speaks to the other."[47] Indeed, the *institutions* of religion and their various descriptive and prescriptive discourses presuppose the eventful situation in question here: the fundamental relationship of self and other that is "my pre-originary *susceptiveness* [to the other] which chooses me before I welcome it" and that is thus the basis for the socio-political transformations of the relationships that occur in everyday life.[48] Levinas's phenomenology of existence is meant to expose the workings of this relationship which, as noted above, he describes as dialogical.

This description may generate confusion, given Levinas's earlier stated claim that "intersubjective space is initially asymmetrical." A genuine dialogue encourages the "two-wayness" of reciprocity, not the "one-wayness" of asymmetry. And as Levinas is fond of repeating, human existence is structured so that "I am responsible for the Other without waiting for his reciprocity, were I to die for it. Reciprocity is *his* affair."[49] We *are* a being-for others; human existence is marked by an openness to and a movement toward otherness. This openness defines its "goodness," its deconstructive way of being a constant interruption that raises a moral issue: Are you being just in all that you say and do? The face speaks: "Where art thou?" Goodness makes it possible to say "Here I am!" and thus to speak and act on behalf of others. We can call all of this a dialogue once the response has been made. And that, I believe, is Levinas's point. The response is already in the making given that the self (ontologically and ethically speaking) is by nature open to the otherness of other selves. Levinas writes about a certain dialogical relationship that lies at the heart of existence and that can be read as an ethical directive: Open yourself to others and welcome their differences—what it is about them that calls your freedom into question. Only by doing this can you provide the necessary space, the requisite dwelling place, that is needed to create and maintain the moral ecology of human fraternity, resting on a relationship whose asymmetry is what it is only as it encourages reciprocity between the self and others.

So Levinas speaks to us of "a philosophy of dialogue that cannot not be an ethics." He further justifies his description in a more "practical" way by considering how the self, in its everyday existence, must contend not only with a specific other but also with "the third party"—all those others who may be affected by what we say and do. Here, writes Levinas, the self's ethical obligation to others doubles back on itself. "The relationship with the third party is an incessant correction of the asymmetry of proximity in which the face it looked at"; for in the company of others, the face of the self also demands attention and respect. Or, as Levinas puts it, "It is only thanks to God that, as a subject incomparable with the other, I am approached as an other by the others, that is, 'for myself.' 'Thanks to God' I am another for the others."[50] The saying of the face, which speaks of otherness, can be heard coming from the self who is other than other selves and who may at any moment take issue with their meanings, values, and actions. Levinas tells us that, owing to its otherness, "the other must be closer to God than I."[51] In its being an other to others, however, the self also assumes this "holy" position, which exists before the dogma of any institutionalized religion is created.

Owing to this positioning of the self and others, salvation can be found in everyday life. We seek to be saved from the pain and suffering of Being, we desire better tomorrows, we hope for a time and place of pardon. Steeped though it is in the empirical and ontological orientation of phenomenology, Levinas's philosophy points us in the direction of metaphysics; it follows the lead of our temporal existence that opens us to the otherness of others, the future, infinity, and even perhaps, to the absolute alterity of an Other whose question to Moses and others—"Where art thou?"—also came with a promise for acknowledgment: "Here I am!"

Although I feel confident in saying that Levinas would have his readers go this far in thinking about the direction of their lives, it must be stressed that he in no way mandates this theological option for defining "the good life." Remember, for Levinas, goodness is rooted in empirical circumstance: the self's openness to otherness. Goodness is the way that human existence is fundamentally structured as a being-for others, as a caress, as a "saying" that calls the self out of itself and that thereby poses the challenge of personal responsibility. Goodness is the ongoing call for acknowledgment that relates the self to others and relates others to the self. "Goodness in the subject is anarchy itself," deconstruction, a constant "interruption" that raises the moral issue of justice.[52] We need not appeal further to God for "proof" of such goodness. We need only remain open to something that is before us everyday and that should be as plain as the nose on our face: the other, whose presence is always saying "Where art thou?" Remember, everyday life is a preoccupation with salvation. In our being open to the other's pain and suffering, we are creatures capable of being instructed about the moral importance of serving the needs of others, of being good neighbors, and of building communities in rhetorically competent and morally just ways. But can we speak of such things in a sensible manner without making at least an implicit reference to some divine intelligence standing behind it all? Is goodness just a lucky, accidental happening that took form sometime and somewhere in the evolution of the universe?

As a religious Jew, Levinas is compelled to take issue with such a suggestion. After all, Judaism defines a way of being that, owing to and in the name of the wholly Other (*Ein Sof*), is awed by the otherness of others and by all that this otherness requires in order to maintain its well-being.[53] Jews have been conditioned to be especially sensitive to this feeling of otherness because for over three thousand years they have been forced to know themselves not only as an "other," but also as an other whom others would marginalize, silence, and even exterminate because of their differences. To be a Jew is to know the tragedy and horror of "anti-Semitism, which is in its essence hatred for a man who is other than oneself—that is to say, hatred for the other man."[54] At the heart of Judaism lies both a keen awareness of what otherness is all about and a rhetoric that tells its story.

Levinas's Rhetoric

This rhetoric is employed throughout Levinas's philosophical writings as he develops a phenomenological description of how human existence offers moral direction to a self that *is*, first and foremost, a being-for others. With this description we are therefore given something of a "religious" take on the matter. For, as Levinas reminds us, we are indeed our "brothers' keepers" and thus we ought to remain open to the presence (the face) of others who, like the "widow, orphan, and stranger" referred to in the Old Testament, are in need of heartfelt acknowledgment. "I will give them a heart to know Me, that I am the Lord" (Jeremiah 24:7). This "gift," as discussed in chapter 1, is the capacity of conscience (Fr. *conscience moral*), which enables us to be awed by the happenings and mysteries of life. In moments of awe, we are made to wonder. And wonder, we should recall, is the state of our being asked, that state where we are addressed and acknowledged and thereby given the opportunity to respond and be accountable. The self, our ego, takes form in light of this opportunity, which comes to us from something that is wholly Other and whose presence, which can never be totally comprehended by a finite creature, still leaves what Levinas terms a "trace" of itself in what is other than one's self. From a Judaic and Levinasian perspective, "there is something more important than my life, and that is the life of the other." For here, in the otherness of other people, in the presence and difference of their pained and joyful faces, lies empirical evidence of what it is that challenges the selfish ways of egoism, that calls on us to recognize the importance of going beyond the limitations of our "personal" interpretations of the world, and that thereby indicates the genuine value of "transcendence"; hence, Levinas's remark: "It is as if God spoke through the face."[55]

Moreover, Levinas would have us understand that the essential truth being spoken here echoes the Sixth Commandment found in the Old Testament: "You shall not commit murder." The face speaks. "This first saying," writes Levinas, "is to be sure but a word. But the word is God."[56] It is a word that commands acknowledgment, the responsible response of commitment whereby we can say "Here I am!" and really mean it. God speaks to us through the identity of the other as this identity is presented in the uniqueness, the sheer difference or alterity, of the other's face. "Thou shalt not kill" this presence, for to do so is to eliminate what the self needs to be itself: the other, that being who is capable of offering the life-giving gift of acknowledgment. Killing others starts a process that is actually suicidal in nature. The self could not exist without the other. And this being so, Levinas hears the commandment of the face as being more than a prohibition only against the sin of intentionally stopping another's heart from beating. "Thou shalt not kill" is a saying whose true meaning speaks against *any* "murderous" deed that threatens the well-being of others. Death is something that is not only associated with physiological functioning but also happens in a "social" way. Thus the previously mentioned phenomenon of social death: a fate people suffer whenever they are marginalized, denied freedom of speech and educational opportunities, forced to live in abject poverty, refused decent medical care, or otherwise left to live a hellish existence that defaces the human spirit. According to Levinas, the original saying of the face speaks against this "evil of suffering" and thereby poses "the inevitable and preemptory ethical problem of the medication which is my duty. ... Wherever a moan, a cry, a groan or a sigh happen there is the original call for aid, for curative help from the other ego whose alterity ... promises salvation."[57]

Owing to the way Levinas intertwines his phenomenological discourse with the rhetoric of his Judaic heritage, it is oftentimes quite difficult to distinguish his philosophical endeavors from what he terms his interest in "understanding the word 'God' as a significant word."[58] Levinas, however, is not bothered by this confusion. As a phenomenologist interested in how human existence is structured as a caress and how this interest necessitates a consideration of such related matters as Being, love, otherness, and ethics, Levinas sees himself as being steeped in and influenced by various long-standing concerns of Western philosophy. But, asks Levinas, "Are not we Westerners, from California to the Urals, nourished by the Bible as much as by the Presocratics?"[59]

Levinas points to the ancient myth and well-rounded narrative of Ulysses returning home to Ithaca as an indication of how Western philosophy operates: it seeks adventure and knowledge of a wide range of topics while holding fast to the expectation that a welcomed homecoming (a privileging of its own understanding and importance) lies in its future. For Levinas, however, the Old Testament story of "Abraham leaving his homeland forever for a still unknown land and even forbidding his son to be brought back to his point of departure" provides an equally compelling and revealing depiction of how the temporal structure of human existence opens the self to the otherness of "what is yet to come."[60] Abraham hears and heeds a call: "Where art thou?" "Here I am!" So begins a life of nomadic wandering, of being for an Other whose mystery is beyond comprehension as it continues to call human understanding into question. Abraham remains steadfast in acting upon his ethical responsibility to answer the call without ever knowing for sure what to expect and where his new home might be. As it holds us in its caress, life offers no guarantee of being a well-rounded narrative, for its way of being, of calling, is more interruptive and deconstructive than that. Otherness is a constant presence in human existence that allows for hope, the possibility of pardon, and the anxiety and joy of expectation, but that makes no promises other than that speaking of the indispensable need for acknowledgment, of being-for others. Hence, the trajectory of Levinas's philosophy, whose rhetoric is offered as a way of demonstrating and thereby reminding us how a moral impulse that lies at the heart of human existence continually raises a question that warrants untiring attention: Are you being just in all that you say and do?

Granting that everyday life *is* a preoccupation with salvation, it is not unwise to hope, and perhaps even to pray, that people ask and honestly answer this question on a daily basis. The well-being of human community is made possible by the doing of this ethical deed, by a simple "reality check" in which people take the time to respect their neighbor by determining to what extent their thoughts and actions are "repulsing, excluding, exiling, stripping, killing" or otherwise contributing to social and/or biological death. Remember, the face speaks a commandment: "Thou shalt not kill." We are creatures who know all too well what life would be like if nobody cared enough to acknowledge our existence, to say "Here I am!" when our love of life, burdened by the pain and suffering of Being, makes us cry out "Where art thou?" Thus begins and continues the ongoing ethical and dialogical relationship between the self and others. This is a relationship that Levinas considers to be "miraculous" and "holy," for it is here that the imperfect human being learns to set the grounds for "peace" by respecting the "plurality" of life that shows itself with every face in the crowd.

Is this showing (saying), in fact, a fundamental way that "God" communicates with us? Levinas addresses this question with the help of a rhetoric that begs the question more than it answers it. This ancient and religious rhetoric is given over to the task of describing what its advocates understand to be a Mystery, something that is "indescribable": absolute alterity, an otherness that is always beyond our grasp and whose presence is always there to interrupt and call into question whatever we think we "know" for sure. This is the way the face speaks; with its otherness it evokes consciousness. As noted earlier, this saying of the face is the original "showing-forth" of humanity's nakedness, a vulnerability that is covered up by the make-up and fashion we put on to give a "good showing" in our daily social activities. Commenting further on this rule-governed realm of decency, Levinas writes:

> Man is a being that has already taken some elementary pains about his appearance. He looked at himself in the mirror and saw himself. He has washed, wiped away the night, and the traces of his instinctual permanence, from his face; he is clean and abstract. Life in society is decent. The most delicate social relationships are carried on in the forms of propriety; they safeguard the appearances, cover over all ambiguities with a cloak of sincerity and make them mundane.

... Social life in the world does not have that disturbing character
that a being feels before another being, before alterity.[61]

Indeed, for Levinas, social life is a preoccupation with salvation, a seeking of
relief from the pain and suffering of Being, an essential form of "habitation" constructed to make us feel at home as much as possible. "The privileged role of the
home," claims Levinas, "does not consist in being the end of human activity but in
being its condition, and in this sense its commencement."[62] As creatures whose
own existence works deconstructively to call our everyday way of being with
things and with others into question, we at the same time are creatures who are
destined to engage in what was described in chapters 4 and 5 as the reconstructive
task of home-making, of creating dwelling places that are livable, meaningful,
worthwhile, enjoyable, and, most importantly for Levinas, "welcoming." A home
that is welcoming displays respect for creatures whose existence is structured as a
caress and, hence, a being-for others. In a move that has incited much controversy
over his philosophy, Levinas equates this welcoming nature of the home with the
"feminine alterity" of "the Woman."[63] This move warrants some discussion, especially because it will play a role in the case study of the caress that is presented in
the next chapter.

In a Talmudic reading entitled "And God Created Woman," Levinas offers a
hint of why he thinks of the Woman in the way that he does. Recalling the last
chapter of Proverbs and the woman who is praised there, he writes: "she makes
possible the life of men, she is the home of men." The "husband," on the other
hand, "has a life outside the home: He sits on the Council of the city, he has a public life; he is at the service of the universal; he does not limit himself to interiority,
to intimacy, to the home, although without them he could ... [do] nothing."[64] Indeed, this woman in the last chapter of Proverbs exemplifies the cherished idea of
what a "home-maker" ought to be, at least from the patriarchal standpoint of the
Old Testament. For example: "The heart of her husband doth safely trust in her, so
that he shall have no need of spoil. She will do him good and not evil all the days
of her life. She seeketh wool, and flax, and worketh willingly with her hands"
(31:11–13); "She riseth also while it is yet night, and giveth meat to her household
... She considereth a field, and buyeth it: with the fruit of her hands she planteth a
vineyard" (31:15–16); "She stretcheth out her hand to the poor; yea, she reacheth
forth her hands to the needy" (31:20); "She maketh fine linen, and selleth it; and
delivereth girdles unto the merchant. Strength and honor are her clothing; and she
shall rejoice in time to come. She openeth her mouth with wisdom: and in her
tongue is the law of kindness. She looketh well to the ways of her household, and
eateth not the bread of idleness" (31:24–27). In short, she is a God-fearing and du-
tiful soul who serves her husband and children in accordance with "His" (God's)
laws (31:30).

Feminist writers such as Simone de Beauvoir, who are critical of Levinas's characterization of the Woman, caution against thinking of her in this way of "masculine privilege." For beginning with the story of Eve in Genesis, "humanity is made and man defines woman not in herself but as relative to him; she is not regarded as an autonomous being. . . . She is defined and differentiated with reference to man and not he with reference to her; she is the incidental, the inessential as opposed to the essential. He is the Subject, he is the Absolute—she is the Other."[65] Levinas does, in fact, write that "the feminine is the other."[66] But this description is intended to connote something more than a class of people who, because of their gender, are fated to live on the margins of society in a state of social death. Rather, Levinas associates "feminine alterity" with what he terms the "voluptuosity" of the future: the ever-more of what is yet to come in our lives; that which makes possible "the pursuit of an ever richer promise"; that dimension of otherness whose truth, although it can be spoken about, remains ungraspable in its wholeness for finite beings; that which maintains the purity of "virginity" even as it is approached and touched by the present and all the human actions that take place in this immediate moment of time.[67]

Although Levinas's employment of sexual metaphors develops a rhetoric that willingly carries the baggage of masculine privilege, this rhetoric, given its association with a dimension of otherness that Levinas relates to an understanding and appreciation of the word "God," also elevates the feminine alterity of Woman to a position that forever remains beyond the height and the story of *man*kind. Remember, the woman who is praised in the last chapter of Proverbs is someone whose home-making activities, generosity, and wisdom make the doings of her husband possible. When Levinas writes about how "the other must be closer to God than I," he can be read as heaping praise on what man has long called the "weaker sex." In Proverbs one reads: "Who can find a virtuous woman? For her price is far above rubies" (31:10). "Give her of the fruit of her hands; and let her own works praise her in the gates" (31:31). Indeed, more than the everyday doings of man, it is "her own works" that find great expression in Levinas's philosophy of the caress and in the event of home-making that this philosophy entails.[68]

The happening of this event is crucial if human beings are to find salvation from the burdens of everyday life. But there is a danger here, warns Levinas, for the homes we create and inhabit can breed immorality. Enjoyment can become so self-satisfying and addictive that, as it nourishes our personal desires and egos, it makes us forgetful of others and of how our behavior might be adversely affecting them. Levinas has this state of forgetfulness in mind when he writes of how social life lacks that disturbing character that we feel before the nudity, vulnerability, and alterity of another being whose suffering is left to happen outside our home and whose call of "Where art thou?" is thereby muted. This muting of the other's call, according to Levinas, is also facilitated by the rhetorical ornamentation or eloquence of our dwelling places. "Rhetoric," writes Levinas, brings into the meaning in which it culminates a certain beauty, a certain elevation, a certain nobility and an expressivity that imposes itself independently of its truth. Even more than verisimilitude, that beauty we call eloquence seduces the listener. . . .

Clearly in our time the effects of eloquence are everywhere, dominating our entire lives. There is no need to go through the whole sociology of our industrialized society here. The media of information in all forms—written, spoken, visual—invade the home, keep people listening to an endless discourse, submit them to the seduction of a rhetoric that is only possible if it is eloquent and persuasive in portraying ideas and things too beautiful to be true.[69]

Such an assessment of rhetorical eloquence dates back to Plato and, as noted earlier, also finds expression in modern architectural theory's critique of decoration and ornamentation. In both cases, we are warned of how the aesthetic (rhetorical) function of a work of art can obscure and distort what the rational function of the work ought to be, *in truth*. Although Levinas acknowledges that rhetorical *praxis* is by its very nature *other-oriented*, he also holds a very narrow understanding of "eloquence." He equates it with the ideological use of language to manipulate and exploit one's interlocutor or audience, which inhibits our ability to hear the one true discourse that never goes away: the "saying" of existence and its otherness—a saying that, for human beings, is most pronounced in the evocative presence, the epideictic display or the primordial rhetoric of another's "face."[70]

It would seem that, for Levinas, the art of rhetoric is fated to lose its saying power of truth once it is transformed from evoking the epiphany of the face and converted into the social and political discourse of everyday life whereby it becomes a vehicle for "ruse, emprise [entertainment], . . . exploitation" and "deceit." Still, Levinas does speak of how such "art," in fulfilling its primary moral function, "seeks to give a face to things," thereby helping others to grasp something of the truth of some matter.[71] This is certainly how Levinas intends his own rhetoric to be read—as one given over to the epideictic task of evoking and showing-forth the truth and the ethical nature of the caress that is human existence. Perhaps, then, one might characterize the competence of Levinas's rhetorical efforts as being an effort in eloquence, at least as this phenomenon is more genuinely and charitably defined throughout the history of rhetoric (than it is in Levinas's writings). For indeed, the true nature of this art "is made up of the methods which reflection and experience have evolved to make a discourse such as to establish the truth and to arouse a love for it in the hearts of [human beings]. Things which strike and arouse the heart . . . eloquence is just that."[72]

And this being the case, I would also amend what has been said so far about the way in which the face speaks, for the epideictic discourse that silently flows from its lips is not without eloquence. On the contrary, whether it is attractive or not, whatever the face expresses behind the public masks meant to put on a "good showing" is itself such a showing, a magnificent and moving discourse that reveals an awe-inspiring truth. The face speaks, interrupts, and evokes a call for acknowledgment. The "saying" going on here is not a rhetoric without eloquence, especially if, as Levinas suggests, this saying speaks of something that is "closer to God than I." The other's face, in all its nudity, vulnerability, and alterity is a most revealing and fitting work of art that speaks of the importance of accountability, responsibility, and justice. The discourse at work here commends a habit of thinking and acting that keeps us open to differences of opinion and lifestyles, invites collaborative and moral deliberation, and evokes in others a sense of wonder and awe for the matter at hand. Whenever discourse is working this way, as Henry Johnstone, Jr. reminds us, it admits a rhetorical function: *Rhetoric is the evocation and the maintenance of the consciousness required for communication.*[73] And that, again, is how Levinas describes what is going on as the "epiphany of the face" unfolds before us: the face evokes consciousness and conscientiousness; it offers a moving (eloquent) discourse that makes us think and care about what we say and do as it holds us in its caress and calls for acknowledgment in the midst of our everyday ways of being with others.[74]

In this social and political environment, those who would answer the call must assume the additional responsibility of discerning how their response might best be performed in order to ensure its effectiveness and desired outcome. Recall that this matter is central to the rhetorical enterprise. The rhetor aims at finding *to prepon*—what is right, fitting, and appropriate for the situation. Rhetorical competence facilitates the caress that is offered to others in need of help. Owing to the ontological and metaphysical orientation of his philosophy, as well as to the biases he holds against the rhetorical techniques of the orator, Levinas is extremely vague when considering this practical matter of "appropriateness." He thereby omits a crucial existential aspect of the phenomenon's bonding function from his philosophy of the caress. In the next chapter, and with the help of a case study (the film *Ordinary People*), I take a closer look at how the appropriateness of the caress plays a crucial role in the dynamics of everyday existence. I introduce the study with some additional comments concerning the centrality of appropriateness to the rhetorical enterprise. Here, too, I appeal once again to both religion and science for directives that confirm the phenomenon's importance.

Chapter Seven

Appropriateness

By responding to another's call for acknowledgment, we secure and strengthen the ontological structure of the caress that forms the fundamental ethical and rhetorical relationship between the self and the other. The last chapter was intended to promote an understanding of this many-faceted phenomenon, which became an issue for us following a discussion of Robert Frost's "The Death of the Hired Man." Recall that, with this poem, Frost not only refers to the caress but also practices it with his rhetorical competence, using words in a certain way to open us to the subject matter of his story and to open this subject matter to us. Frost designs a discourse meant to "touch" us and to arouse our interest in a matter of importance: acknowledgment, the opening of dwelling places that invite us to feel at home and experience a loving caress. Frost is both a poet and a rhetorical architect who invites us to join him in the noble task of home-making.

Levinas, too, offers this invitation, although his is more ontologically and metaphysically oriented. He wants us *to go as far as we can* in understanding the all important basis of a simple directive: "I welcome the Other who presents himself in my home by opening my home to him," and saying "Here I am!"[1] Mary did this for Silas when she took him to her kitchen and defended him against Warren's instrumental outlook. And Warren did this for Mary when he opened himself to her caring words and held her hand in grief. With such responses of "loving-kindness," they were being true to the caress that is human existence, a caress whose ontological and metaphysical workings encourage us to think about otherness and its "absolute" state—what humans commonly call "God." Recall that there is a "religious" quality to "The Death of the Hired Man," although the word "God" is never spoken by any of its characters.

Frost's artistic talents provide an illustrative dimension of concreteness to Levinas's philosophy of the caress, which certainly takes us further than Heidegger in revealing the comprehensive nature of the phenomenon. Still, there is at least one additional step that must be taken beyond Levinas (and Frost) in coming to terms with the burdens, benefits, and overall goodness of the caress. Yes, with the caress come pain and suffering and the medicament of love. In the quest for salvation in everyday life, however, the workings of the caress are not so straightforward, especially when it comes to the rhetorical matter of *appropriateness*. Imagine, for example, a much-revised ending of Frost's poem. Warren returns to the porch, utters his last word ("Dead"), sits down next to Mary to hold her hand, and then, after however long its takes for this caress to work its wonders, refuses to let go of Mary even after she gives clear indication that "enough is enough already." The scene could become pitiful or even comical. Warren has lost it; his pain and suffering force him to hold on to Mary for dear life, although Mary's hand is starting to hurt by now as her grimacing facial expressions make clear. Warren, nevertheless, squeezes even harder as his pain and suffering refuse to subside.

A loving caress can become a suffocating embrace. The overly possessive husband or wife, father or mother, friend or lover, provide cases in point. "The Death of the Hired Man" does not deal with the issue. Levinas makes a brief reference to this issue of "possession," but his mixture of philosophical, poetical, and rhetorical prose is so dense (and one might argue "inappropriate") that only the most interested and hermeneutically charitable readers are likely to recognize his stance on the issue, which seems to be this: The overly possessive person does a disservice to others by not respecting their right and obligation to stand on their own two feet and to assume as much responsibility as possible in directing their own lives.[2] It would seem that, despite the way in which existence is structured as a caress and despite how this structure obliges us to-be-for-others, not every call for acknowledgment that happens in everyday life warrants an unrestrained "Here I am!" Welcoming another person into our home for an unlimited stay does not guarantee the growth of his or her moral character.

But how do we know where to draw the line between being too welcoming and not being welcoming enough? It is a judgment call, to be sure—one that requires competence in talking out decisions in an appropriate and just manner. Such competence is rightly recognized as being rhetorical. The goal of rhetoric is the appropriate production of a dwelling place where sound judgment can be fostered in and through collaborative deliberation. Rhetorical competence enables human beings to advance nature's law of the survival of the fittest in the sense that it reinforces the value of supporting those who are ethically the best.[3]

Levinas is not in the habit of offering careful assessments of this process in the form of detailed case studies; rather, he remains content to speak philosophically about specific ethical matters and comment on how rhetorical eloquence too often deafens us to these matters' instructive teachings. In the remaining pages of this chapter, I focus on a case study that not only deals with the unresolved issue of the appropriateness of the caress in everyday life but does so in what I take to be a rhetorically competent and eloquent manner. The case is that of the novel-based film *Ordinary People*—a work of art and entertainment that holds its audience in a caress while at the same time telling a moving story about this very phenomenon and its relationship to the life-giving gift of acknowledgment. Levinas's critical assessment of the rhetorical fashioning of everyday life by the mass media does not offer much encouragement for attending to such an entertaining artifact. With this case study, I also wish to call into question such a lack of support that, since Plato, has too often allowed philosophy to cast a scornful eye at popular culture and its world of entertainment.[4]

Considering the various meanings associated with the term, entertainment can refer to something "diverting" *or* "engaging." So, for example, people are entertained by things and activities that are stupid but funny, an enjoyable way to waste time, and mindless. And they are also entertained by things and activities that are serious, difficult but still enjoyable, worthwhile, intellectually stimulating, and perhaps even awe-inspiring. Owing to the plethora of dis(at)tractions that are offered by today's mass-mediated and show-business culture, entertainment is more often associated with what is diverting rather than engaging, playful rather than compelling, shallow rather than deep, vacuous rather than full of significant meaning. Hence, such nationally televised tabloid "news" shows like *Entertainment Tonight* that provide the "scoop" about the ups and downs of celebrities, thereby offering viewers an "escape" from their own trying days.[5] But again, a given experience need not be merely a source of diversion to qualify as a source of entertainment. The profession of teaching certainly provides a case in point. The "true" educator is forever facing the challenge of finding ways to make his or her presentations interesting enough such that others are willing to *entertain* ("show hospitality to"; "keep hold, or maintain in mind"; "receive and take into consideration") all that is being said about some relevant matter. Such an act of entertaining requires the attention and attunement of consciousness, which must be evoked and maintained in order to cultivate the acknowledgment that the teacher seeks from students. The goal here requires some degree of rhetorical competence on the part of the teacher. For remember: "Rhetoric is the evocation and the maintenance of the consciousness required for communication."

I will have much more to say about the vocation of teaching and its relationship with acknowledgment in the next chapter. The analysis of *Ordinary People* offered below will help set the stage for assessing that relationship. With this film we have a work of art that, as the expression goes, "puts a human face" on the existential workings of the appropriateness of the caress and thereby brings to life an issue of existence that we dare not forsake in our everyday being-with-and-for-others.

The Appropriateness of the Caress: A Case Study

The opening credits are presented without a sound. The film's theme song is then played as viewers are shown some of the beachfront, woods, and parks of Lake Forest, Illinois, one of the most exclusive upper-middle-class and upper-class communities on the North Shore of Chicago. It is early fall. The colors add to the magnificence of an already picture perfect environment where big homes are situated on big lots of manicured property. Lake Forest has style and a carefully displayed sense of decorum.

I lived on Chicago's North Shore for thirteen years, although not in Lake Forest. I drove through the community, however, to view its beauty and to marvel at its homes. I imagined that the inside of the homes looked like pages from *Architectural Digest* or from eye-catching coffee table books like Beverly Pagram's *Home & Heart: Simple, Beautiful Ways to Create Spirit, Harmony & Warmth in Every Room*. As Pagram writes in her introduction:

> This book is about making sure our living spaces offer a warm emotional landscape and reflect the individuality of the people who spend so much time in them. That they offer the right psychic climate to generate the sharing, continually learning and caring home-culture which makes happy, healthy children and well-balanced grown-ups. Ways of making this possible are mostly simple. They rest on encouraging personal creativity, satisfying effort and self-expression for everyone in the household; as well as meaningful, security-enhancing daily and seasonal ritual and celebration for individuals and groups. Most important in the home sanctuary is the concept of "bringing the outside in" and "taking the inside out"—an environmental shift in lifestyle-thinking, setting everyday lives in harmony with the natural world.[6]

Pagram's book instructs readers on how to design a well-ordered, charming, and awesome dwelling place, one whose rooms, furnishings, hallways, nooks, crannies, and landscaped exterior all display an elegant presence, an "appropriateness" that caters to and caresses your body, mind, and moral well-being. Envy aside, you feel good—at home and at peace in the universe—as you read the author's prose and view her book's pictures. All of the windows she displays (with the exception of one bathroom window) are vertical. This is significant because, as James Kunstler points out,

> vertical windows frame the standing human figure. They represent *the idea* of people standing erect inside the house. This appeals to our minds. Horizontal windows are rather disturbing at a subconscious level. If they frame the human figure at all, they do so in ways

that make us vaguely uncomfortable: they suggest that the inhabitants are either sleeping, having sex, or dead.

Now, sleeping, sex, and being dead are all obviously part of the human condition, but as casual observers we don't want to project them onto the house and its denizens. Most of the time, the people inside are strangers to us. Our minds want to conceive them in the most dignified condition possible. That's what standing signifies. It is generalized, formal, composed, and dignified, like a portrait. The convention of vertical windows . . . is a device for regulating a house's sense of dignity.[7]

Indeed, as its Latin root *dignitas* suggests, dignity speaks to us of "worthiness," "elevation," "honor," "height"—in short, of "excellence" or "virtue." A house's sense of dignity orients its inhabitants and onlookers toward the heavens. It functions aesthetically and rhetorically to lift the human *spirit* and thus to make us feel *alive*.[8]

The family whose story is told in *Ordinary People* lives in a house that oozes dignity. Lake Forest, indeed: a large, two-story white dwelling with eleven vertical windows in the front. The interior of the house, which appears throughout the film, is also, of course, most properly and tastefully designed. Nothing is out of place. Everything is neat and clean. Elegance every which way you turn. It is a picture book habitat that, to say the least, speaks of the "good" life. But all is not well for the family that dwells there. The Jarretts—Beth (mother; thirty-nine-year-old socialite), Calvin (father; forty-one-year-old tax attorney), and Conrad (son; seventeen-year-old high school student)—are in a state of crisis, desperately seeking salvation from the horrors that currently haunt them and call into question the life that their dignified dwelling place is meant to sustain. Being around or at home with the Jarretts is a tension filled experience.

The crisis came about when the small boat that Conrad and his fourteen-month older brother Buck were sailing in Lake Michigan capsized in a storm. Hanging on to the boat, the boys screamed directives and encouragement to each other. Conrad appeared far more terrified than his brother during the ordeal. And this terror grew even more intense for Conrad as Buck eventually lost his grip on the boat, on Conrad, and drowned.

The actual scene of the boating accident is presented in flashback footage near the end of the film. The audience knows nothing of its occurrence when the film begins, although the psychological and social consequences that the accident has had on the Jarrett family are evident in every preceding scene. Although this way of editing the film is not a novel technique for Hollywood filmmakers trying to tell a "good" story, it certainly is an effective rhetorical strategy for gaining the interest of an audience. For it invites you to take a more active role in making sense of a story-line whose narrative remains incomplete even after you acquire a more coherent understanding of why things are happening the way they are. Some degree of audience participation is a prerequisite for the success of any work of art; thus the value of the filmmaker's and actors' rhetorical competence. This skill is a mainstay of good storytelling and is a necessary ingredient for attending to the needs of those beings who are, among other things, *homo narrans*: creatures who find it appropriate to tell stories as a fundamental way of bringing order to and thereby feeling at home with their existence.[9]

The Jarretts no longer feel completely at home with their everyday lives. The unexpected death of a loved one is a heart-ripping and gut-wrenching experience, an existential interruption that disrupts and breaks down everyday habits of living and thinking and thereby brings us face-to-face with the pain, suffering, and challenge of responsibility that accompanies Being. Action and a love of life are necessary in order to gain some freedom from this suffocating embrace of Being's caress. Conrad fails the challenge at first, for we learn shortly after the film begins that, overwhelmed by grief and guilt, he attempted suicide by slitting his wrists in his bathroom. He has only recently returned home from a psychiatric hospital. He is a picture of unfitness, of weariness and fatigue: disheveled hair, dark rings under his eyes, sloppy clothing. This is how he appears at home and at school. His presence bothers and embarrasses his mother, who tells him as much in both words and actions that are always sharp, cold, and dismissive.

Beth is described in the book as someone who is "All elegance and self-possession. So beautiful in every detail that men and women both like to look at her." Moreover, her husband Cal "emphatically does not own her, nor does he have control over her, nor can he understand or even predict with reliability her moods, her attitudes."[10] He is, however, well aware of Beth's obsession with perfection, which showed itself early in their marriage, when the boys were just toddlers. Cal remembers some episodes:

> Her figure, tense with fury as she scrubbed the fingermarks from the walls; her bursting suddenly into tears because of a toy left out of place, or a spoonful of food thrown on to the floor from the high chair. And it did not pay him to become exasperated with her. Once he had done so, had shouted at her to forget the damned cleaning schedule for once. She had flown into a rage, railed at him, and flung herself across the bed, in hysterics. Everything had to be perfect, never mind the impossible hardship it worked on her, on them all; never mind the utter lack of meaning in such perfection, weighed as it was against the endless repetition of days, weeks, months. They learned, all of them, that certain things drove her to the point of madness: dirt tracked in on a freshly scrubbed floor; water-spotted shower stalls; articles of clothing left out of place.[11]

Although these specific recollections are not presented in the film, there is no mistaking who and how Beth is as we watch her character on screen: stunning, neat, calculating—like her house—and "rotten with perfection."[12] During one scene, for example, she shows more concern for a dinner plate she has broken in the kitchen than she does for her son whom she has just refused to have her picture taken with during a family gathering and who has recently begun seeing a psychiatrist.

It was Calvin's idea to have Conrad make an appointment with the psychiatrist, Dr. Berger. Calvin is a loving father who worries a lot about his son. He thinks that it would be wise to cancel their yearly Christmas vacation so that Conrad need not disrupt his sessions with Dr. Berger. But Beth is strongly opposed to the idea. The scene in which this disagreement unfolds makes it clear that Calvin and Beth are on opposite ends of the spectrum when it comes to being-for others. A later scene is especially telling of this point. Calvin and Conrad are setting up a Christmas tree in the living room when Beth appears with a look of anger that freezes both her husband and son:

> Calvin: "What's wrong?"
> Beth: "Why don't you ask him what's wrong? Then maybe you wouldn't have to hear it from Carol Lazenby."
> Calvin: "Hear what?"
> Conrad: (after a long pause) "Dad, I quit the swim team."
> Calvin: "What?"
> Beth: "Carol thought I knew. Of course, why wouldn't I? It happened over a month ago."
> Calvin: "Quit! When? Where have you been every night?"
> Conrad: "Nowhere. Around. The library mostly."
> Calvin: "Why didn't you tell us, Connie?"
> Conrad: "I don't know. I didn't think it mattered."
> Calvin: "What do you mean? Why wouldn't it matter? Of course it matters."
> Beth: "No, that was meant for me, Calvin."
> Calvin: "What was meant for you?"
> Beth: "It's really important to try to hurt me, isn't it?"
> Conrad: "Don't you have that backward?"
> Beth: "Oh? And how do I hurt you? By embarrassing you in front of a friend? Poor Beth, she has no idea what her son is up to, he lies and she believes every word of it."
> Conrad: "I didn't lie!"
> Beth: "You did. You lied every time you came into this house at six-thirty. If it is starting all over again, the lying, the covering up, the disappearing for hours, I will not stand for it. I can't stand it. I really can't."

Conrad: "Then don't then. Go to Europe."

Calvin: "Connie, now . . ."

Conrad: "The only reason she cares, the only reason she gives a fuck about it is cause someone else knew about it first."

Calvin: "Just stop it, Connie!"

Conrad: "No, you tell her to stop it. You never tell her a goddamn thing. And I know why she never came to the hospital. She was busy going to goddamn Spain and goddamn Portugal. Why should she care if I am hung out by the balls out there?"

Beth: "Maybe this is how they sit around and talk at the hospital but we are not at the hospital now."

Conrad: "You never came to the hospital . . ."

Calvin: "Connie. . ."

Conrad: "How do you know about the hospital?"

Calvin: "Now you know that she did, she had the flu and she couldn't come inside, but she came to the hospital."

Conrad: "Yeah, but she wouldn't have had the flu if Buck was in the hospital. She would have come if Buck was in the hospital."

Beth: "Buck never would have been in the hospital."

(Conrad, in exasperation, grabs his head and hurries upstairs to his room.)

Calvin: "That's enough. That is enough."

Beth: "I wouldn't do it again, I really wouldn't do it."

Calvin: "What in the hell has happened? Somebody better go up there."

Beth: "Oh God yes, that's the pattern isn't it. He walks all over us and then you go up and apologize to him."

Calvin: "I am not going to apologize . . ."

Beth: "Yes, of course you are, you always do. You have been apologizing to him ever since he got home from the hospital, only you don't *see* it."

Calvin: "I am not apologizing, *I am trying to goddamn understand him.*"

Beth: "Don't talk to me that way. Don't you talk to me the way he talks to you."

Calvin: "Beth . . . (gently holds her shoulders), let's not fight, okay? No fighting, okay? Please let's go upstairs."

Beth just stares at Calvin and does not move. Calvin turns and walks up to Conrad's room, where he finds his son face down on the bed. "I want to talk to you," says Calvin. Without looking up, Conrad replies, "I didn't mean it. Please don't be mad." Calvin emphasizes that he is not mad and Conrad pleads, "Just tell her I am sorry." When Calvin asks why Conrad will not apologize personally to his mother, Conrad replies, "Oh God, no I can't. Don't you see I can't talk to her?" In a caring tone, Calvin asks, "why not?" And his son answers: "Cause it doesn't change anything. It doesn't change the way she looks at me." Calvin admits that he doesn't understand and begs for an explanation.

> Conrad: "I, I can't. Everything is jello and pudding with you, dad. You don't see things."
> Calvin: "What things? What things? Please, I want you to tell me."
> Conrad: "That she hates me. Can't you see that?"

It is not so much that Calvin does not *see* things; rather, he does not *observe* them. When he tries to remain open to the crisis that engulfs his family, it proves to be too complex, too frustrating, and too sad. Calvin has a big heart. As Conrad puts it during one of his sessions with Dr. Berger: Dad "loves everybody." But when Calvin attempts to figure things out, he lacks the stamina for deep thought, remains at a loss for words, lacks rhetorical competence, and thereby ends up offering rather deficient statements about what is going on in his mind. He is a "jello and pudding" type of guy and a husband who is ill-prepared for confrontations with his wife, a woman who rarely budges an inch and whose mere facial expressions are intimidating and breath-taking.

Indeed, all of the acting in *Ordinary People* is truly awe-some. I would go so far as to say that there is not a single scene in the book whose "realistic" description of things hateful, loving, tearful, or puzzling are not made more vivid and wonder-ful by their portrayal on film. Of course, this is the way it should be in an award-winning film that seeks to be evocative and honest about its subject matter while at the same time being entertaining. It is a matter of rhetorical competence, of rhetorical eloquence, of knowing how to awaken and maintain the interest (consciousness) of others so that they can better identify with and be moved by what is being disclosed through skillful acting, directing, writing, filming, editing, and other related artistic talents. A film whose epideictic power for showing-forth its material proves insufficient in helping others to both see and observe, for example, what it means for "ordinary people" to be going through a crisis, is a film destined to lose its hold (caress) on its audience.

And this is certainly what *Ordinary People* is about: a family in crisis; a mother, father, and son desperately seeking to accomplish something that they fear—opening themselves to each other so that they might dwell in peace again. Beth, Calvin, and Conrad are failing in the ethical and rhetorical task of home-making. Beth is too selfish and defensive; Calvin is too loving and giving. Beth is too distant; Calvin is too close. Although for different reasons, neither of them wants to suffocate their son with an overly caring embrace. Beth keeps insisting that Conrad needs to maintain more control and responsibility for his life in order to survive the tragic circumstances at hand. Calvin does not disagree, but he is more sensitive to the fact that sometimes surviving requires a more heart-felt and welcoming way of being-for others than that allowed for by his wife. In terms of Levinas' philosophy, Calvin displays more of a "feminine" or caressing alterity than does Beth. In dealing with this continuing situation, Conrad's problem is that he both values and loathes the perfectionism of his mother *and* the loving-kindness of his father; both parents work against him as they try to help him. It is a classic double-bind: caught in the tension between his mother and father, Conrad cannot win for losing. Still, an appropriate solution must be found. The potential destructiveness of staying in a double-bind for too long is well known.[13]

To be or not to be? The question was once simple for Conrad. He chose the second option but was given another chance when his parents found him and called an ambulance in time. Having reestablished something of a love of life, Conrad must now struggle to find some balance between two other extremes: To be loved (caressed) too little or to be loved (suffocated) too much. Neither will do. The either/or logic of the bind poses a major problem, as Dr. Berger makes clear in his ongoing sessions with Conrad. During the session that followed the last scene described above for example, Conrad tells Berger that he does not blame his mother "given all of the shit [he] pulled." Berger asks for clarification, but tells Conrad not to focus once on the suicide episode. Conrad's response is noteworthy:

> Listen, I am never going to be forgiven for that. Never. You know you can't get it out, all the blood in her towels and her rug. Everything had to be pitched. Even the tile in the bathroom had to be re-grouted. Christ, she fired the goddamn maid because she couldn't dust the living room right. If you think I-am-going-to-forgive-she-is-going-to-forgive-me . . . .

This last slip of the tongue works as a rhetorical interruption that gives Conrad long pause for thought. "What?" asks Dr. Berger. Walking silently toward the office window, Conrad replies: "I think I just figured something out." Berger again asks the question. To which Conrad answers: "Who it is who can't forgive who."

Beth's "positive" influence on Conrad's life involves an appreciation for survival, self-control, and perfectionism; hence, the tragic irony of his suicide attempt. In seeking control over his imperfect life by trying to end it in what he thought was a perfect way, he actually made matters much worse by further soiling his mother's world, which only encouraged her to become more rotten with perfection. And Calvin's "positive" influence on Conrad's life serves mostly to increase Conrad's susceptibility to his mother's obsessive and hurtful ways. Dr. Berger suggests that the problem between Conrad and his mother might not be her *refusal to love him* but rather her *inability to love him enough*. "Maybe,"

Berger continues, "she can't express it the way you would like her to. Maybe she is afraid to show you what she feels." The issue of "appropriateness" is thus put on the table. Conrad, however, does not understand. "What do you mean?" he asks. Berger answers, "I mean there is someone besides your mother you have to forgive." Conrad looks puzzled and again asks for clarification: "You mean me? For trying to off myself? Don't just sit there and stare at me! What for?" Berger remains enigmatic: "Why don't you give yourself a break. Let yourself off the hook." "What did I do?" asks Conrad. *"What did I do?"* But time is up. Berger tells him to think about it until their next meeting and, over Conrad's objections, ends the session.

The question of the caress: What would life be like if no one acknowledged your existence, if no one took the time to open a space, a dwelling place, for you in their life? With Levinas we learned that the ontological and metaphysical importance of this question lies in how human existence itself is structured as a caress that makes the self's most genuine way of being one of being-for others. It is in large part a "feminine" matter. Dr. Berger calls on Conrad to be better, more perfect ("feminine") than his mother by being far more welcoming toward her than she is toward him. Perfection need not necessarily be rotten in its workings. Berger's request, as Levinas teaches, makes the situation "religious" in the deepest and holiest sense of the word. After all, we are creatures who dwell in the presence of Otherness which, among other things, calls us into question and allows for hope and pardon. The face speaks: Thou shalt not kill! Is there a God who *listens* to our prayers ("Where art thou?") and responds ("Here I am!")? Perhaps it is simply a case of vibrating strings. But even if it is, Conrad is still faced with the reality of a terrible situation in need of an appropriate response.

Conrad admits to Jeannine (a female classmate who is kind to him and whom he has a crush on) that he does not believe in God. Much like Dr. Berger, this teenage girl is especially interested in Conrad's depression, why he attempted suicide, and what it felt like. And like Berger, she is willing to listen to what Conrad has to say. Listening is a moral act that, according to Levinas, defines "the first ethical gesture," for this is how we, in our being-for others, open ourselves to all that others have to say about who and how they are and what they need in order to be saved from the pain and suffering of Being.[14] The entire process constitutes a primordial ethical happening that, for Levinas, is not reducible to a survival of the fittest mentality. It can manifest itself even in "the smallest and most commonplace gestures, such as saying 'after you' as we sit at the dinner table or walk through a door."[15] Listening helps set the stage for the goodness of acknowledgment; it is a capacity for welcoming and that thus aids salvation. There is something fundamentally "feminine" about it, and sacred, too. Listening is what God is supposed to do when no one else will.

Conrad wants to be saved. He needs the kind of acknowledgment that Dr. Berger and Jeannine provide: an appropriate caress—one that is caring, loving, but not suffocating. Owing to the help he receives from these individuals, Conrad's psychological state shows some noticeable improvement. Calvin, who continues to be pained by Beth's cold treatment of Conrad, also decides to set up an appointment with Dr. Berger. During their session, which is only shown in part, Calvin admits many things in a hesitating and confused sort of way. He talks about how Beth was more affectionate toward Buck ("her favorite"; her "first born") than toward Conrad, how Conrad sometimes displays his mother's obsessive tendencies, how neither Beth nor Conrad cried at the funeral, and how his talking with Berger about these matters is helpful. Berger is a good listener, a sort of "feminine" and "holy" character if you will. The scene ends as Calvin says "I think I know why I came here. I came here to talk about myself." The therapeutic quality of such expression is indicated by Gusdorf when he notes:

> Not all men write, but all resort to the power of expression in speech or in action to overcome inner threats, to check the idle temptations of care or suffering. Speaking here indicates a stepping-back. The decision to express marks the threshold between the passivity of eating one's heart out and creative activity. To speak, to write, to express is to act, to survive crisis, to begin living again, even when one thinks it is only to relive one's sorrow. Expression is a kind of exorcism because it crystallizes the resolve not to let oneself go.[16]

And as long as our expression is listened to, there exists the possibility of hope and improvement.

Indeed, to be listened to, caressed, helped, and respected is to receive the life-giving gift of acknowledgment. Calvin seeks salvation; he wants to feel at home with his self and his surroundings. Returning home from his session with Berger, he gathers the courage and enough rhetorical competence to ask Beth about something that happened right before Buck's funeral and that had been on his mind ever since. Beth is adamant about avoiding the topic, but Calvin pushes on, reminding her of how she insisted that he change his socks before the funeral because they didn't match. Why did she even care about such a trivial matter given the circumstances? Her behavior, to say the least, was inappropriate.[17] But Beth offers no answer as she hugs her distraught husband and assures him that he will be all right. In a later scene, however, Beth and Calvin have another major argument over his showing more concern for Conrad's welfare than he does for Beth's desire to stay mentally and physically fit in order to survive and forget the past, and be happy.

This second argument takes place in public while Beth and Calvin are visiting her brother and his wife in Texas. During this time, Conrad suffers a major setback after attempting to call Karen, a young girl who was also a patient in the psychiatric hospital. She told him after they both returned home that she was doing "great" and he promised to stay in touch. But Karen's father informs him that she has committed suicide. Conrad freaks out and begins to recall (through a series of flashbacks) what happened when Buck drowned. In desperation he calls Dr. Berger in the middle of the night, asking to meet at his office to talk out this crisis. During the special session, Conrad realizes what Berger meant when he told Conrad that there was someone he had to forgive besides his mother.

Sitting down with Berger and crying hysterically, Conrad says that "something happened" but does not specify what it was. As Berger tries to get him to be more specific, Conrad shouts, "I got to get off the hook for what I did to him." He is referring to Buck. In a moment of psychiatric transference, Berger becomes Buck in Conrad's mind. Berger (Buck) is then scolded by the teenager for not hanging on to the boat and to Conrad. That should not have happened. Buck was the stronger and more perfect son; he should have survived. "Why did he let go?" cries Conrad. Berger suggests that maybe Conrad was, in fact, the "stronger" of the two and asks him, "How long are you going to punish yourself? When are you going to quit?" Berger then asks Conrad what he was referring to when he said that something happened. Conrad tells him about Karen and admits feeling "really bad" about not being able to help her. Berger again argues that Conrad is being too hard on himself. "It's not fair," complains Conrad. "You just do one wrong thing . . ." Berger interrupts: "And what was the one wrong thing you did? You know!" Sobbing, Conrad replies, "I hung on. I stayed with the boat."

Berger confirms the importance of this action. Conrad is "alive!" There is nothing "wrong" with that. "It doesn't feel good," replies Conrad. "It *is good*," insists Berger. "Believe me." With tears still flowing down his face, Conrad asks, "How do you know?" Berger replies, "Because I'm your friend." Conrad admits that he doesn't know what he would have done if Berger had not been there for him. "Are you really my friend?" he asks. "I am. Count on it," says Berger. The scene, which is highly emotional and brilliantly portrayed, ends with the two wrapping their arms around each other. This caress may not seem like the "manly" thing to do, but it is quite right, fitting, and just. The situation calls for rhetorical competence—an appropriate response that can aid Conrad in his struggle to be a good home-maker.

The pain and suffering of Being, the challenge of responsibility, the love of life, and being-for others: all of these things are at work in the scene. There is also one additional factor that, as far as I can tell, is not emphasized in Levinas' philosophy of the caress: the need to be able to caress ourselves at times, to let ourselves off the hook for things that are not our fault. The lesson is not lost on Conrad. After his parents return from their trip, he walks into the den looking more relaxed than ever before. He tells them that he is glad they are back home and walks over to his mother and gives her a big hug before going upstairs. From then on the only two people that we see in the scene are Beth and Calvin. Beth is not welcoming; she does not return Conrad's caress and her face displays more of a catatonic expression than one of compassion and joy. Staring at his wife, Conrad's sad eyes show forth a heartbreaking degree of disappointment at yet another inappropriate response from Beth. The face speaks: Thou shall not kill! The rhetorical competence of the actors brings a most important rhetorical and life-giving phenomenon to life in a stunning and eloquent way.

The next two scenes continue to emphasize the workings of the caress as they bring the film to its conclusion. Beth wakes during the night and finds that Calvin is not beside her. She walks downstairs and finds him sitting at the dining room table, crying. Standing at the doorway with a look of confusion, she speaks: "Calvin? . . . Why are you crying? . . . Can I get you something? . . . Tell me!" Calvin eventually looks up and responds. It is a moment of truth and rhetorical competence:

> Calvin: "You are beautiful. And you are unpredictable. But you are so cautious. You are determined, Beth, but you know something, you're not strong. And I don't know if you are really giving. Tell me something! Do you love me? Do you really love me?"
>
> Beth: "I feel the way I've always felt about you." (More tears flow down Calvin's face with this specific and somewhat cold reply)
>
> Calvin: "It would have been alright if there hadn't been any mess. But you can't handle mess. You need everything neat and easy. I don't know. Maybe you can't love anybody. It was so much Buck. When Buck died it was as if you buried all your love with him and I don't understand that. I just don't know. I don't . . . Maybe it wasn't even Buck. Maybe it was just you. Maybe finally it was the best of you that you buried. But whatever it was, I don't know who you are. I don't know what we have been playing at. So I was crying. Because I don't know if I love you anymore and I don't know what I am going to do without that."

Beth's eyes are watering ever so slightly as she listens to Calvin. She says nothing. When he finishes she merely turns around, goes back upstairs to their bedroom, and closes the door behind her. She walks to the closet, pulls out a suitcase, places it on the bed, and opens it. She then goes back to the closet and picks up a small carrying-case. This time, however, she hesitates. She gasps as if someone has just hit her in the stomach. She begins to shake and cry. It is hard not to feel for Beth at this moment. She is doing what any good-hearted person might expect her to do. Her behavior is right, fitting, and appropriate. But then, in a somewhat chilling instant, she resumes her survival of the fittest way of being, closes her eyes, and composes herself as the scene ends.

We then see Conrad lying in his bed. It is early morning. He hears a car door close, walks to his window, and sees a taxi-cab departing from the front of the house. Puzzled, he walks downstairs and looks in various rooms. He notices that his father is standing outside in the backyard. Putting on a jacket, he joins him.

Conrad: "Dad?"

Calvin (looking out over the landscaped and large backyard): "The yard looks smaller with these leaves."

Conrad: "Dad, what happened?"

Calvin: "Your mother is going away for a while."

Conrad: "Where? Why?"

Calvin: "Back to Houston. I don't know."

Conrad: "Why? What? I know why. It's me, isn't it?"

Calvin: "No."

Conrad: "Yeah it is, it's my fault."

Calvin (in a stern voice): "Don't do that, don't do that to yourself. It's nobody's fault. Things happen in this world. People don't always have the answer for them you know . . . I don't know why I am yelling at you for."

Conrad (sitting down next to his father whose sad eyes are watering): "No, that's right. You ought to do that more often . . ."

Calvin: "Oh yeah?"

Conrad: "Yeah, yeah. Haul my ass a little, you know. Get after me. The way you used to for him."

Calvin: "Oh, he needed it, you didn't. You were so always so hard on yourself, I never had the heart."

Conrad: "Oh dad, don't . . ."

Calvin: "No, well, it's the truth. I never worried about you. I just wasn't listening."

Conrad: "I wasn't putting out many signals then. I really don't think you could have done anything."

Calvin: "No, no. I should have got a handle on it somehow."

Conrad: "You know I use to figure you had a handle on everything. You knew it all. I knew that wasn't fair but you always made us feel that everything was going to be alright. I thought about that a lot lately. I really admire you for it."

Calvin: "Well, don't admire people too much. They'll disappoint you sometimes."

Conrad: "I'm not disappointed. . . . I love you!"

Calvin (starts to cry as he and Conrad hug each other): "I love you, too."

Ordinary People ends with a caress, a love of life, a being-for others, and a wonderful moment of acknowledgment and salvation. Two very vulnerable souls are there for each other with no pretensions whatsoever. Sitting together outside a very dignified house whose perfect climate had grown rotten, they finally feel at home . . . at least for the moment. For as the credits roll, we are left to wonder about the fate of the family, whose crisis is not yet over. What about Beth? Will she return? Can life ever be "perfect" again for the Jarrett family?

Ordinary People, working rhetorically, calls the meaning of (male and female) perfection/fitness into question. It leaves us with an unfinished story. The journey is fated to continue. *Ordinary People* is more Jewish than Greek, more Abraham than Ulysses.[18] The father and the son's homecoming is not yet completed. The ethical and rhetorical task of home-making is still at hand, as is the issue of appropriateness that is part of this task, especially when keeping Beth in mind. We can only hope that all will turn out well, that the members of the Jarrett family will be successful in their continuing struggle to be just in all that they say and do with, to, and for each other. Still, for the moment, a person who was rotten with perfection and who, despite her stunning looks, was not "feminine" enough in her relationship with her son and her husband is gone and the simple event of a parent and child joined in an appropriate caress is comforting, as it should be. For it is the nakedness of the face, not its manufactured look, that reveals its truth in the ethical happening of its eloquent, epideictic, "feminine," and rhetorical presentation.

Of course, being a Hollywood film, *Ordinary People* is a manufactured thing itself. Its presence, its face, is strategically made up to be eloquent and entertaining, to put on a good showing. Levinas, recall, points to this process as being a major cause of the "deceit" of art, but he also allows for the potential of the process to "put a face on things" so that witnesses might be taken with and awed by the truth at hand. In this analysis, I have suggested how *Ordinary People* does exactly that: how it speaks of things that lie at the heart of existence, things that are identified in Levinas' philosophy of the caress. In both cases, the life-giving gift of acknowledgment is very much an issue. "Where art thou?" "Here I am!" With *Ordinary People,* however, the related and practical issues of the appropriateness of the caress, the therapeutic act of self-acknowledgment, and the way that a man, to his credit, can sometimes act like "a woman" while a woman, to her discredit, can sometimes act like "a man," are more carefully observed and skillfully treated. Philosophy is known to inform great art. And great art, with its rhetorical competence, is known to return the favor. It is the appropriate thing to do.[19]

Have I given the film too much credit? Have I slighted Levinas by simplifying—"dumbing-down"—his teachings too much? These teachings, according to their author, are intended to disclose what he takes to be the source of all "teaching": the ethical speaking of the face, of otherness, of something that was never a human creation in the first place, as is *Ordinary People.*[20] Still, I do not hesitate to nominate this ethical and rhetorical artifact from popular culture as an outstanding teaching tool for discussing the workings of a certain life-giving gift in a practical and entertaining way. Teaching and acknowledgment ought to go hand in hand. In the next chapter, I continue to clarify and expand on this claim.

Chapter Eight

Teaching

By answering their calling in front of their students and colleagues, teachers make a "profession." They "declare aloud" that they have special knowledge that they believe is worthy of being communicated because of its value to those who are willing to listen (and to respond) for the good of themselves and others. As Edmund Pellegrino and David Thomasma point out, "That is what entering a profession means—not simply becoming a member of a defined group with a common education, standards of performance, and a common ethic. These are all accidental to the central act of profession, which is an active, conscious declaration, voluntarily entered into, and signifying a willingness to assume the obligations necessary to make the declaration authentic."[1] Although these obligations will vary with the specific expertise and discipline being professed, there is at least one obligation that *must* be met by any and all who would call themselves teachers: acknowledgment.

The tasks before the dedicated teacher always include finding a way to transform space and time into a dwelling place where people can open themselves to each other, take an interest in whatever is being said, and come to know together its reasonableness, worth, and how perhaps to make it more enlightening, revealing, truthful, accurate, and applicable to people's lives. Teaching, in other words, is an ethical activity requiring rhetorical competence. When you observe the great teacher at work, you should be witnessing an event where, among others things, a life-giving gift is being shared in an appropriate and awe-inspiring manner. You might even see what the teacher is doing as being entertaining.

If you have never had the pleasure of working with such a teacher, then your education remains incomplete. I was fortunate enough to experience this pleasure throughout my masters and doctoral programs. I worked with teachers who knew how to read their students like they would a much cherished book: with care and devotion. Sure, there were times in seminars when they would give a clear indication that they were not "comfortable" with what some student was arguing. But these teachers would still go out of their way to make it clear that, despite "the possible error in one's thinking" (a.k.a. stupidity), the student still warranted respect as a member of the class. You feared being wrong in the presence of these teachers because it felt so bad when you thought you were disappointing them. They were committed to helping others cultivate their conscience. They were models for learning how to say "Here I am!" to those in need of acknowledgment, guidance, and friendship. They were, without a doubt, very gifted souls who welcomed the challenge of authenticity that faces every true teacher: the challenge of putting yourself on the line and running the risk of learning that you have yet to get things right.

Beginning at least with Socrates, teachers have associated this risk with the development of moral character (both in themselves and in their students). Moreover, it is a risk that can become a source of instructive entertainment in the give and take environment of the hospitable classroom, where people learn that effort, devotion, offering a helping hand, and showing respect for others even when they make mistakes can all lead to an enjoyable educational experience. This is not to say, of course, that every moment of the teaching experience must generate amusement. Teaching is a serious calling, but that does not preclude it from being appropriately entertaining: that is, engaging.

The computer industry makes much of this fact as it advertises and sells its wares to schools, colleges, and universities. I know a number of teachers who, borrowing a phrase from Neil Postman, find the computer's increasing presence in the classroom to be, for the most part, just another way of "amusing ourselves to death."[2] Later on (chapter 10), when I offer a critical assessment of the computer as a tool for acknowledgment, I will address this assessment.

Here, however, I intend to take another small step in developing the claim that, as suggested in my discussion of *Ordinary People*, entertainment has a significant role to play in the teaching experience. I make this move as I elaborate on the larger issue of how teaching and acknowledgment are related.[3] This elaboration is structured with two additional sub-topics in mind: teaching as a "religious" activity, and the teacher as a giver and receiver of gifts. I will eventually offer a case study on the relationship between teaching and the life-giving gift of acknowledgment in order to continue to promote a concrete understanding of the workings of acknowledgment—an understanding rooted in that existential domain where the art of rhetoric makes its living: the everyday world of practice. I will speak again about this art and such related matters as consciousness, dwelling places, home, the caress, appropriateness, and self-acknowledgment. I will also be focusing on a related topic that has been mentioned in previous chapters but that has yet to be analyzed carefully as a feature of the workings of acknowledgment: death. This specific type of "ending" fuels the life-giving quality of acknowledgment. The experience of teaching offers itself as an exemplar of this fact of life.

Teaching as a "Religious" Activity

In light of the earlier discussion and critical assessment of Levinas's philosophy of the caress, it should make sense to speak of the "religious" nature of teaching. Recall that Levinas understands the source of teaching, its most original enactment, to be rooted in the otherness or alterity that marks human existence, awakens and provokes consciousness, and directs thought beyond any "totality"—any human-made conceptual system for understanding society, the world, or the universe. The Other speaks to us of infinity and more. In doing so, notes Levinas, it "does not offend like an opinion; it does not limit a mind in a way inadmissible to a philosopher." Rather its "mastery" shows itself in what it has *to say* about how we are held in a caress by something whose "height" transcends the most extended reach of human understanding and thereby encourages us to look forward and upward as we seek salvation from the burdens of everyday life. Institutionalized religion (which is not what is being referred to here) presupposes the workings of this saying, for this is how the notion of "God" comes to mind. Hence, Levinas maintains that "Teaching," in its most genuine, honorable, and sacred sense, "is not a species of a genus called domination, a hegemony at work within a totality [some institutionalized religion, for example], but is the presence of infinity breaking the closed circle of totality."[4]

To speak of the "religious" nature of teaching is to note how this vocation is dedicated to *opening* people to what is perceived to be the "truth" of some matter of interest so that they might better understand the matter, discuss it, and perhaps take issue with any claim being made regarding the matter and related concerns. The teacher is called to do this first and foremost by the otherness of existence, by that which is always calling us into question as temporal beings who are on their way to what is not yet, the future. The ethic of scientific inquiry and research that advocates the related obligations of being open-minded and self-critical when seeking the "truth" of whatever is under investigation is certainly a result of people paying homage and being responsive to this fundamental existential calling of the otherness of existence. The same can be said, of course, about the ethic of religious inquiry. In Judaism, for example, we find a particularly nuanced assessment of the matter.

Consider, for a moment, the words of Rabbi Abraham Heschel:

> Everything depends on the person who stands in the front of the classroom. The teacher is not an automatic fountain from which intellectual beverages may be obtained. He is either a witness or a stranger. To guide a pupil into the promised land, he must have

been there himself. When asking himself: Do I stand for what I
teach? Do I believe what I say? He must be able to answer in the af-
firmative.

What we need more than anything else is not *textbooks* but
textpeople. It is the personality of the teacher which is the text that
the pupils read; the text that they will never forget.[5]

These words echo the teachings of a three-thousand-year-old religion that would
have us be especially clear about what is meant here by the words "textpeople" and
"the personality of the teacher."

In Judaism, the importance of the text cannot be overemphasized. For such
holy texts as the Torah and the Talmud record how a people of faith engaged in
the hermeneutical and rhetorical process of hearing, interpreting, and communicating the Word of God. In Judaism, it is this Word—which includes the teaching
of how necessary it is to keep the process going for truth's sake—that comes before everything else. Levinas, for example, puts it this way:

> The Bible clarified and accentuated by the [Talmudic] commentar-
> ies from the great age that proceeds and follows the destruction of
> the Second Temple, when an ancient and uninterrupted tradition
> finally blossoms, is a book that leads us not toward the mystery of
> God, but toward the human tasks of man. Monotheism is a human-
> ism. Only simpletons made it into a theological arithmetic. The
> books in which this humanism is inscribed await their humanists.
> The task for those who wish to continue Judaism consists in having
> these books opened.[6]

The words of these books that must be read and interpreted over and over
again are the traditional refuge of the Jewish people. Jonathan Rosen expands on
this point in his discussion of the Talmud:

> The Talmud offered a virtual home for an uprooted culture, and
> grew out of the Jewish need to pack civilization into words and
> wander out into the world. The Talmud became essential for Jewish
> survival once the Temple—God's pre-Talmud home—was de-
> stroyed, and the Temple practices, those bodily rituals of blood and
> fire and physical atonement, could no longer be performed. When
> the Jewish people lost their home (the land of Israel) and God lost
> His (the Temple), then a new way of being was devised and Jews be-
> came the people of the book and not the people of the Temple or
> the land. They became the people of the book because they had no
> place else to live.[7]

A sense of Diaspora—a feeling of being everywhere and nowhere, homeless—is very much a part of Jewish life. It motivates a textpeoples' longing for community; hence, the practice of studying the Talmud "in pairs"—*hevruta*. Rosen, again, states the matter well: "The Aramaic word for a Talmudic study partner, has the same root as the word *haver*, which means 'friend.' Out of these study pairs a community is born and out of that community a society, and out of that society a whole world. The Talmud isn't read like a book but studied aloud, chanted, lived."[8]

In Judaism, *to live* the teachings (the Word) of God is to take them "to heart," embody them, grant them a dwelling place in one's being, provide them with a *person*-ality and an active character so that they can be seen, heard, understood, and perhaps even appropriated by others. This hermeneutical and rhetorical process marks the ultimate way to acknowledge that which is beyond description (*Ein Sof*) but still calls for symbolic effort on the part of human beings. For as Heschel notes, "The Bible speaks not only of man's search for God but also of God's search for man. 'Thou dost hunt me like a lion,' exclaimed Job (10:16). . . . This is the mysterious paradox of Biblical faith: *God is pursuing man*. It is as if God were unwilling to be alone, and He had chosen man to serve Him."[9] Levinas, we have seen, asks us to consider the possibility of how this choice shows itself in the way human existence is structured as a caress, a being-for others, and a call to share the life-giving gift of acknowledgment by assuming the vocation of being a teacher of good will, loving-kindness, and civic virtue. In the presence of such a person, we expect to see a robust amount of acknowledgment taking place between the teacher, his or her texts, and his or her students.

All academic disciplines that I am aware of pride themselves on having members who are textpeople, that is, teachers and scholars who are devoted to maintaining an openness towards their texts, students, and research endeavors. Although the type of personality that these people are supposed to display is likely to vary with the rules of decorum operating in their specific disciplines and in their own minds, the "textperson" is still recognized as possessing that "special something" that aids an audience in taking an interest in the topics and materials under consideration. The "famous" scholar/researcher who is so boring in the classroom that it is nearly impossible to remain open to the value of what is being taught is rightly called a "bad" teacher. Students sometimes associate the discomfort of having to listen to or read the words of such a teacher with the unpleasant experience of "chewing on a mohair sweater." Indeed, teachers can be "awfully dry" when they have yet to find a way to make their presentations interesting enough such that others are willing to *entertain* ("keep hold, or maintain in mind") all that is being said.

My way of phrasing this last point is important in that it obviously provides me with a way of returning to the issue of how entertainment has a significant role to play in the teaching experience. Teaching is a matter of being *engaging* rather than merely being *amusing*. The goal here thus requires some degree of rhetorical competence on the part of the teacher if he or she intends to be as effective as possible in getting others to reflect on and take seriously what she or he is explaining, discussing, critiquing, or maintaining to be the case. Teaching involves one in a process of evocation—a showing-forth of what is. The teacher/rhetor is obliged to demonstrate some command of epideictic discourse in order to open and move people to ideas and ideas to people.

"Where art thou?" In the classroom, the lecture hall, or the laboratory, this question comes silently from students and colleagues who are there to learn, seek help and direction in their studies, or just get their "money's worth." For any and all of these reasons, they thus await a response from the teacher: "Here I am!" The challenge before the teacher is one of acknowledgment, of transforming space and time in order to create a dwelling place where learning can happen in a caring (caressing) environment and where people can feel at home. Recognizing the importance of this task for the orator, Aristotle devoted book 2 of his *Rhetoric* to a discussion of the *pathe* (the emotions) and the ways in which they serve to attune our interests to our surroundings: According to Aristotle, the emotional character of human beings plays a crucial role in their development; it constitutes a person's spirited potential for coming to judge what is true, just, and virtuous. A moving of the passions is the sine qua non of critical judgment and persuasion; truth alone is not sufficient to guide the thoughtful actions of human beings.[10]

The teaching environment is energized and actualized by the emotional involvement that people have with each other and with their subjects of study. If engagement is to have priority over diversion, ideas need to be presented in an interesting way so that they will be taken seriously by students who await acknowledgment from a teacher who is obliged to give it. Teaching requires a commitment to being-for others. Therein lies its "religious" nature, which can and should be quite "entertaining" in the most awesome sense of this term: engaging others in an activity believed to be life-giving. The teacher is someone who must enter the scene bearing gifts and who, as will be discussed below, has the right to expect something worthwhile in return.

The Teacher as a Giver and Receiver of Gifts

The philosopher Calvin Schrag speaks of the "genuineness" of gift-giving as something that must be taken seriously if humankind is to cultivate a temperament of grace.

> A gift, to be genuinely a gift, is given without any expectation of return. There can be no expectation of a "countergift," for such would place the giving within the context of a contractual rather than a gift-giving relation. Certainly, if there is to be any countergift, a species of "gift exchange" if you will, the same gift that was given cannot be returned without annulling the very conditions of gift-giving, and

in the end amounting to a refusal of the gift. . . . *Mutatis mutandis*, from the side of the gift-reception, the receiver of a gift in accepting the gift needs to be freed from any obligations to reciprocate, for such would transform the gift into an incursion of a debt that requires repayment.[11]

Schrag would thus have us understand that the genuineness of the gift comes from "outside the economy, both economy in the narrower sense of monetary management and in the broader sense of motivating forces and requirements of reciprocity and exchange in the culture-spheres of scientific, artistic, ethico-moral, and religious-institutional endeavors."[12] Human beings are gifted with the capacity to be gift-givers, but the power (*dynamus*) of this capacity, according to Schrag, draws its authenticity from the even greater capacities of *caritas* and *agape* and the fundamental expression of "love" that they make possible—"a love that issues from a power to love in spite of rejection, a love that loves for the sake of loving," and hence a love that "is construed as freely given and nonpossessive in nature."[13]

Love is a gift that should be given with no catches and caveats. Schrag draws support for this claim by turning to such religious thinkers as Augustine, Kierkegaard, Tillich, and Levinas. It thus might be said that the gift of which Schrag speaks is one that is best understood by turning to the Holy Scriptures. Here it is told how a loving God, who at times could become quite angry, called us into being with a "Word" of acknowledgment that brought forth the truth of all that is. By way of this most glorious gift, God created the place wherein all other such gifts could be given by creatures with the capacity to do so. Schrag never explicitly states that he wants us to be god-like when it comes to giving gifts, although he would have us use "the measure of the gift of love" when determining how best to craft a "fitting response" to the exigencies of life. He thus tells us that the "fitting response, using the measure of the gift of love, responds by apprehending space as a habitat for deeds that *can be done*, concretely illustrated in random acts of kindness and mercy, in which one exemplifies the virtuous deed of a Good Samaritan, as well as in the collaborative social projects of selfless charity, institutionalized, for example, in the Habitat for Humanity program."[14]

Recalling his reading of Philip Hallie's *Lest Innocent Blood Be Shed: The Story of the Village of Le Chambon and How Goodness Happened There*, Schrag emphasizes the "sacrificial love" that the people of the village performed during World War II as they risked their own lives in order to help hide and thus save thousands of Jews from the Nazi horde. As Schrag puts it: "In this isolated village in Southern France there was a display of a gift that was unconditional, with its reward residing in the act of its being given." Schrag then goes on to note: "The story of Le Chambon, and others like it, stands as a reminder of the need to consult local narratives and case studies to illustrate how the gift can be given and received and how goodness can happen and justice be done within the economy of our civil societies."[15]

With all this in mind, I must take issue with my "teacher's" position.[16] Schrag speaks to us of a gift that ought to be given "without any expectation of return." With the Old Testament in mind, I must admit that I have a difficult time accepting this prescription. For, as Heschel reminds us with his reading of this holy text, it is not only God who acknowledges us, but we who, in turn, must acknowledge God.[17] From the very beginning, if you will, the loving gift of acknowledgment was given with an expectation of return. The gift thus brings with it an obligation to reciprocate. Schrag would have us see matters otherwise. The *giving* of the gift of acknowledgment defines an asymmetrical operation: the only thing that counts is the saying of "Here I am!" to those who call out "Where art thou?"[18] My much loved and respected teacher, Professor Schrag, is known for his belief that, when all the teaching and writing are done, "it is our students that should matter the most." As a student, however, I submit that those who have devoted themselves to their calling as much as this generous soul certainly deserve at least some small gift in return. Great teachers warrant heartfelt acknowledgment and remembrance, for that is how we keep them alive so that their wisdom and dedication can educate future generations of students.

Contrary to Professor Schrag, I maintain that reciprocity should be at work in the teaching situation. The teacher should be a giver *and* a receiver of the gift of acknowledgment. Students and colleagues who seek this life-giving gift from a teacher have an obligation to at least try to return the favor as a way of contributing to the dynamics and instructive potential of the classroom, thereby adding to the confidence, passion, and feeling of self-worth of the teacher. Schrag's theory of the gift emphasizes the importance of pure altruism on the part of the teacher. Although I commend this take on the matter, I do not think it is realistic given where we are on the evolutionary scale today. Pure altruism has not yet become a basic and inheritable trait of the human species. We have only advanced to the biological stage of being capable of feeling good when we do a good deed or at least think a good thought. Owing to our intellectual and psychological capabilities, we are also capable of cultivating this good feeling in our social and political environments. Billions of years after the Big Bang, we have reached the stage where we can ask the question and value (if not dread) its answer: What if no one cared enough to take the time to open himself or herself to you and acknowledge your existence?[19]

Human beings need acknowledgment; and those with academic egos, perhaps, need it more than most. Working under the credo of "the teacher/scholar" model, teachers must display a high degree of competence in the classroom (as measured by student and peer evaluations) while also registering their wisdom in peer-reviewed publications that are meant to demonstrate expertise in specific areas of research and scholarship. This is how teachers keep their jobs and advance their careers. I know of no teacher who does not feel "good" when he or she succeeds in these tasks. The feeling of "self-worth" that accompanies this feeling of goodness, I think it is fair to say, adds fuel to the teacher's desire to continue to improve on the performance of his or her vocation so that, among other things, he or she will become more competent in enacting acknowledgment. In the classroom, whenever possible, acknowledgment should beget acknowledgment for the benefit of all.

I say this as someone who, in trying to answer the call of teaching in a professional way for the past twenty-eight years, has not only benefited from the lifegiving gift of acknowledgment offered by students and colleagues, but has also experienced the horrible feeling of failure that comes with the realization that I am not being a good enough teacher/scholar for a lot of people who are paying a lot of money to be in my classroom so that they can learn what I contend is important. Fueled by the embarrassment that can accompany this failure, the feeling can be so overwhelming at times that, as the saying goes, "I just want to die." Yet, despite the dread it imposes, the feeling is not without positive potential. For it is this feeling that attests to the teacher's biological and intellectual ability to care enough about what he or she is doing that a sub-par performance will be recognized for what it is and remedied by someone who, through an act of self-acknowledgment, has become quite aware of what it takes to do a better job. Theologians and scientists have long attempted to trace these related abilities back to a Big Bang and what instigated it. My task here is just an attempt to make sure that we remember how a certain life-giving gift is central to such praiseworthy endeavors and to the teaching associated with them.

"Where art thou?" Teachers and students must ask this question of each other and respond in kind: "Here I am!" In the teaching situation, acknowledgment is not a one-way street. Support for this claim is found in Professor Mark Edmundson's candid essay "On the Uses of a Liberal Education: As Lite Entertainment for Bored College Students."[20] Edmundson, who teaches in the Department of English at the University of Virginia, begins his essay with this observation:

> Today is evaluation day in my Freud class, and everything has changed. The class meets twice a week, late in the afternoon, and the clientele, about fifty undergraduates, tends to drag in and slump, looking disconsolate and a little lost, waiting for a jump start. To get the discussion moving, they usually require a joke, an anecdote, an off-the-wall question—When you were a kid, were your Halloween getups ego costumes, id costumes, or superego costumes? That sort of thing. But today, as soon as I flourish the forms, a buzz rises in the room. Today they write their assessments of the course, their assessment of *me*, and they are without a doubt wide-awake. "What is your evaluation of the instructor?" asks question number eight, entreating them to circle a number between five (excellent) and one

(poor, poor). Whatever interpretive subtlety they've acquired during the term is now out the window. Edmundson: one to five, stand and shoot. . . .

[The students are] playing the informed consumer, letting the provider know where he's come through and where he's not quite up to snuff. (39)

Edmundson goes on to explain that "chances are the evaluations will be much like what they've been in the past—they'll be just fine." He will be credited with being "interesting," "relaxed and tolerant," "humorous," and "capable" when it comes to connecting "the arcana of the subject matter with current culture." But Edmundson is still "distressed" by the moment:

> I have to admit that I do not much like the image of myself that emerges from these forms, the image of knowledgeable, humorous detachment and bland tolerance. I do not like the forms themselves, with their number ratings, reminiscent of the sheets circulated after the TV pilot has just played to its sample audience in Burbank. Most of all I dislike the attitude of calm consumer expertise that pervades the responses. I'm disturbed by the serene belief that my function—and, more important, Freud's, or Shakespeare's, or Blake's—is to divert, entertain, and interest. Observes one respondent, not at all unrepresentative: "Edmundson has done a fantastic job of presenting this difficult, important & controversial material in an enjoyable and approachable way."
>
> Thanks but no thanks. I don't teach to amuse, to divert, or even, for that matter, to be merely interesting. When someone says she "enjoyed" the course—and that word crops up again and again in my evaluations—somewhere at the edge of my immediate complacency I feel encroaching self-dislike. . . . I want some of [my students] to say that they've been changed by the course. I want them to measure themselves against what they've read. . . . Why are my students describing the Oedipus complex and death drive as being interesting and enjoyable to contemplate? And why am I coming across as an urbane, mildly ironic, endlessly affable guide to this intellectual territory, operating without intensity, generous, funny, and loose?
>
> Because that's what works. On evaluation day, I reap the rewards of my partial compliance with the culture of my students and, too, with the culture of the university as it now operates. (39–40)

The remainder of Edmundson's essay is devoted to a discussion of how the student culture brings "a consumer *weltanschauung* to school, where it exerts a powerful, and largely unacknowledged, influence." Edmundson, however, is very much into acknowledgment. He writes to reveal how and why on "good days" his students "display a light, appealing glow; on bad days, shuffling disgruntlement. But there's little fire, little passion to be found."(40). And why should there be? The students were attracted to a university whose "marketing department" learned from the students themselves what sells and what does not. "Is it surprising," writes Edmundson, "that someone who has been approached with photos and tapes, bells and whistles, might come in thinking that the Freud and Shakespeare she had signed up to study were also going to be agreeable treats?" (44).

Edmundson has "some" praise for his students. "At their best," they are "decent." They believe in "equality." They "volunteer to tutor poor kids to get a stripe on their resume" and "they also want other people to have a fair shot. . . . If I were on trial and innocent," admits Edmundson, "I'd want them on the jury" (42). Still, Edmundson is distressed. His students and university are too caught up in the "cool consumer culture" whose "laid back" style maintains a "whatever" attitude, at least until something happens that is not advantageous to making it big in the marketplace after graduation. Edmundson mentions the "Socratic method" being used in class as an example of this type of interruption. For this method

> —the animated, sometimes impolite give-and-take between student and teacher—seems too jagged for current sensibilities. Students frequently come to my office to tell me how intimidated they feel in class; the thought of being embarrassed in front of the group fills them with dread. I remember a student telling me how humiliating it was to be corrected by the teacher, by me. So I asked the logical question: "Should I let a major factual error go by so as to save discomfort?" The student—a good student, smart and earnest—said that was a tough question. He'd need to think about it. (45)

Edmundson wants more from his students than such a disappointing response. He wants genuine acknowledgment. He wants students in his classes who are there to learn, not those who just stroke his ego and only do what it takes to get an "A." No, he wants passionate students who are rhetorically competent and who are willing to put themselves on the line in order to defend and critique important matters like "democracy" and "genius." For Edmundson, the two go hand in hand: "A democracy needs to constantly develop, and to do so it requires the most powerful visionary minds [genius] to interpret the present and to propose possible shapes for the future. . . . If we teachers do not endorse genius and self-overcoming, can we be surprised when our students find their ideal images in TV's latest persona ads?" (49).

Yes, Edmundson is distressed. His students joyfully inhabit a university that offers itself as "a cross between summer camp and lotusland" and whose administrators are pleased by how content the students are with their entertaining sur-roundings and interactions (46). Campus life defines a dwelling place where asking "Where art thou?" is most welcomed and expected by students as long as no strenuous demands accompany their saying of "Here I am!" But this is not the way it is supposed to be, especially if the teaching experience is to produce genuine acknowledgment that allows students and their teachers to dwell together, know together, and reap the rewards of giving and receiving a life-giving gift. Edmundson thus asks his colleagues to join him in an important task: "We professors talk a lot about subversion, which generally means subverting the views of people who never hear us talk or read our work. But to subvert the views of our students, our customers, that would be something else again." And as a way of taking the lead, Edmundson ends his essay by sharing what he specifically intends to do.

> As for myself, I'm canning my low-key one-liners; when the kids'
> TV-based tastes come to the fore, I'll aim and shoot. And when it's
> time to praise genius, I'll try to do it in the right style, full-out, with
> faith that finer artistic spirits (maybe not Homer and Isaiah quite,
> but close, close), still alive somewhere in the ether, will help me out
> when my invention flags, the students doze, or the dean mutters
> into the phone. I'm getting back to a more exuberant style; I'll be
> expostulating and arm waving straight into the millennium, yes I
> will. (49)

Notice that Edmundson's plan for self-improvement includes the development of rhetorical competence ("the right style"). I will return to this point shortly.

Edmundson's essay is an assigned reading in my undergraduate/graduate seminar on communication ethics. The students love it for multiple reasons. First, in their opinion, he speaks the truth. His description of students is "right on"; they recognize themselves in much of what he has to say about their "whatever" attitudes and "consumer mentality." As one student put it: "It's kind of cool and admittedly refreshing to enjoy being embarrassed by who you are, at least sometimes." This admission is encouraging because it signals that students are open to the possibility of improving their ability to give (and not merely receive) acknowledgment. Second, they like the way Edmundson is wise enough to recognize that the problem is not just their fault but is also fueled by university officials and parents who have an overly economical view about what it means to get their money's worth. They especially appreciate his honesty in admitting, in a moment of self-acknowledgment, how he has also contributed to the problem. He is practicing what he preaches. Third, the students enjoy Edmundson's rhetorical competence, his way with words. He makes the topic interesting, captivating, and engaging by having the guts to speak his mind in a "perceptive," "creative," "instructive," sometimes "brilliant," and "entertaining" way. Now "that's entertainment!" Of course, I agree. Edmundson's essay is a "must read" for anyone interested in the student-teacher relationship and the acknowledgment that should hold it together.

Finally, the students take special pleasure in pointing out a paradox in Edmundson's way of expressing his thoughts. To quote one student: "Edmundson's entertaining style of writing appears to be the very thing that he professes he wants to eliminate in himself, his colleagues, and his students. And notice how this style is employed as a padding through which he softens his 'offensive' message. In doing this, however, he becomes offensive to his own ideals." The paradox would not exist, however, if Edmundson was more careful in his understanding and use of the word "entertainment," which, as I have tried to suggest, refers not only to amusing and mindless things but also to a phenomenon that, by way of rhetorical competence, can help promote the expression and reception of a life-giving gift.

Yes, "the right style"—a fitting and appropriate way with words that helps to transform space and time into a dwelling place, a habitat of learning where we can feel at home in our being-with-and-for others. The teaching experience lives and dies on how well acknowledgment is cultivated in the classroom, lecture hall, and laboratory between people, their topics, and their texts.

Life and Death

The phrasing of this last point is important for my purposes. Related as it is to the cultivation of acknowledgment, teaching *is* a matter of life and death. Edmundson is distressed over something that is dying in his students, his university, and himself. Bringing it back to life calls on the rhetorical competence of the teacher who, among other things, is an instructor of this art for his or her students and colleagues. What would your life be like if no one acknowledged your existence? Teachers and students most likely know the hurt of that sinking, life-sapping feeling that wells up when acknowledgment is being snuffed out by the ideas and actions of uncaring others. The power of the life-giving gift of acknowledgment lies in its ontological status, the way human existence is structured as a caress that is fated to break down sooner or later and eventually lose its hold altogether on the lives of we finite beings.

Acknowledgment, teaching, life, and death: From Adam to Moses to Jesus, the Bible is filled with stories that instruct us about the relationship that holds between these phenomena. Within the teaching profession, Socrates provides the most famous exemplar.

Socrates associates his call to teach with a "prophetic voice" that first came to him in early childhood and remained his "constant companion."[21] The voice commanded his "service to God" (23b), which he took to mean that his life's calling must be that of "leading the philosophical life" (28e), of "elucidating the truth" for others (29d), and encouraging them "not to think more of practical advantages than of . . . [their] mental and moral well-being" (36c). To those who accused him of corrupting the minds of the youth, Socrates said, "I am . . . a gift from God" (31a). He could not say this if he did not believe it to be true, he said, for the voice always spoke up and prevented him from committing any wrongdoing (40a–b). When the call came, lying was out of the question. Although he accepted being called an "orator" as long as the term was defined to mean "one who speaks the truth" (17b), Socrates "would much rather die" as the result of his philosophical ways and commitments than engage himself in the unethical maneuvers of sophistry (38d–e). The voice, his constant companion, never balked at this decision. In the *Phaedo*, he explains how it is "natural that a man who has really devoted his life to philosophy [and hence to the struggle of finding out what it means to live and to teach the good life] should be cheerful in the face of death, and confident of finding the greatest blessing in the next world when his life is finished."[22] After he was found guilty of corruption and just before he drank the hemlock at an earlier hour than was necessary, Socrates informed his friends that "I should only make myself ridiculous in my own eyes if I clung to life and hugged it when it has no more to offer" (117a). Again, no objection came forth from his inner voice. A life without philosophy and teaching is supposedly not worth living. Socrates had lived a good life. Now it was time to die a good death, surrounded by loved ones and true friends who, according to Socrates, should realize that although "it is not legitimate to do oneself violence," putting "an end to ourselves" is justified whenever "God sends some compulsion like the one which we are facing now" (61d–62c).

From the standpoint of the Judeo-Christian tradition, Socrates' words and actions make sense. For in this tradition it is taught that

> Our greatest problem is not how to continue but how to return. "How can I repay unto the Lord all his bountiful dealing with me?" (Psalm 116:12). When life is an answer, death is a home-coming.
>
> The deepest wisdom man can attain is to know that his destiny is to aid, to serve [to be for others]. . . . This is the meaning of death: the ultimate self-dedication to the divine. Death so understood will not be distorted by the craving for immortality, for this act of giving away is reciprocity on man's part for God's gift of life. For the pious man it is a privilege to die.[23]

Socrates was a teacher to the very end, dedicating himself to assisting others in giving birth to ideas. Commenting on the dialectical method that Socrates used to elicit, draw out, and evoke these ideas, Levinas emphasizes how this method is faithful to "the openness of the very dimension of infinity" that leaves a trace of itself in the otherness or alterity that marks human existence and that calls for acknowledgment.[24] Socrates opened himself and his students to this call. Heidegger speaks of Socrates as "the purest thinker of the West" and emphasizes the importance of his contribution to an understanding of the difficult demands placed on those who are called to teach:

> Teaching is even more difficult than learning. We know that; but we rarely think about it. And why is teaching more difficult than learning? Not because the teacher must have a larger store of information, and have it always ready. Teaching is more difficult than learning because what teaching calls for is this: to let learn. The real teacher . . . is ahead of his apprentices in this alone, that he has still far more to learn than they—he has to learn to let them learn. The teacher must be capable of being more teachable than the apprentices. . . . If the relation between the teacher and the taught is genuine, therefore, there is never a place in it for the authority of the know it all or the authoritative sway of the official. It is still an exalted matter, then, to become a teacher—which is something else entirely than becoming a famous professor.[25]

To say that the teacher has to learn to let students learn is to emphasize how acknowledgment *must* take place in the teaching situation. Recall that for Heidegger, "acknowledgment lets that toward which it goes come toward it"—which is to say that the teacher must remain *open* to his or her students and what they are saying and not saying about the issues at hand. Learning presupposes the openness that acknowledgment makes possible between teachers and students, their texts and topics, and their own selves (e.g., being able, in a moment of self-acknowledgment, to recognize our own faults and shortcomings). Moreover, the teacher has the additional responsibility of finding ways to encourage and cultivate this openness by way of his or her rhetorical competence. Remember, it is the "art of eloquence" that instructs us on how to present knowledge of a subject in such a way that it can assume a publicly accessible form, and function effectively in the social and political arena. Rhetoric offers itself as a tool for opening people to the teachings of philosophy, religion, science, or whatever discipline is on the line and whose members seek acknowledgment for what they have to say about the worth of their endeavors.

The so-called "bottom line" for such worthiness is inevitably tied to how well some domain of expertise contributes to the *ethos* and quality of life of human beings so that these beings can do a better job in taking care of themselves, others (be they human or not), and their environments. Acknowledgment *is* a life-giving gift. Whether it is given or received inside or outside of the classroom, this gift must always be appreciated against the backdrop of that which is also a necessary part of life: its ending, our Being-towards-death. It is life's ending that makes anything that comes before it worthwhile and thus worth teaching to and for others. Teaching, acknowledgment, and death go hand in hand. Teachers and students must do their jobs before it is too late.

As a way of bringing together all that has been said so far about the relationship between teaching, acknowledgment, and death, I now offer a brief case study in which these three phenomena are right before us, at work in the true story of a teacher and one of his students. The case has all of the ingredients of acknowledgment that have been covered in the previous chapters: the attunement of consciousness, the transformation of space and time into dwelling places, the home, the caress, and the related rhetorical issues of appropriateness and entertainment. The element of death will be obvious in this case; it concerns a much loved college teacher who is dying and a one time student of his who tells the story of their last "class" together. The story *Tuesdays with Morrie: An Old Man, A Young Man, and Life's Greatest Lesson*, by sports columnist and national best selling author Mitch Albom, continues to receive much acclaim from its readers.[26] I begin the case study by sharing some of my initial reactions to the book.

A Case Study

Many students, colleagues, and friends encouraged me to read *Tuesdays with Morrie* before I took the time to do so. They eagerly raved about the book to me mainly because they thought it spoke to issues raised in my teaching and writing, such related topics as rhetoric, conscience, medicine, and the euthanasia debate. Still, I was not particularly interested in reading the book for two reasons. First, having been told what this nationally best selling book was about, I did not think at the time that it would have much to say that was new. I was already quite familiar with the scholarly and popular literature on "living the good life and dying the good death." I had been keeping up with this literature since 1981, the year my greatest teacher, my father, suffered complete kidney failure. For the next four years he lived a hellish life: his body and mind never took kindly to the required regimen of high-tech medicine and psychiatric care. He died in 1984. Although not as much as my mother, I journeyed with him as things continued to get worse. Hence, my second reason for ignoring the suggestions of others: I didn't need yet another author telling me about the experience of being with a loved one who is dying; I had already lived the experience and carried the psychological scars to prove it. When I finally did read the book, I was not disappointed, although there was something about the story that bothered me.

There was Morrie Schwartz, the professor of sociology, dying and confined to his house, but remaining happy and inspirational as his body was slowly being overwhelmed by the progression of Lou Gehrig's Disease (amyotrophic lateral sclerosis or ALS). And there was Mitch who, upon finding out about Morrie's illness, traveled seven hundred miles by plane and rental car to his house every Tuesday for fourteen weeks so that he, alone, could take one more class from his famous and favorite college professor. The topic of the class was "The Meaning of Life," which "was taught from experience."

> No grades were given, but there were oral exams each week. You were expected to respond to questions, and you were expected to pose questions of your own. You were also required to perform physical tasks now and then, such as lifting the professor's head to a comfortable spot on the pillow or placing his glasses on the bridge of his nose. Kissing him good-bye earned you extra credit. . . . Although no final exam was given, you were expected to produce one long paper on what was learned. (1–2)

From this class came *Tuesdays with Morrie*, a book intended to acknowledge the life and times of a great acknowledger.

What bothered me about this book emerged in the context of the memories of my father's illness; the years of fieldwork I had spent in hospitals and intensive care units; and the interviews with doctors, nurses, theologians, medical ethicists, patients and their family members, who were all willing to share with me and members of my research team their stories about winning and losing the "battles" with serious illnesses and accidents. The war metaphor looms large in the history and practice of medicine and also in the lives of those who medicine is obliged to serve. It is awesome to witness and hear first hand accounts of the joy that accompanies the winning of these battles. Some people even talk about how their outcomes were "miracles." But with war also comes casualties and haunting memories.

I found it hard to believe that Albom's professor could continue to be so joyful and inspirational with full knowledge of all that ALS was destined to do to him. Inspired by his teacher, Albom spoke of the disease this way:

> ALS is like a lit candle; it melts your nerves and leaves your body a pile of wax. Often, it begins with the legs and works its way up. You lose control of your thigh muscles, so that you cannot support yourself standing. You lose control of your trunk muscles, so that you cannot sit up straight. By the end, if you are still alive, you are breathing through a tube in a hole in your throat, while your soul, perfectly awake, is imprisoned inside a limp husk, perhaps able to blink, or cluck a tongue, like something from a science fiction movie, the man frozen inside his own flesh. (10)

Albom then goes on to relate how his

> old professor had made a profound decision, one he began to construct the day he came out of the doctor's office with a sword hanging over his head. *Do I wither up and disappear, or do I make the best*

of my time left? he had asked himself.

He would not wither. He would not be ashamed of dying.

Instead, he would make death his final project, the center point of his days. Since everyone was going to die, he could be of great value, right? He could be research. A human textbook. *Study me in my slow and patient demise. Watch what happens to me. Learn with me.*

Morrie would walk that final bridge between life and death, and narrate the trip. (10)

As I have elsewhere admitted (when writing about an ALS patient who exhibited similar resoluteness), I find such a devoted and courageous attitude to be the source of a heroism that is necessary if the moral consciousness of humanity is to prosper.[27] Still, Morrie's story sounded too perfect. Here was a person who dreaded the fact that, owing to his disease "one day soon, someone's gonna have to wipe [his] ass" (22). That day had come and, for Morrie, it was "the ultimate sign of dependency. Someone wiping your bottom." But Morrie was determined: "I'm trying to enjoy the process." Albom was surprised. "Enjoy it?" he asked cynically. "Yes," replied Morrie. "After all, I get to be a baby one more time" (49). *Really?*

I remember my father telling me how complication from his dialysis treatments sometimes resulted in him becoming so "impacted" that a nurse would have to stick her hand far up into his anal cavity and "pull out all the shit" that he couldn't push out himself. My father was a proud and great man. He died a hero. But because of the "humiliating" situations that plagued him throughout the four years of his illness, he sometimes required psychiatric treatment. The first time I visited him in the psychiatric ward, he stared at me and cried: "Look what they've done to your Daddy." It was the saddest moment I ever shared with my father.

Throughout his book, Albom makes sure that we know that Morrie's situation was grueling and sad. We also learn that Morrie's suffering would sometimes lead the professor to cry because he felt bad for himself. Albom writes about the day the "seventy something" Morrie and his wife, Charlotte, received the diagnosis of ALS. "Charlotte had a million thoughts running through her mind: *How much time do we have left? How will we manage? How will we pay the bills?*" As for Morrie, he was "stunned by the normalcy of the day around him. *Shouldn't the world stop? Don't they know what has happened to me?*" "But the world did not stop," writes Albom, "it took no notice at all . . . [and Morrie] felt as if he were dropping into a hole" (8). Indeed, such lack of acknowledgment can be both painful and terrifying.

The same thing happened to my mother and father when he was rushed to a hospital's intensive care unit for dialysis treatment after his kidneys first shut down. But their questions never stopped as the days, weeks, months, and years went by. My father—despite periods marked by calm, hope, and a lot of love from family and friends—continued "dropping into a hole." Like ALS, renal failure and its physiological, psychological, social, and economic consequences go on every hour of the day; they are not things that can be carefully observed, acknowledged, and fully appreciated by being in the presence of the dying patient for only one day a week.

I cannot believe that *Tuesdays with Morrie* tells the whole story of this man's battle with ALS. Albom is a wonderful writer and story-teller and his weekly visits to his teacher's home say much about who he is as a caring soul, loving friend, and devoted student. But I am certain that his work has holes in it. Yet, for my purposes, that makes it all the more relevant.

Albom's work defines an effort in epideictic rhetoric: he writes in praise of a teacher who helped change his life for the better. As will be discussed in greater detail below, this change is rooted in Morrie's powers of acknowledgment. Albom writes in order to return the favor with the same life-giving gift, thereby helping to secure his teacher's wisdom and loving-kindness in the minds and memories of others. Human beings like to think that they will be remembered after they are gone for whatever good they have done. They are fated to develop this desire because of the ontological structure of their existence, be it a result of the mysterious workings of God or of the more scientifically and mathematically grounded theories of the Big Bang and evolution.

Morrie is dying as he teaches a course on "The Meaning of Life" to one student, someone who has heard him say "I want to tell you about my life. I want to tell you before I can't tell you anymore. . . . I want someone to hear my story. Will you?" (63). Morrie, who wants his tombstone to read "A Teacher to the Last" (134), is seeking acknowledgment. With tape-recorder in hand, Mitch is there to hear and respond to the call so that he can complete the course's final assignment of writing "one long paper" on all that he has learned. The issue of rhetorical competence is thus at hand: How is Albom to construct and compose his paper so that it tells, thereby showing-forth, the story of a wonderful human being? Acknowledgment and rhetorical competence are, indeed, related. Thus another necessary and related question: What is the most fitting and thus most appropriate way to speak of both Morrie's life and death?

As orators like Pericles and Lincoln made abundantly clear in their respective and famous eulogies of their fallen comrades, it takes talent to speak about those who have passed away but who still warrant heart-felt acknowledgment (no matter what shortcomings they may have displayed while alive). Pericles and Lincoln spoke about courage against the backdrop of war. Albom must also consider the war that Morrie is fighting yet losing against a horrible disease. But with this rhetorical situation the main character wants to be known as nothing less than a devoted teacher trying to inspire moral consciousness. Consider this exchange between Morrie and Mitch.

"Mitch," he said, "the culture doesn't encourage you to think about such things until you're about to die. We're so wrapped up with egotistical things, career, family, having enough money, meeting the mortgage, getting a new car, fixing the radiator when it breaks—we're involved in trillions of little acts just to keep going: So we don't get into the habit of standing back and looking at our lives and saying, Is this all? Is this all I want? Is something missing?"

He paused.

"You need someone to probe you in that direction. It won't just happen automatically."

I knew what he was saying. We all need teachers in our lives. And mine was sitting in front of me. (64–65)

Mitch must figure out a way to write a story about a teacher and a student who knew him to be a model for educators and students alike. In telling the story, Mitch also must take on the role of being a good teacher—one who can write a story that is moving and memorable. In order to perform such an act of acknowledgment, we might expect Mitch to have a host of related concerns in mind, topics that have been addressed in earlier chapters and that his professor was supposedly a master of: attuning consciousness, creating dwelling places, making others feel at home, holding on to people in appropriate and entertaining ways. The problem of saying too much or too little about Morrie and his ongoing situation thus demanded attention. In order to tell the truth about his subject, must Albom disclose *everything* about Morrie's life and times, his disease, and his good and bad moments during the class? Clearly, this is not what epideictic rhetoric is supposed to do. When its evocative power is directed toward saying something good about a person, such rhetoric is only obligated to express matters in such a way that something of their truth remains memorable as a source of wisdom, inspiration, justice, and moral integrity. Albom was called on to be a rhetorical architect, not a medical scientist. He had to display an artistic sense of knowing what to emphasize and what not to emphasize, what to speak of and what to remain silent on, and how to tell a moving story that is not so moving that it becomes too difficult to continue reading. I should not fault Albom for leaving things out of his story as long as these omissions, if added to the narrative, would not call his assessment of the truth of his subject matter and the competence of his rhetorical skills into question. Such competence definitely informs Morrie's story—the story of one student's hero.

We live in a world that places high value on being a celebrity, where "career advisors" teach us that "it really doesn't matter if your good famous or bad famous" as long as you can become a well-recognized "face" and a source of entertainment.[28] Albom considers Morrie a hero, a man of great dignity and integrity, not a mere celebrity seeking fame by being amusing. When first remarking on his professor's presence, however, Albom does depict Morrie as being a source of amusement:

> He is a small man who takes small steps, as if a strong wind could, at any time, whisk him up into the clouds. In his graduation day robe, he looks like a cross between a biblical prophet and a Christmas elf. He has sparkling blue-green eyes, thinning silver hair that spills onto his forehead, big ears, a triangular nose, and tufts of graying eyebrows. Although his teeth are crooked and his lower ones are slanted back—as if someone had once punched them in—when he smiles it's as if you'd just told him the first joke on earth. (3–4)

With this description of Morrie's presence, face, and the expressiveness of his being, Albom begins the rhetorical feat of bringing his teacher back to life so that readers can believe that, yes, this character is real, somebody who they can identify with, admire, and fondly remember. Morrie is a hero, although he does not look like one. But, as Levinas reminds us, the "face" of a hero encompasses more than the body's physical attributes; it is also informed by a person's moral character.

The demonstration of moral character in everyday life prompts the dawning and attuning of consciousness in others. With a person's heroic actions, we learn of ways of acknowledging and being-for others. Moreover, the hero has much to teach us about a fact of life and death: *Ars moriendi* is *ars vivendi*—the "art of dying" is the "art of living." Morrie makes much of this fact in his class with Mitch: "To know you're going to die, and to be *prepared* for it at any time" encourages you to "be more involved in your life while you're living"; for "[t]he truth is . . . once you learn how to die, you learn how to live" (81–82). Dr. Sherwin Nuland, in his award-winning book *How We Die: Reflections on Life's Final Chapter*, makes the point rather well: "The honesty and grace of the years of life that are ending is the real measure of how we die. It is not in the last week or days that we compose the message that will be remembered, but in all the decades that preceded them. Who has lived in dignity, dies in dignity."[29] Morrie has lived a dignified life and now intends to die a dignified death. It is altogether the right, fitting, and thus appropriate thing to do—something that certainly warrants acknowledgment in the most appropriate way possible.

Albom's ability to be appropriate when writing about his professor is most evident in his talent for telling what I have termed elsewhere a good "person story" rather than an expert "body story."[30] Both types of stories are always called for when treating and speaking about those who are under the ontological assault of some disease. Physicians are obligated, first and foremost, to construct an expert body story, for it is the body—the place where a disease happens—that must assume priority as a matter of interest to those who hope to find a cure. Body stories are designed to cut through the personhood (the everyday, existential trials and

tribulations) of the patient like a scalpel, leaving intact only those portions of the
patient's history that can be used to make a good case about some disease, in some
body, in some bed. Medical case histories mark out an effort in dissection directed
toward offering a depersonalized perception and account of the patient. They are
prized for their self-effacing objectivity and efficiency, both of which are communicated via the antiseptic language of "disease theory" and what it has to say about
the sick body. As for the person who owns this body, that, again, is a different
story. For such a person (at least if he or she is not in a persistent vegetative state)
is more than the flesh, bone, and blood of their body; they are also a living history
filled with memories, meaningful relationships, fears, hopes, dreams, and other
subjectively valued things. This is the stuff of person stories, material that is
known to get in the way of a well-told, analytic, and unambiguous body story.

With the progression of a currently incurable disease such as ALS, however,
the two types of stories can easily merge, resulting in a horrific "illness story" that
is extremely difficult to watch or read. Standing face-to-face with someone whose
body speaks so readily of wounded humanity, we must acknowledge and come to
terms with our own finitude. As soon as we are born, we are old enough to die.
Being reminded of this fact of life, of how our bodies are fated to break down, we
are likely to undergo the psychological experience of "annihilation anxiety," where
the future is known primarily by a sorrowful if not terrifying name: death. People
like Morrie are not ready to die, but reactions to their presence can often make
them feel that their life "is not worth living."

Albom has to find a way of speaking about Morrie that is engaging, not
overwhelming; entertaining, not merely amusing. The closest he comes to telling a
pure body story is when he describes, as noted above, how "ALS is like a lit candle;
it melts your nerves and leaves your body a pile of wax. . . ." Morrie is not mentioned in this description. Here, however, is an example of what happens to the
narrative when Morrie enters the scene:

> Since my last visit, a nurse had inserted a catheter into his penis,
> which drew the urine out through a tube and into a bag that sat at the
> foot of his chair. His legs needed constant tending (he could still feel
> pain, even though he could not move them, another one of ALS's
> cruel little ironies), and unless his feet dangled just the right number
> of inches off the foam pads, it felt as if someone were poking him
> with a fork. In the middle of conversations, Morrie would have to ask
> visitors to lift his foot and move it just an inch, or to adjust his head so
> that it fit more easily into the palm of the colored pillows. Can you
> imagine being unable to move your own head? (130–131)

The scene is pitiful and becomes even more distressing when you recall how ALS
eventually works its way up the body, making simple things like hand gestures and

speaking impossible. Morrie admits feeling a sense of dread: "What am I going to do without my hands? What happens when I can't speak? . . . They're such an essential part of me. I talk with my voice. I gesture with my hands. This is how I give to people" (70).

Morrie is a very giving person, an acknowledger second to none. To speak of this aspect of Morrie's being is to begin telling a person story, and this is mostly what Albom's book is: a story about a person who loves giving a certain gift to others even as he is losing control of his body. "[G]iving to other people is what makes me feel alive," says Morrie, "not my car or my home. Not what I look like in the mirror. When I give my time, when I can make someone smile after they were feeling sad, it's as close to healthy as I ever feel" (128). "If I can't give them the right attention, I can't help them" (132). Albom elaborates on his teacher's generosity: "When Morrie was with you, he was really with you. He looked you straight in the eye, and he listened as if you were the only person in the world. How much better would people get along if their first encounter each day were like this—instead of a grumble from a waitress or a bus driver or a boss?" (135). Albom remembers being taught this idea by Morrie back in college and admits that it was "more important than almost everything" else he learned in any of his other classes. Albom writes: "I believe many visitors in the last few months of Morrie's life were drawn not because of the attention they wanted to pay him but because of the attention he paid *to them*. Despite his personal pain and decay, this little old man listened the way they always wanted someone to listen" (137–138).

Human beings are in need of acknowledgment and, in their "goodness," are capable of returning the favor. Happiness is associated with the certainty of being needed. Morrie has a life-giving gift for others: he listens to them and makes them feel needed. It is not until the sixth Tuesday meeting that we learn that Morrie, too, has this need, although it is not Morrie himself who admits it. Rather, it is his devoted wife who acknowledges this fact when she explains to Mitch how his presence is helping her husband: "He looks forward to your visits. He talks about having to do this project with you, how he has to concentrate and put the time aside. I think it's giving him a good sense of purpose . . ." (101). Indeed, human beings are purposeful creatures. When they have nothing to do they get bored. When they wake up in the morning and see no reason for getting out of bed they are in trouble. We need to be needed. Morrie is no exception. That Albom does not explicitly admit as much may be the result of Morrie never saying it directly "for the record." The closest the professor comes to acknowledging this personal need is when he is explaining to Mitch how one "really" gains "satisfaction" in life by "Offering others what you have to give." In responding to Mitch's cynical reply—"You sound like a Boy Scout"—Morrie goes on to explain: "I don't mean money, Mitch. I mean your time. Your concern. Your storytelling. It's not so hard. . . . There are plenty of places to do this. . . You play cards with a lonely older man and you find new respect for yourself, because you are needed" (126–127). In the eyes of students and friends like Mitch, Morrie may be a saint, but remember how Heschel puts it: even "God is in search of man." Perhaps Mitch chose not to expand on the matter because he thought that the need to be needed represented a weakness in people, and given what Morrie was willing to endure, the word "weakness" was not appropriate.

Before commenting further on this possibility, it is important to make sure (especially given the purpose of the present chapter) that the reader appreciates the significance of Morrie's way of being-for others. Morrie is a dedicated teacher. Even in his deteriorating state, he is a living response to a question: "Where art thou?" Morrie says "Here I am!" by giving others "the right [appropriate] attention," listening and remaining open to them, and thereby creating a dwelling place where he and others can feel at home as they consider and discuss matters of importance and learn to care for each other's ideas. Genuine acknowledgment requires nothing less than this entertaining process of engagement. Morrie puts it this way to Mitch:

> So many people walk around with a meaningless life. They seem half-asleep, even when they're busy doing things they think are important. This is because they're chasing the wrong things. The way you get meaning into your life is to devote yourself to loving others, devote yourself to your community around you, and devote yourself to creating something that gives you purpose and meaning. (43)

Recalling Levinas's teachings, we might describe the philosophy being espoused here as genuinely "religious," although I have heard some of my students call it "corny" and refer to it as "chicken soup for the soul."

I do not dismiss such assessments because similar words popped into my mind a time or two when I first read the book. As indicated earlier, I was bothered by how it sounded too good to be true at times. Albom, however, helps to temper such cynicism by explaining how Morrie's goodness did not simply spring from within. It was rooted in his being raised by a loving family and by his decision after completing a master's degree and Ph.D. from the University of Chicago to reject the professions of medicine, law, and business and, instead, do research at a mental hospital—"a place where he could contribute without exploiting others." Here, Morrie learned in a very practical way how human beings are in desperate need of the life-giving gift of acknowledgment. For in working with patients, writes Albom, Morrie observed that most of them "had been rejected and ignored in their lives, made to feel they didn't exist. They also missed compassion—something that staff ran out of quickly. And many of these patients were well-off, from rich families, so their wealth did not buy them happiness or contentment. It was a lesson he never forgot" (110–111).

Indeed, it is a lesson that no one should forget. Still, in my first reading of

Tuesdays with Morrie, I was bothered by the perfection of its central character. And Albom admits that he, too, found Morrie's story hard to believe at times. Late in the book, for example, Albom explains how he once tried to imagine Morrie healthy: "I tried to imagine him pulling the covers from his body, stepping from that chair, the two of us going for a walk around the neighborhood, the way we used to walk around campus" (175). Albom then asked Morrie, "What if you had one day perfectly healthy . . . What would you do?" Morrie's answer included such things as getting up in the morning and doing his exercises, having "a lovely breakfast of sweet rolls and tea," being with friends and talking about "how much we mean to each other," going for a walk in a garden where he could enjoy watching trees and birds, having a great dinner once again with friends, dancing the night away until he was "exhausted," and then going home and having "a deep, wonderful sleep." "That's it?" asks Mitch. "That's it," answers Morrie. Albom admits being "disappointed" with the answer. "It was so simple. So average. . . . I figured he'd fly to Italy or have lunch with the President or romp on the seashore or try every exotic thing he could think of. After all these months, lying there, unable to move a leg or a foot—how could he find perfection in such an average day?" But then, admits Albom, "[he] realized this was the whole point" (176).

I find this to be a fascinating realization. Albom writes about a person who, in facing death, is so down to earth that his story at times sounds too corny, too good to be true, too perfect. But the story, according to the author, is nevertheless true: Perfection is something pure and simple, although, as discussed in the last chapter, it can be transformed into something egotistical, selfish, and even rotten. Morrie warns about this transformation. Albom realizes that this warning is fundamental to his teacher's personal and professional calling. By the time readers arrive at page 176, and given all that Albom has disclosed about Morrie up to that point in the book, such a realization should be obvious. When the author shares his realization, you almost want to respond: Did it really take you this long to figure it out? Or, as some of my students put it: "*Duh.*" The question brings me back to an issue that I promised to address: the possibility that Mitch was stacking the cards a bit when he didn't clarify how his teacher/hero needed to be needed.

Morrie's story is also Mitch's story, and the story of this student is confessional and self-critical throughout most of the narrative. Albom acknowledges, for example, that when he graduated from college, Morrie hugged him goodbye and asked if he would stay in touch. "Of course," Mitch replied. But he broke this promise as he got caught up in his profession: ". . . I was not only penning columns, I was writing sports books, doing radio shows, and appearing regularly on TV . . . I was part of the media thunderstorm that now soaks our country. I was in demand" (16). Albom goes on to tell how he immersed himself in a yuppie existence: "I made more money than I had ever figured to see." He married after a seven-year courtship and told his wife that they "would one day start a family, something she wanted very much." But that day never came. "Instead, I buried myself in accomplishments, because with accomplishments, I believed I could control things, I could squeeze in every last piece of happiness before I got sick and died" (16–17).

Mitch's story is much different from Morrie's, for it tells of a person whose quest for perfection is steeped in egotistical and selfish behavior. When first learning of Morrie's illness while watching a TV news show, Mitch admits that he was both "impressed" and "envious" of all the friends that Morrie had who were still in touch with him. Mitch had been too busy with work to know or care about where *his* friends from college had gone. This is not to say, however, that Mitch had no need to be needed. On the contrary, Mitch thrived on acknowledgment. He admits as much as he shares an experience he had when the unions at his newspaper went on strike: "I felt confused and depressed. Although the TV and radio work were nice supplements, the newspaper had been my lifeline, my oxygen; when I saw my stories in print in each morning [edition], I knew that, in at least one way, I was alive." The strike was killing him. "There were sporting events each night that I would have gone to cover. Instead, I stayed home, watched them on TV. I had grown used to thinking readers somehow needed my column. I was stunned at how easily things went on without me" (44–45). Yes, it hurts not to be acknowledged for who you are and what you have done, especially when you believe that it is worthwhile.

Morrie may not actually be as perfect as he is made out to be in a story that has very little to say about his need to be needed, but he certainly has a much greater capacity of being-for others than Mitch does. And in an epideictic work like *Tuesdays with Morrie*, which seeks to make "life's greatest lesson" clear, it is this capacity that must capture and direct our attention. Throughout the book, Mitch thus continues to confess his shortcomings as they disclose themselves in the presence of someone who, despite his weaknesses, still evokes an awareness of "goodness" in others. The contrast is *rhetorically* striking; it makes for a good and entertaining read—one that holds our attention as we wait to see how a teacher's ability to share the life-giving gift of acknowledgment will affect a student who has yet to become totally rotten with perfection. Will Mitch ever feel at home with himself? We must finish reading the book to know. Are there any readers who are so perfect that they never had to or never will need to ask this question of themselves?

My students sometimes say "duh" to Albom on page 176 because he has demonstrated the appropriate amount of rhetorical competence in directing them toward that moment in the story where it is hard for any reader with a heart not to raise the question. *Tuesdays with Morrie* is a book about acknowledgment, about a life-giving gift that the book itself, in the way it is written, is designed to share with others who, like both Morrie and Mitch, have a need to be needed. Mitch may have other problems, but he is no dummy when it comes to constructing a story that, even at the expense of its author's reputation, would have us move closer to the goodness of a gift that lies at the heart of human existence. *Tuesdays with Morrie* is a "religious" story.

That said, I have one more piece of evidence to share in support of my reading. In one of his confessional moments, Mitch tells of how, during his first visit with Morrie, he was shaken by his teacher's appearance and the "faintly sour" smell of his frail body.

Moreover, Mitch was disturbed by a realization that was evoked by Morrie's presence: "I knew, deep down, that I was no longer the good, gift-bearing student he remembered" (28). When Morrie first began to explain to his student how he was dying from ALS and was "sunk," Mitch was at a loss for words: "I had no idea what to say, so I said, 'Well, you know, I mean . . . you never know'" (36).

Mitch's problem here is a common one for people who are not used to being in the presence of a friend or loved one who is dying. Zygmunt Bauman speaks of this problem when he notes:

> We do not know what to tell the dying, though we gladly and easily conversed with them before. Yes, we feel embarrassed, and to avoid feeling ashamed we prefer not to find ourselves in the presence of the dying, though before they came to be dying we avidly sought their company and enjoyed every moment of togetherness. . . . Indeed, we have nothing to say to a person who has no further use for the language of survival. . . . We may offer the dying only the language of survival; but this is precisely the one language which cannot grasp the condition from which they (not unlike us, who may still desert them and look the other way) can hide no more.[31]

The face of a dying person speaks to us of a fact of life that most people would rather forget. In avoiding their presence, we deny them the respect of acknowledgment and thereby run the risk of contributing to the pain and suffering of their social death. If, on the other hand, we do pay them respect with our presence but do not know, beyond uttering the language of survival, what to say to them, we still promote their social death by not providing them with an environment where their voice can be heard and responded to in a genuine way. A person who is dying and, for his or her "peace of mind," wants to talk about his or her death, is not being authentically acknowledged if all that is afforded the person are words like "Well, you know, I mean . . . you never know."

As the story moves on, however, the problem here is slowly remedied by a student who, with the help of his professor, learns to cope with and talk about the sadness of losing a dear and much loved friend. So, for example, in an attempt to develop a sense of how Morrie stood with God as he approached death, Mitch asks him what he thinks about the biblical story of Job and all the pain and suffering it entailed. Mitch reports that Morrie coughed violently and his hands quivered as he dropped them by his side. But then, with a smile on his face, he replied: "I think God overdid it" (151). Still, Morrie later admitted that he was willing to bargain with God so that he might "get to be one of the angels" (163).

And then there was the related lesson about forgiveness:

> It's not just other people we need to forgive ... We also need to forgive ourselves. ... Yes. For all the things we didn't do. All the things we should have done. You can't get stuck on the regrets of what should have happened. That doesn't help you when you get to where I am.
>
> I always wished I had done more with my work; I wished I had written more books. I used to beat myself up over it. Now I see that never did any good. Make peace. You need to make peace with yourself and everyone around you. (166–167)

Recall how this same lesson played a crucial role in *Ordinary People*. In *Tuesdays with Morrie*, the lesson is equally significant.

Mitch made peace with Morrie up until the very end. He no longer felt "embarrassed or squeamish" about his teacher's deteriorating condition and, having learned to avoid the inappropriate language of survival when conversing with Morrie, Mitch was no longer afraid of saying good-bye. "*After I'm dead, you talk. And I'll listen*," Morrie promised (170). This promise was based on the teaching that "Death ends a life, not a relationship" (174). Language like this was once alien to Mitch. No longer. And so when the day came to say good-bye, Mitch was ready to act appropriately. The teacher and student expressed their love for each other. They both *needed* to do this. Then, according to Mitch, Morrie's

> eyes got small, and then he cried, his face contorting like a baby who hasn't figured how his tear ducts work. I held him close for several minutes. I rubbed his loose skin. I stroked his hair. I put a palm against his face and felt the bones close to the flesh and the tiny wet tears, as if squeezed from a dropper. ... I leaned in and kissed him closely, my face against his, whiskers on whiskers, skin on skin, holding it there, longer than normal, in case it gave him even a split second of pleasure. (186)

"Where art thou?" "Here I am!" Acknowledgment. The need to be needed. It was all there, as were the tears in Mitch's eyes that Morrie had always wanted to see as an indication that his student's heart was open to life, to those in need of help, and to death. "I like to think it was a fleeting moment of satisfaction for my dear old professor," writes Albom: "he had finally made me cry" (186). The last several sentences of the book are especially fitting: "Have you ever really had a teacher?

One who saw you as a raw but precious thing, a jewel that, with wisdom, could be polished to a proud shine? If you are lucky enough to find your way to such teachers, you will always find your way back. . . . The teaching goes on" (192).

Summary

Students need devoted teachers. Teachers need devoted students. Such devotion, whether it happens inside or outside the school, college, or university, presupposes the event of acknowledgment, a life-giving gift that involves the attunement of consciousness, the transformation of time and space, the creation of dwelling places, and the appropriate rhetorical competence that can make such places into homes known for the caring people who live and visit there. In this chapter, I have attempted to further an understanding of acknowledgment by showing how this event, especially as it takes form in the various classrooms of life, functions in both a "religious" and "entertaining" manner. The teacher is a "textperson" who must hear, answer, and raise the call in an engaging way: "Where art thou?" "Here I am!" "Where art *thou?*" The student is obligated to do the same. Both the teacher and the student must learn to open themselves to each other so that they can be the givers and receivers of an essential gift that helps to make life worth living.

Living the worthwhile life necessarily unfolds in the face of death. Life, let alone one that is worthwhile, would not be what it is without its ending. We *are* a Being-toward-death, mortals who are capable of thinking about and being awed by the finitude of our existence coupled with the otherness that marks it and encourages us to think beyond its boundaries. *Tuesdays with Morrie* speaks of all of this. It is a story that is designed to acknowledge acknowledgment by way of the appropriate use of epideictic rhetoric: that type of discourse that is dedicated to disclosing and showing-forth the truth of some matter of importance. Epideictic rhetoric evokes an awareness of the faces of people and of things—who, what, and how they are. This is how Mitch brings Morrie back to life so that readers might acknowledge a great teacher who wanted to be remembered for a gift that he gave to and received from many people, including students like Mitch. It took Mitch awhile to put what he learned from his teacher about the workings and wonders of acknowledgment into practice. The longer we wait to do this, the greater the chances that the role played by death in the process will be clearly recognized. Sooner or later, death has its way.

Morrie was lucky. While his body was dying, his personhood was fortified by the presence and caress of loving family members and friends. At least as his story is told by Mitch, Morrie never had to experience the hurt of social death, of being forsaken and forgotten by others who would place him on the margins of their interests and activities so that his presence would not interfere with their daily progress and he would not remind them of their own vulnerability. Social death takes place in schools, colleges, and universities everyday as teachers and students fail to fulfill their professional and social obligations both inside and outside the classroom. As suggested in my earlier discussion of the Columbine High School Massacre, the consequences of social death can be catastrophic. In the next chapter, I take a closer look at how this phenomenon infects and causes dis-ease in communities that are struggling to receive the life-giving gift of acknowledgment.

Chapter Nine

Social Death

It was around eleven on a Saturday evening and David and I were sitting on the floor of his dormitory room, drinking Jack Daniels, and worrying about our graduate student existence at Purdue University. We were enrolled in the masters degree program in the Department of Communication at the time. It was 1973. We were both twenty-two years old. Most of our teachers were excellent, but the workload and competition were intense. With the whiskey flowing, we were relaxed enough to share our fears about making it through the program and perhaps then going on for a doctorate. We were discussing his class on "media and culture" when David—who was especially interested in how members of his race, African American, were typically depicted on television—launched into a critique of media's biased take on and misrepresentation of "people of color." I remember thinking and saying that, at times, he came off as being too insecure and defensive about his peoples' status. I also remember a move he made in support of his argument that I would never forget.

He began by asking me if I watched much television when I was a little kid growing up in the 1950s and '60s. "Of course," I said, and then we started to recall the "good old days": Saturday morning cartoons with all their advertised toys, *Lassie, Sky King, Hop-A-Long Cassidy, Leave It to Beaver, Father Knows Best, The Mickey Mouse Club.* The list grew at a fast pace and David occasionally threw in a question such as: Did you really like these shows? Did your parents buy you the toys you saw on the tube? Where any of the stars your heroes? My replies were simple: Yes. You bet. Absolutely. I even recalled how my mother would sit me in front of the TV, in a special kids' "TV chair" that had a movable table designed for eating "TV dinners" attached to it. "And while you were chomping away," asked

David," "did you ever see any cartoon character, or toy, or star, or hero who was black?" "Nope, not a one," I admitted, realizing at that moment that I was about to be checkmated. "Indeed," continued David, "all the stuff that you watched on TV, thought was good, and desired was the same color that you saw when you looked in the mirror. It's good and desirable to be white. But what do you think went through a little black kid's mind when he or she was in front of the mirror and saw a face that was noticeably different than all that was good and desirable on TV?" "Good move!" was my sincere and embarrassed response, coupled with my hope that "certainly things had improved at least a little bit since then." Another drink went down as I continued to listen carefully to related experiences having to do with what I eventually came to call "social death."

Social death takes place in any culture where people are slighted and marginalized because of their race, gender, religion, age, sexual orientation, or physical and mental status. A student once asked me to imagine what my life would be like if I were, say, a black-female-Jewish-old-lesbian who was physically handicapped and confined to a wheelchair. My students sometimes laugh when I repeat the example, although I do not raise it for humorous purposes. Rather, I offer an "extreme" case in order to present a host of options that students can think about regarding the general dis-ease in question. And then, as a way of being more specific and making it "easier" on the students, I might ask them, for example, to consider the words of Larry McAfee, a quadriplegic: "[a disabled individual is] looked upon as a second-rate citizen. People say 'you're using my taxes. You don't deserve to be here. You should hurry up and leave.' You reach a point where you just can't take anymore."[1] I have never had a student who admitted that he or she thought about the disabled in this way, although students *are* willing to admit that they know *other* people who do think this way—be it about the disabled or about blacks, Hispanics, Jews, Catholics, feminists, gays, or whatever group of "undesirables" come to mind.

Social death thrives in environments where people are marginalized; their treatment defaces the human spirit. With Levinas, we should recall that the original saying of the face speaks against this "evil of suffering" and thereby poses "the inevitable and preemptory ethical problem of the medication which is [our] duty. . . . [W]herever a moan, a cry, a groan or a sigh happen there is the original call for aid, for curative help, for help from the other ego whose alterity . . . promises salvation." With the face there comes a call for acknowledgment, a call whose interruption "is the original opening toward what is helpful, where the primordial, irreducible, and ethical, anthropological category of the medical comes to impose itself."[2] The face calls its witnesses to demonstrate a "physicianship" in their everyday dealing with others. The Hippocratic code puts it this way: "Do no harm." While attending to those who seek the curing and caring ways of medicine, the physician must avoid having a hand in either the social or physical death of another person. The same is true for any human being standing face-to-face with a presence that, without even opening its mouth, calls out, "Where art thou?"

Acknowledgment is a necessary ingredient in the antidote for social death. For with acknowledgment comes the relief of having a place to dwell, with people who are caring and willing to help others in need. Acknowledgment clears space and makes time for others who want to feel at home but whose life on the margins of society brings with it a feeling of homelessness instead. As the last chapter demonstrated, Morrie did not have to suffer this feeling. If he had, *Tuesdays with Morrie* would most likely read differently. The rhetorical competence that informs the book would have to include a rhetoric of social death, a rhetoric that shows itself as the result of people both seeking the life-giving gift of acknowledgment *and* preventing the giving of this gift.

In this chapter, I focus on the workings of social death as it showed itself in a recent and much publicized controversy regarding the justifiability and social acceptability of flying the Confederate battle flag over the statehouse in Columbia, South Carolina. The flag, seen as a reminder of slavery for some and a tribute to Southern heritage for others, flew atop the Statehouse dome for thirty-eight years before it was removed and placed atop a Confederate memorial in front of the Statehouse on July 1, 2000. Investigating this controversy will continue to keep us in touch with the world of practice, where the workings of acknowledgment actually show themselves and where rhetorical competence is needed not only to facilitate acknowledgment but also to impede it. Although I have pointed to the presence of the rhetoric of social death in my discussions of Annie Dillard's "A Hill Far Away," the Columbine High School Massacre, Robert Frost's "The Death of the Hired Man," and the Hollywood film *Ordinary People*, I have yet to present a specific, in-depth assessment of its nature and its threat to the life-giving capacity of acknowledgment.

With the controversy over the flying of the Confederate battle flag, we have a case that not only unfolds as a struggle over the right to receive the gift of acknowledgment, but that also forces a consideration of what I take to be one of the most pressing and depressing issues facing our country today: the status of race relations between whites and African Americans. Before beginning to unravel and critically assess the controversy, it will be helpful to briefly return to the rhetorical artifacts just mentioned in order to recall certain things that they teach us about the rhetoric of social death.

Acknowledgment and the Rhetoric of Social Death

The rhetoric of social death that is at work in Dillard's "A Hill Far Away" is also a rhetoric that allows for acknowledgment. Its presence is symbolized in an illuminated eight-foot aluminum cross in the front yard that reads "CHRIST THE LORD IS YOUR SALVATION." This rhetoric commands those who embrace it to assume the role of Christian witness and thereby to greet strangers with a question: "Do you know the Lord as your personal savior?" One acknowledges others by way of God, by asking a question that immediately acknowledges God and that at the same time opens a space where others can take the time to do the same. God and community go hand in hand. But, of course, it is not that simple; hence, Dillard's concern for a young boy living under the influence of a rhetoric that, as in the case of the boy's mother, makes its speakers quite nervous and cautious while at the same time contributing to the cultivation of a lonely existence (unless the company you keep is hard-core "fundamentalist" and is always there with you). As seen in the boy's interaction with Dillard, he has yet to be totally indoctrinated by this rhetoric. He may utter words about salvation, but he has yet to be saved from the loneliness that these words can foster. The boy is being programmed by a rhetoric that promises that the loneliness will cease (for God is always with you) but only as he continues to isolate himself within the well-marked boundaries of a world-view that teaches how people are going to Hell if they are not really good Christians. The rhetoric of social death is alive and well in that part of the child's world that is home to his parents and that offers a clear view of those who, owing to their sacrilegious ways, are more on the margins than at the center of God's realm.

I suspect that there are many people who would take exception to the association between religion and the rhetoric of social death being made here. Still, I see no way around acknowledging the association as long as we are talking about some institutionalized religion that, by definition, must create a discourse intended to argue for the sacredness of some Deity. When we take on this task, manipulation and marginalization are necessarily at hand, no matter how perfect we attempt to be. For, as Kenneth Burke so often reminds us, although definitions constitute vocabularies intended to be "reflections" of reality, they also at the same time are "selections" of reality. And any selection of reality must function as a "deflection" of reality, whereby the beginnings of manipulation and marginalization begin to form.[3] Of course, this is not to say that the rhetoric of religion is void of any positive potential for improving peoples' lives. Perhaps the Columbine Massacre would not have happened if Harris and Klebold thought more in terms of religious rhetoric than in terms of Nazi rhetoric. Armed with the hatred and "Übermensch" mentality of this rhetoric, they placed no limits on the revenge that was their goal. They killed people who, at least for them, were contributors to a rhetoric of social death that made sure that people like Harris and Klebold recognized themselves as outsiders, freaks, troublemakers, and losers.

In Frost's "The Death of the Hired Man," the rhetoric of social death informs Warren's ideological, instrumental, and survival of the fittest outlook. He sees Silas first and foremost only in terms of his "use" value, his being a means to Warren's desired end of keeping his farm going. The logic here is not unlike the one that is at work when the "cool" kids who make up the "in crowd" assess the worth of outsiders and find them useless, worthless, and undeserving of acceptance. Heidegger, recall, warned of the dangers of such a "calculative rationality." Warren's wife, Mary, helps to remedy the problem here by being rhetorically competent enough to open Warren to Silas's presence (face) as a person, not just as a hired hand. Mary is touched by this presence and wants to return the favor of its caress by making Silas feel at home. She would substitute the rhetoric of social death with the life-giving gift of acknowledgment that, at least in Frost's poem, excludes and marginalizes no one. In her conversation with Warren, Mary speaks a rhetoric that simply says "Here I am!" Following Levinas, we are taught to understand that such a rhetoric is what enables any institutionalized religion to come into being. There is something truly religious going on when Warren caresses Mary as the poem ends.

The rhetoric of social death caresses only those who are willing and able to remain within its prescribed boundaries of "right," "good," and "just" behavior. Questioning the standards here can be life threatening. Look at what happens to Conrad in *Ordinary People* when he fails to adhere to his mother's perfectionist tendencies: he gets so depressed that he tries to "off" himself. The only caress Conrad receives from his mother is words and actions demanding more perfection. The rhetoric of social death can be brutal. Worse yet, it can kill, unless its strangle hold on people is removed by the caring help of others. But *Ordinary People* also tells the story of how such help, if not performed with the appropriate rhetorical skill, can become a suffocating embrace itself. Conrad's father, Calvin, dearly loves his son, yet this love also has a significant role to play in the ongoing crisis that confronts the Jarrett family. The very thing that is intended to halt and reverse the motion of some rhetoric of social death can, ironically and tragically, fuel its momentum. If not given and received in the appropriate way, the life-giving gift of acknowledgment can bring with it potential pitfalls. Educating others about how to avoid these pitfalls is an essential task of the teacher.

With this last point in mind, I must admit that the case that will be considered in this chapter makes me feel somewhat uneasy. I am neither a born and bred Southerner nor an African American. What I have to say (and teach) about the case is not rooted in the type of "lived experience" that gives credibility to the strong feelings that fuel the arguments over the "true" meaning of the Confederate battle flag. Yet, in a work dedicated to enhancing an appreciation of a certain life-giving gift, the controversy is too good of a teaching tool to pass up. The rhetoric of social death that permeates this controversy both confirms and extends what has been said so far about the matter by focusing on a case of public moral argument.

A Case Study

In 1962, the Confederate battle flag was raised over the Statehouse in Columbia, South Carolina, to commemorate the Civil War's centennial, celebrate the state's heritage, and remember the sacrifices made by its natives during the war. The year also marked a time of heightened racism throughout the South, as many whites continued to react angrily to the court-ordered school desegregation that had begun in the 1950s when the Supreme Court of the United States announced its original integration decision in *Brown v. Board of Education of Topeka, Kansas* (1954). This decision actually led to a renewed passion for displaying the battle flag as a symbol of Southern pride and resoluteness.

During its 1991 national convention, the National Association for the Advancement of Colored People (NAACP) passed the following resolution:

> . . . WHEREAS, the tyrannical evil symbolized in the Confederate Battle Flag is an abhorrence to all Americans and decent people of this country, and indeed the world and is an odious blight upon the universe; and, WHEREAS, African-Americans, had no voice, no consultation, no concurrence, no commonality, not in fact nor in philosophy, in the vile conception of the Confederate Battle Flag or State Flags containing the ugly symbol of idiotic white supremacy, racism, and denigration; and, WHEREAS, we adamantly reject the notion that African-Americans should accept this flag for any stretch of the imagination or approve its presence on State Flags; NOW THEREFORE BE IT RESOLVED, that the national office of the NAACP and all units commit their legal resources to the removal of the Confederate Flag from all public properties.

South Carolina was not moved by the rhetoric of this resolution. So in October 1999, the NAACP's national board approved a tourism boycott of the state until elected officials agreed to remove the Confederate flag from the Statehouse dome. On January 10, 2000, approximately 6,000 people attended a pro-flag march and rally in front of the Statehouse. Three bagpipers led the march, followed by a group of ministers carrying a banner that read "No King but Jesus." Behind them were a group of women dressed in period costume and widow's black garb. Ranks of Confederate soldier re-enactors followed with shouldered muskets and bayonets. The rest of the marchers stretched more than six blocks. Speakers at the Statehouse rally derided the NAACP as "outsiders" and "agitators." When State Senator Arthur Ravenel told the crowd that an out-of-state reporter had recently asked him "Aren't you people in South Carolina worried about what the people in the rest of the country think about you?" the crowd shouted back with a resounding "No!" Ravenel also declared that lawmakers should not bow to the "National Association for Retarded People." Responding two days later to reports about his derogatory reference to the NAACP, Ravenel said he "apologized to the retarded folks of the world" for equating them with an organization that warranted no apology from him.[4]

On the following Saturday (January 18, 2000), an estimated 46,000 people, black and white, from all across the United States, gathered in Columbia, South Carolina for a march and a rally against the continued flying of the flag. The gathering coincided with the birthday of Dr. Martin Luther King, Jr., a day which had yet to become a sanctioned state holiday. During the march, the massive crowd chanted "The flag is coming down today" in an updated version of the civil rights song "We Shall Overcome." At the rally in front of the Statehouse, speaker after speaker derided the battle flag flying far above their heads as a symbol of slavery and hatred. James Gallman, president of the South Carolina chapter of the NAACP, proclaimed: "Not everyone in South Carolina is still living in the 18th century. . . . We are going to send a clear message to those who have the authority to deal with the placement of the Confederate battle flag. Let it be clearly understood that we live in the sovereign state of South Carolina, and not in the Confederate States of America." Reverend John Hurst Adams, bishop of the regional district of the African Methodist Episcopal Church, noted that "The Civil War's been over a long time. We know you got an inferiority complex because you lost, but you compensated for that a long time ago." Kweisi Mfume, National President of the NAACP and the main speaker at the rally, also made his point clear: "We stand under this symbol of bigotry to say that Jim Crow Sr. is dead, but Jim Crowe Jr. is alive and well." Many in the crowd waved posters of Dr. King and carried signs that offered a response to the "Heritage, Not Hate" message that had been emphasized by sign carrying supporters of the flag a week earlier (and that was once again in view). Their response read: "Your Heritage Is My Slavery."

People warrant credit for their rhetorical competence when they come up with an economical and catchy slogan that condenses the entire meaning of an involved argument into just a few words. The appropriateness of these words is determined by how well they are true to, convey, and get others to remember what the argument is supposedly *all* about; hence, the evocative power and "genius" of slogans. "Heritage, Not Hate" is easy to remember given its use of alliteration. Moreover, as will be discussed in greater detail below, the slogan does have a ring of truth to it. "Your Heritage Is My Slavery" is also easy to remember and truthful. But with this second slogan, the all important and praiseworthy notion of "Heritage" is co-opted and made to admit that there is more to its story than just "goodness."

Indeed, the controversy over the Confederate battle flag is more complex than what either of the two slogans allow for with their rhetoric. In a moment of "either-or" thinking, each side would have us appropriate *the-honest-to-goodness-truth* of *its* slogan. As I hope to demonstrate, however, if there is any "rational" way of resolving the controversy it must, at the very least, be approached with a "both/and" rather than an "either-or" mentality. I say this for two related reasons. First, the history that supports these separate and competing slogans also calls them into question. Second, a just resolution of any controversy presupposes the presence and openness of acknowledgment—an openness whose "logic" commends "both/and" thinking. In elaborating on these two reasons, I begin with the second, more philosophical one.

A Philosophy of Controversy

We are fated to dwell rhetorically as we remain open to others, to how their thoughts and actions may be different from ours, and to how this difference, especially if it evokes serious controversy, requires moral and collaborative deliberation aimed at establishing a sense of what is good, just, and truthful given the situation at hand. Such open communication encourages people to become thoughtful and respectful of the rights, circumstances, and feelings of others by allowing them the time to share their interpretations of the issues under consideration. This is what the self must do if, as Heidegger would have it, it is "to let Others who are with it 'be' in their own most potentiality-for-Being" so that they can play a genuine role in the building of "authentic community." And this, in turn, might require great patience on the part of the self because what others have to say in response may indicate that they do not understand, that they misunderstand what they are being told, or that they even find the self to be "guilty" of maintaining an incorrect point of view. Indeed, trying to build an authentic community can be a time-consuming task filled with controversy.[5]

Still, for those who want to be true to the way in which existence is always calling them into question (and thus always speaking of the importance of being open-minded), the struggle must go on. The self must remain open to the personhood of others and to their discourse, which tells of this personhood by giving some indication of how people are faring in their relationships with things and with each other. Being open to others, listening carefully and taking what they have to say seriously, is how the self counters the egotistic tendency of becoming so engrossed in figuring out what it wants to express next that it misses what others are expressing. Authentic community is not built on egoism—on individuals demanding that "it is *either* my way *or* no way"—but on the altruism of being-for others and on the empathy that this altruism makes possible. In their communicative struggle to ascertain the truth of some disputed matter and to advance their community's *ethos* and moral consciousness, *both* the self *and* others are responsible for making sure that the life-giving gift of acknowledgment and the openness it fosters are cultivated and shared as much as possible.

A History of a Controversy

The controversy over the flying of the Confederate flag in South Carolina showed little evidence of this "both/and" mentality, and when it was advocated it was not without its problems. Consider, for example, how John Shelton Reed, professor of sociology at the University of North Carolina and co-editor of the quarterly

Southern Cultures, deals with the matter in a piece in the *Wall Street Journal*. Noting that the meaning of the flag "has, notoriously, been deployed by groups ranging from Dixiecrats to the Ku Klux Klan as a symbol of white supremacy, and for a racist fringe of Southern whites it still has that meaning," Reed also notes that

> Most white Southerners . . . see the flag as representing what they sincerely believe to be an honorable Civil War legacy of duty, valor and sacrifice. Some (I am among them) question whether a state government should display a symbol so demonstrably offensive to a large minority of citizens, but that doesn't mean we see the flag as solely, or even primarily, a racist symbol. When defenders of the flag print T-shirts and erect billboards that say the flag stands for "Heritage, Not Hate," they're not being disingenuous.[6]

Indeed, as Reed continues to point out: "In 1989 the Sons of Confederate Veterans passed a resolution denouncing 'extremist political groups and individuals who seek to clothe themselves in respectability by misappropriating the banner under which our Southern ancestors fought for a cause which was as noble as much latter day use is ignoble.'"

Reed concedes that Black protestors "have a point" when they say "Your Heritage Is My Slavery." He writes: "If 'heritage' refers to the South's political and economic history, then that history—like that of most peoples—is a sorry stage of conflict, division, oppression and exploitation. Slavery was an important part of that history, and undeniably part of what secession [was] all about, as any honest reading of the secession debates in various Southern states will reveal. This is not to say [, however,] that individual Confederate soldiers were fighting for slavery . . ." But the word "Heritage," Reed contends, can also refer to something much different. To give just a few examples, " 'heritage' means food, music, speech, religion, humor." With these meanings of the term in mind, it can be argued, according to Reed, "that black and white Southerners share a great deal." Reed thus maintains that

> The challenge is finding symbols of the South's cultural history, which from the start has been a story of borrowing, copying and blending, producing a flavorsome Creole stew. If Southerners can ever get past the political history that divides them and simply enjoy a culture whose making they have shared and still do—if they can 'forget the bad and keep the good' (as country singer Tanya Tucker put it)—the South might really rise again.

In concluding his essay, Reed would have his readers consider this possibility in light of the following facts:

In 1994, when the University of North Carolina's Southern Focus Poll asked residents of 13 Southern states whether the flag was 'more a symbol of racial conflict or of Southern pride,' only 26% of blacks chose Southern pride, compared to 75% of whites. But in response to another, perhaps more telling, question, one-third of whites and half of blacks said that they 'don't care much about [the flag] one way or the other.' I suspect that many Southerners of both races are profoundly bored with the subject and would welcome even another celebrity murder trial or presidential sex scandal if it would just get the flag off their front pages and TV screens.

I have no doubt that Professor Reed writes with the best of intentions, for he is certainly not an advocate of "either/or" thinking. Still, I find his presentation wanting, for "the challenge" he speaks of entails more than simply finding symbols that recall how both blacks and whites contributed to and share a common cultural history or "heritage." Yes, the term can refer to "food, music, speech, religion, [and] humor," but even if it does the problem at hand is not necessarily remedied. On the contrary, it may intensify.

As historian William Miller notes, slavery is a "tragic evil" that is never entirely forgotten when racism lives as it still does today.[7] Moreover, of the five options that Reed offers for rethinking the meaning of "heritage," the one that I believe might be most relevant for the Southern whites and blacks whose history is deeply rooted in the nation's "bible belt" is "religion." In the pre–Civil War South, religion served as a major justification of slavery as a "positive good"; hence, the words of South Carolina Congressman James Henry Hammond, who in 1836 declared to his colleagues in the House of Representatives that slavery was "the greatest of all the great blessings which a kind Providence has bestowed upon our glorious region."[8]

This certainly was not a view shared by slaves, who also sought support and hope from religion. A telling illustration of the contradiction that existed between the "master's" and the slave's take on the topic is provided by James H. Cone in his landmark study of the development of Black Theology. Writing about how slaves used folkloric tales to express how their existing state of oppression contradicted their real humanity as defined by God's future, Cone shares the tale entitled "Swapping Dreams":

> The master told Ike: "I dreamed I went to Nigger Heaven last night and I saw there a lot of garbage, some torn-down houses, a few old broken down, rotten fences, the muddiest, sloppiest streets I ever saw, and a big bunch of ragged, dirty Negroes walking around." But rather than accept the master's perspective about himself and his community, Ike responded with a comment that was deceptive and

full of humor but liberating in its rejection of the present white values system. "Umph, umph, Massa," said Ike, "yah sho' musta et de same t'ing Ah did las' night, 'cause Ah dreamed Ah went up ter de white man's paradise, an' de streets wuz all ob gol' an' silvah, and dey was lost of o' milk an' honey dere, an' putty pearly gates, but dey wuzn't uh soul in de whole place."[9]

According to Cone, with such a folkloric tale "black people created liberated structures of the future wherein they were able to encounter freedom's essence even though they were slaves."[10] I would put it somewhat differently: Freedom's essence lies at the heart of human existence in the way in which human beings— be they white, black, or any other color—are open to the future and are therefore confronted with the ethical responsibility of making choices. "Where art thou?" "Here I am!" Freedom is always caught up in the ontological workings of acknowledgment, of the self and others finding ways of being-for each other. In the above story, the master's use of religion degrades the slave's presence on earth *and* in "Nigger Heaven"; at best, it offers only negative acknowledgment. The slave's rebuttal returns the favor, thereby suggesting that "de white man's paradise" is too good of a place for the white man to dwell. The Lord calls out "Where art thou?" and the white man's immoral system of slavery is in no way a fitting and just response. Heaven is not a home for those whose "good" existence is made possible by the harshness of slavery.

Abolitionists like Frederick Douglass never tired of making this point in identifying the principle cause of the Civil War and the hell on earth it created: "It has sprung out of a malign selfishness and a haughty and imperious pride which only the practice of the most hateful oppression and cruelty could generate and develop. No ordinary love of gain, no ordinary love of power, could have stirred up this terrible revolt. . . . The monster was brought to its birth by pride, lust and cruelty which could not brook the sober restraints of law, order and justice."[11] The Bible, of course, speaks against such vices, which dehumanize, demoralize, and deface the human spirit. The face speaks: "Thou shalt not kill!" The institution of slavery disregarded this holy command as its rhetoric continued to foster a life of social death.

"Heritage Not Hate." Religion does not settle the controversy associated with the supposed truth of this claim. This is not to say, however, that white southerners never employed religion as an argument against the misery of slavery. Mary Boykin Chesnut, the wife of James Chesnut, Jr., an aide to President Jefferson Davis and a brigadier-general in the Confederate Army, is perhaps the most famous southern aristocrat whose diaries record a revulsion with the degrading and unholy "institution." Part of her diary entry of June 12, 1862, for example, explains how she "tried to read [*Uncle Tom's Cabin*] and could not. It was too sickening. A

man sent his little son to beat a human being tied to a tree." Mrs. Chesnut compared the feeling to the "pulling out of eyeballs in Lear."[12] Indeed, although she
never directly challenged the "orthodox assumption" about the innate inferiority
of the black race, the religious Mrs. Chesnut nevertheless spoke of slaves not as
chattel but as *human beings*. According to her biographer, Elizabeth Muhlenfeld,
Mary "loved the serenity and panoply of church services and attended church
regularly. Although she felt allegiance for no particular church, she was partial to a
Negro church on Mulberry Plantation. Mary often attended these services and
sometimes felt they brought her closer to the pure meaning of Christianity than
did the more reserved churches of the gentry."[13] Writing about Mrs. Chesnut and
other "southern white women who where unhappy about slavery" even though
their families owned slaves, Robert Durden notes that "the situation was much
like that with the miserable weather of January and February: one could only suffer and wish that it would somehow go away."[14]

The situation Durden refers to entailed more than a disagreement over the
pure meaning of Christianity and the brutal institution of slavery. This institution
was inextricably tied to the economic and social well being of the South. In the
same address he gave to the House of Representatives in 1836, South Carolina
Congressman Hammond not only extolled slavery as "the greatest of all the great
blessings" that God had bestowed upon the South, but he also emphasized how it
"rendered our southern country proverbial for its wealth, genius, and its manners." The South ought to be proud of its "aristocratic" nature, argued Hammond:

> I accept the term. It is a government of the best. Combining all the
> advantages, and possessing but few of the disadvantages, of the aris-
> tocracy of the old world, without fostering to an unwarrantable ex-
> tent the pride, the exclusiveness, the selfishness, the thirst for sway,
> the contempt for the rights of others, which distinguish the nobility
> of Europe, it gives us their education, their polish, their munifi-
> cence, their high honor, their undaunted spirit. Slavery does indeed
> create an aristocracy—an aristocracy of talents, of virtues, of gener-
> osity and courage. In a slave country every free man is an aristocrat.
> Be he rich or poor, if he does not possess a single slave, he has been
> born to all the natural advantages of the society in which he is
> placed, and all its honors lie open before him, inviting his genius
> and industry.[15]

With this argument for white supremacy, even "poor white trash" could see
themselves as having a place in the social hierarchy. They could consider themselves above and beyond a race of people who, according to those like South Carolina Senator John C. Calhoun, were existing in an environment that was far more
civilized, comfortable, and respectable than anything that existed in Africa. Slavery

was a "positive good," argued Calhoun, one that assured that the white race would continue to advance economically and socially, thereby supplying a better world for those of the black race who were the purchased and legal property of their Southern masters.[16] As will be discussed in greater detail shortly, the Constitution could certainly be read as affording protection of such "property" in its affirmation of the sovereignty of states rights. In his last speech in the Senate (March 4, 1850), Calhoun advanced his argument further by using this reading of the Constitution to maintain that the growing controversy between the North and the South was fueled primarily by Northern aggressions rather than by Southern obstinacy. According to Calhoun, the North "cannot refuse" to respect the rights of the Southern states

> if she has half the love of the Union which she professes to have, or without justly exposing herself to the charge that her love of power and aggrandizement is far greater than her love of the Union. At all events, the responsibility of saving the Union rests on the North, and not on the South. The South cannot save it by any act of hers [that in turn will not destroy the South's economic and social wellbeing], and the North may save it without any sacrifice whatever, unless to do justice, and to perform her duties under the constitution, should be regarded by her as a sacrifice.[17]

Notice that with the pro-slavery argument advanced by Hammond, Calhoun, and many other Southern politicians, the life-giving gift of acknowledgment becomes an issue. Despite their "inferior" status, blacks had been given a place to dwell in the South where they could reap certain rewards of the region that they, through their labor and devotion, had made possible. The South valued its property, cared for its slaves, and, with the support of the Constitution (and the guiding hand of Providence), had the right to maintain the sanctity of its homeland and thus continue doing a favor for blacks.

As Alice Fahs points out, Southern writers well into the twentieth century made much of the "grace" and "duty" at work here when presenting their view of how the once happy slave, kidnapped by the vile Yankees and forced into the ranks, only wanted to return to his home so that he could "belong to somebody" and thereby maintain his supposedly "natural" state of subservience.[18] The institution of slavery granted whites *and* blacks a place to call "home." According to historian William C. Davis, the South's "natural instinct" to protect this much cherished place and to thereby "promote home and hearth" was the "real" reason why "1 million Southern men" went to war. Slavery had "absolutely nothing" to do with it.[19] Although this claim is certainly debatable, it nevertheless points to a factor—the home—that did maintain a central position in the ideology of the South. Bell Irvin Wiley makes the point well:

The rallying cry of some was "the Union and freedom" and this combination carried unusual appeal. But the men in blue, save for very brief periods of threatened invasion, had no cause so dynamic as that of the Confederates in defending their homes. "John Brown's Body" and "Hail Columbia" were stirring songs, but neither possessed the emotional tug of the Rebel favorite "The despot's heel is on thy shore, Maryland! My Maryland!"[20]

As should be clear from all that has been said so far about the life-giving gift of acknowledgment, the notion of "home" carries much ontological weight for human beings. Home is where the heart is, where comfort and a loving caress are expected. It is where, if possible, we go to die so not to be alone at this most final of earthly moments. Sooner or later life forces the question: "Where art thou?" We are made to feel at home only as long as others are willing to say "Here I am," thereby providing a place we can dwell with them for the time being. Mary Chesnut did not speak of a "nigger slave" tied to a tree; no, she used the term "human being" to describe the "sickening" scene. From the ontological and moral point of view emphasized in this book, the term is certainly a more fitting and appropriate way to express the presence, the face, of someone who is about to feel the whip and perhaps cry out (or at least wonder in silence) "Where art thou?"

How many Southerners acknowledged slaves first and foremost as human beings? How many slaves genuinely felt at home in the South? "The Union and freedom." "The despot's heel is on thy shore, Maryland! My Maryland!" Discussing the attitudes that informed these sayings, Kenneth Stampp notes that

> Sectional partisans . . . invidiously compared their society with the other, and proudly proclaimed the superiority of their own. To Northerners the South was backward, semicivilized, and out of harmony with the [progressive] ideals of the nineteenth century. To Southerners the North was a hotbed of radical "isms" (feminism, abolitionism, and socialism, among others), of puritan hypocrisy, and of crude parvenus. Each section reduced the other to a cultural stereotype and made it an object of hatred.[21]

Reducing others to a cultural stereotype necessarily diminishes their humanity and contributes to their social death. The process defines a rhetorical version of "calculative rationality" that, as seen in the war between the states, associated the color of a person's skin and uniform—white, black; blue, gray—with ways of being which were fated for a brutal confrontation. Sometimes the worst can happen when people get caught up in a struggle to feel at home with themselves and with each other.

Such a struggle was at work as the nation's Founding Fathers composed a document, the Constitution, meant to express, among other things, the holiness and thus the greatness of liberty and equality that was first articulated in the pre-amble of the Declaration of Independence: "We hold these truths to be self-evident, that all men are created equal, that they are endowed by their Creator with certain unalienable Rights, that among these are Life, Liberty, and the pursuit of happiness." The nation was no longer a slave to British rule, but it was a home to the institution of slavery, which existed all across colonial America. When the founders met in Philadelphia in May of 1787, over six hundred thousand human beings (one-sixth of the country's population) were slaves. In the "land of the free and the home of the brave," the institution of slavery was a contradiction begging for a resolution. The founders provided this remedy by composing a document that was ambiguous on the matter of slavery. The Constitution does acknowledge "a right to property," but it does not explicitly relate this right to the owning of slaves. In fact, the word "slave" or "slavery" never appears in the Constitution. William Miller's explanation of this fact is noteworthy:

> The use of elaborate euphemisms and circumlocutory verbal de-vices to avoid the words "slave" and "slavery," at considerable cost at least to brevity and possibly to clarity, had an important purpose. It was explicitly designed to keep the Constitution from recognizing, as James Madison put it, that there could be "property in men." In its silent way it was rather a touching appeal to future generations to do what the framers were not able to do [—eliminate a "tragic evil" that, at the time, was too close to the heart of a newborn nation and that thus posed too much of a risk to be operated on and removed entirely from the body politic].[22]

According to Miller, the problem of slavery was "not only a moral one, but an intellectual one and a rhetorical one." With the above explanation, Miller is emphasizing the rhetorical aspect of the problem. What something means and *how* it means are the results of how authors, when formulating a "fitting response" to some issue, choose to use and not use certain words given the exigencies of the situation at hand. It is a matter of appropriateness: the "truth" of a document is inevitably tied to the words that are present and the words that are absent. The rhetorical operation of discourse is always caught up in this presence/absence phenomenon of language-use, whereby our specific employment of words takes on what Richard Weaver identifies as a "sermonic" function: "We have no sooner uttered words than we have given impulse to other people to look at the world, or some small part of it, in our way. Thus caught up in a great web of inter-communication and inter-fluence, we speak as rhetoricians affecting one another for good or ill."[23]

The Declaration of Independence and the Constitution speak to us of the importance of proper conduct and duty; hence their sermonic function, one that is especially hard at work when the issue at hand is how a people shall be governed. In the case of the founders, as Miller points out, this issue necessarily involved the creation of a "debating society" that enabled and encouraged people to govern "themselves—'self-government'—by the instrument of their chosen representatives. That is to say also that they shall be governed by deliberation—by mutual argument and persuasion. . . . The people were guaranteed freedom of 'conscience,' first of all, and freedoms by which that conscience might be expressed: freedom of speech and freedom of the press."[24] Working together, these freedoms allow for the giving and receiving of the gift of acknowledgment. They are used rhetorically to make space and time for people to dwell together as a community, to entertain each other's ideas and stances, and thereby to know together all that must be done in order to ensure the well-being and just development of the union of their togetherness.

The South, of course, did not feel at home in its union with the North, where so-called "Black republicans" like Abraham Lincoln constantly sounded calls of conscience meant to bring about the abolition of slavery. Without slavery, the South could not be itself. The point was clearly made in the letters and diaries of fallen Confederate soldiers as they expressed their fears about "the ruthless invader who is seeking to reduce us to abject slavery"; or how "The Deep still quiet peace of the grave is more desirable than Vassalage or Slavery"; or how the men in gray must "die as free men or live as slaves." According to James McPherson, these soldiers "were using the word *slavery* in the same sense that Americans in 1776 had used it to describe their subordination to Britain. Confederates claimed to fight for the same liberty their forefathers had won in 1783."[25] In the case of the Confederacy, however, the contradiction between freedom and slavery had evolved into a life-threatening paradox: Only by maintaining the institution of slavery could the South remain free of slavery. Thus Abraham Lincoln's critical assessment of the region: "The perfect liberty they sigh for" is "the liberty of making slaves of other people."[26] Beginning with the secession crisis in South Carolina, however, a rhetoric arose to combat Northern criticism by announcing a "fear appeal": the freeing of slaves, especially those who had been mistreated, would pose a serious threat to the white population. Slavery was thus defended as an "essential" institution for "race control" that, among other things, would prevent abolitionist preachers from consummating the marriage of white southern females to black husbands.[27]

"Where art thou?" The North asked the South this question with the hope of keeping the "Union" together for both God and the nation's sake. The South asked the North the same question with the hope that their way of life, steeped in tradition and in the "blessings" of "a kind Providence," would be allowed to thrive. Although the Declaration of Independence spoke in favor of the North's position, the Constitution could be read to support the South's version of freedom. Moreover, believing in the workings and results of "Providence," the South could also point to the invention of the cotton gin in 1793 as a "sign" of where it was destined to go. This technology made it possible for textile mills to use the short-staple cotton which the Southern states could grow so abundantly and cheaply with slave labor.[28]

Lincoln read the Declaration of Independence and the Constitution as articulations of the founding father's intentions to abolish the institution of slavery, which needed to be placed "where the public mind shall rest in the belief that it is in course of ultimate extinction."[29] He did not see the cotton gin as an indication that his reading was incorrect. On the contrary, as an advocate of the ways and means of civic republicanism, Lincoln held firm to the belief that "public sentiment" must be included in the moral deliberations of government and that someone who is capable of molding such sentiment and directing it toward the truth "goes deeper than he who enacts statutes or pronounces decisions."[30] By the time of his second inaugural address, March 4, 1865, Lincoln had committed himself to the abolitionist interpretation of the human crisis at hand and made abolition the primary goal of the war. Realizing, however, that the strong religious underpinnings of this interpretation were incommensurate with the equally strong religious assessments of the issue of slavery, Lincoln treated the issue with great rhetorical sensitivity:

> Both [the North and the South] read the same Bible and pray to the same God, and each invokes His aid against the other. It may seem strange that any men should dare to ask a just God's assistance in wringing their bread from the sweat of other men's faces, but let us judge not, that we be not judged. The prayers of both could not be answered. That of neither has been answered fully. The Almighty has His own purposes. . . . Fondly do we hope, fervently do we pray, that this mighty scourge of war may speedily pass away. Yet, if God wills that it continue until all the wealth piled up by the bondsman's two hundred and fifty years of unrequited toil shall be sunk, and until every drop of blood drawn with the lash shall be paid by another drawn with the sword, as was said three thousand years ago, so still it must be said, "The judgments of the Lord are true and righteous altogether."[31]

Although I know of no speech given by Lincoln in which he admitted that his stance on the issue of slavery was contradicted by these judgments, he did identify with a position during his debates with Stephen Douglas in 1858 that certainly displayed a racist tone:

> I will say . . . that I am not, nor ever have been in favor of bringing about in any way the social and political equality of the white and black races, that I am not nor ever have been in favor of making

voters or jurors of negroes, nor of qualifying them to hold office, nor to intermarry with white people; and I will say in addition to this that there is a physical difference between the white and black races which I believe will forever forbid the two races living together on terms of social and political equality. And inasmuch as they cannot so live, while they do remain together there must be the position of superior and inferior, and I as much as any other man am in favor of having the superior position assigned to the white race.[32]

Commenting on these remarks, David Zarefsky notes that they "are conveniently 'forgotten' [by Lincoln's admirers], excused as a necessary adaptation to local politics, or disparaged by those wishing to argue that by today's standards the Great Emancipator was actually a racist." Zarefsky goes on to emphasize, however, that "What is collectively remembered from the debates [with Douglas] is . . . Lincoln's masterful statement at Alton: 'The real issue in this controversy—the one pressing upon every mind—is the sentiment on the part of one class that looks upon the institution of slavery *as a wrong*, and of another class that *does not* look upon it as a wrong.'" For Zarefsky, this "unqualified statement of Lincoln's [fundamental] principles is what endures."[33]

I agree with Zarefsky. But Lincoln's remarks are still *on the record* and I cite them here to make a point that was given little attention during the Confederate flag controversy in South Carolina: Before, during, and after the Civil War, racism remained "alive and well" in the North as well as in the South. As seen, for example, in the letter from a young Boston blue blood who wrote his brother from New Orleans in early 1863, this racism could be extreme and incredibly sickening: "As I was going along this afternoon a little black baby that could just walk got under my feet and it look[ed] so much like a big worm that I wanted to step on it and crush it, the nasty, greasy little vermin was the best that could be said of it."[34]

This racism was rooted in a white supremacist world-view that permeated the ranks of the Union soldiers. Disdain for the black race was also (and ironically) fueled by a document that eventually doomed the Confederacy to defeat: Lincoln's Emancipation Proclamation (September, 1862). According to McPherson, "plenty of soldiers believed that the proclamation *had* changed the purpose of the war. They professed to feel betrayed. They were willing to risk their lives for Union, they said, but not for black freedom. The proclamation intensified a morale crisis in the Union armies," leading to threats of desertion as Union troops took exception to fighting what they termed a "nigger war."[35] Realizing as time went on, however, that the emancipation and the enlistment of blacks into the Union army was, in fact, a very *pragmatic* means to a much desired end (winning the war), racism in the Northern ranks became less obvious. When Lincoln ran for reelection in 1864, pledging a constitutional amendment to abolish slavery, he received nearly eighty percent of the soldier vote. Commenting on this change of attitude toward slavery, McPherson shares portions of a letter written by a soldier from Lincoln's state of Illinois: "It is astonishing how things has changed in reference to freeing the Negroes . . . It allwais has been plane to me that this rase must be freed befor god would recognise us . . . we bost of liberty and we Should not be Selfish in it as god gives us liberty we Should try to impart it to others . . .thank god the chanes will Soon be bursted . . . now I belive we are on gods side . . . now I can fight with a good heart."[36]

"The Union and freedom"—and God once again. "Where art thou?" "Here I am!" Was God on the side of the Union and the slaves it emancipated? If this was the case, then God had to forgive a lot of Northerners who, as the historical record makes clear, were not as genuine in their feelings toward black *human beings* as Southern aristocrats such as Mary Chesnut were. In a book on acknowledgment, we *must be open* to this possibility, even when, as in the case of Mrs. Chesnut, our hatred of slavery does not inspire unorthodoxy on race. Perhaps the claim "Heritage, Not Hate" should not be immediately and totally dismissed. The thoughts and actions of all those who allowed themselves to be represented by the Confederate flag may not have been just a mean-spirited source of hate supporting the tragic evil of slavery. Although not advanced in the context of the Confederate flag controversy, Miller's way of making this point is worth noting:

> It is true that the sections were scarred by the war in ways that have not vanished over a century and a quarter later. It is true that the North turned aside and went about moneymaking and (mostly) forgot the plight of freedmen, but nevertheless used the bloody shirt from the war, and the "treasury of virtue" stored up in its alleged moral superiority, to dominate. It is true that the white South, defeated, constructed a new pattern of racial domination. But for all that, the nation did not fall apart, did not abandon republicanism (democracy), did abolish slavery, and did affirm the formal equality of black persons (or rather of all persons born or naturalized in the United States, of all citizens without regard to race, color, or previous condition of servitude). It did strengthen the Union, and make itself more clearly one nation. Winning the war by itself would not have been sufficient to accomplish these things, if the opposition to them had been unconditional, unambiguous, absolute, unified, fueled by a radically contrary philosophy and a bottomless hatred. But it was not.[37]

The "opposition" Miller refers to has much more to do with the South than with the North. Perhaps, then, a certain claim should be amended to read: "Heritage, Not A Bottomless Hatred."

I suggest this amendment not to allow slavery *any* reprieve, but rather in the spirit of fairness (open-mindedness) that is required by acknowledgment and that grants its intended object—in this case the Confederate flag—a chance to disclose all that it symbolizes. As I have tried to suggest so far, in order to appreciate this object's full range of meaning, we must recall and come to terms with a past whose "truth" continues to be a contested issue between Northerners and Southerners, blacks and whites. This rhetorical struggle marks out a long-standing argument over, among other things, definitions: the use of symbols "to draw a line around" (*definire*) something in order to mark its meaningful borders. What exactly *does* the Confederate battle flag mean? As with any object, this one means by way of what is "inside" and "outside" its demarcated borders. The meaning of the flag's being is at one and the same time *both* what it is *and* what it is not. What the South and its flag stood for made no sense without the North and what its flag stood for. There is no "is" without a corresponding "is not." Once the definitions are established and the lines are drawn, however, the conditions for exclusion, marginalization, and social death are set. The reification of these conditions comes about with the human tendency to think in terms of "either/or," black or white—a tendency that eliminates the ambiguity that is allowed for by the "both/and logic" that necessarily informs the workings of any definition.

Conditioned as our thinking is by the many definitions that we employ everyday to make sense of the world, we always run the risk of becoming forgetful of things. The more our definitions become narrow-minded and reified, the more they restrict our ways of appreciating the past, present, and future of all that stands before us. Such forgetfulness is a breeding ground for "indifference," and both of these phenomena are at work in the controversy over the flying of the Confederate flag. In concluding his 1995 book on the Civil War, *What They Fought For*, McPherson offers an example of the problem I am referring to here:

> By the 1890s the road to reunion between men who wore the blue and gray had paved over the issues of slavery and equal rights for freed slaves. Middle-aged veterans in the Grand Army of the Republic and the United Confederate Veterans held joint encampments at which they reminisced about the glorious deeds of their youth. Many of them reached a tacit consensus, which some voiced openly: "Confederate soldiers had not fought for slavery; Union soldiers had not fought for its abolition." It had been a tragic war of brothers whose issues were best forgotten in the interest of family reconciliation. In the popular romanticization of the Civil War, the issue of slavery became almost as invisible as black Union veterans at a reunion encampment. Somehow the Civil War became a heroic contest, a sort of grand, if deadly, football game without ideological cause or purpose.[38]

Indeed, selective memory can foster an unfortunate indifference to the truth of things past.

Resolution?

Recall that, when beginning my discussion of the Confederate flag controversy in South Carolina, I referred to John Shelton Reed's view on the topic. He suggested that the controversy could be resolved if Southerners, white and black, could "get past the political history that divides them and simply enjoy a culture whose making they have shared and still do." He maintained that religion, among other things, defines such common ground. He also suggested that "many Southerners of both races are profoundly bored with the subject and would welcome even another celebrity murder trial or presidential sex scandal if it would just get the flag off their front pages and TV screens." These are good-hearted and well-intended suggestions, but I find them lacking because they seem content with a solution that encourages selective memory and indifference. Such contentment might rest well in the hearts and minds of Southern whites whose ancestors fought a fratricidal war "simply" to protect home and hearth. But what about those whose ancestors were slaves? Are they not right to remain resolute in the belief that "Your Heritage Is My Slavery"? Certainly they have a point. Inside the meaningful boundaries of the Confederate flag lies the fact of slavery—a fact that, as I have suggested above, is right in our face when we consider it from the vantage point of religion.

Recall also the earlier quote from the 1991 NAACP resolution that made the organization's reaction to this fact clear. It spoke of the "tyrannical evil symbolized in the Confederate Battle Flag" that "is an abhorrence to all Americans and decent people of this country and indeed the world" and that is "an odious blight upon the universe." African-Americans "had no voice, no consultation, no concurrence, no commonality, not in fact nor in philosophy, in the vile conception of the Confederate Battle Flag or State Flags containing the ugly symbol of idiotic white supremacy, racism, and denigration." These words speak of slavery as an institution that spoke of God while at the same time condemning a race of people to social and physical death. But these words also show no flexibility, no leniency, in their condemnation of the evil under consideration. They provide no opening for continued dialogue. The rhetoric of the resolution is close-fisted. It does not seek to transform space and time into a dwelling place where people of differing opinions about the Confederate flag can feel at home with each other and know together all that this meaning entails. The resolution offers no caress to anyone who might question its "truth." The judgment has been made. The time for moral and collaborative deliberation is over. The voice of African-Americans will no longer be muted and eliminated by racist rants and the symbols that "deceitfully" grant them legitimacy. In short, as far as the NAACP is concerned, the Confederate flag warrants no positive acknowledgment at all.

Although this judgment is certainly not as harsh as the abject cruelty spawned by the institution of slavery was, it nevertheless is still remarkable for its lack of openness. Receiving the life-giving gift of acknowledgment grants a person at least a momentary reprieve from the misery of isolation, of being forgotten and forsaken. To refuse others acknowledgment is to condemn them to social death and its hell on earth. African-Americans have long suffered the social, political, economic, psychological, and physical consequences of this practice and its death sentence. Extending this sentence to the Confederate flag and its supporters, the NAACP sought to put an end to the evil at work here.

Such moral action is both supported and criticized by the Bible. In the Old Testament, for example, there is the "judgment" of an "Eye for eye, tooth for tooth, hand for hand, foot for foot, Burning for burning, wound for wound, stripe for stripe" (Exodus 21:24–25). In the New Testament, however, the judgment is amended: "That ye resist not evil: but whosoever shall smite thee on thy right cheek, turn to him the other also" (Matthew 5:39). The action of the NAACP adheres, of course, to the first judgment. But what if, as suggested above, the Confederate flag is an artifact whose "true" meaning of "Heritage," although marred by the evil of slavery, should not be aligned only with the "bottomless hatred" of this evil?

This possibility is the only one that offers a genuine excuse for South Carolina's refusal to lower the flag for nine years, until the NAACP's tourism boycott of the state finally achieved victory in 2001. The "emergency resolution" announcing this boycott in 1999, is noteworthy for its rhetoric, which although still close-fisted is not as emotionally hard-hitting in its choice of words (e.g., "tyrannical evil"; "abhorrence to all Americans and decent people"; "odious blight upon the universe"). The resolution speaks of how "the Confederate States of America came into being by way of secession from the war against the United States of America out of a desire to defend the right of individual states to maintain an economic system based on slave labor"; how "the Confederate Battle Flag was raised in the States that comprised the defunct Confederate States of America for the supposed celebration of the Centennial of the War Between the States as an unspoken symbol of resistance to the battle for civil rights and equality in the early 1960's"; how "the Confederate Battle Flag in its present position of display makes a statement of public policy that continues to be an affront to the sensibilities and dignity of a majority of African-Americans in the state of South Carolina"; how "the state of South Carolina possesses a unique linkage of heritage and family which makes South Carolina a prime destination for African-American family reunions, resulting in tourism dollars that benefit the state"; how these dollars spent "by African-Americans, other people of conscience and corporate entities serve to enrich the State of South Carolina, the 'Mother State of Secession', which continues to fly the banner of secession"; and how this banner must be removed and relocated "to a place of historical rather than sovereign context."

Notice that with more historically (rather than emotionally) oriented rhetoric, the NAACP recalls how the raising of the Confederate flag was not simply an act of celebration but also and primarily an act of "resistance to the battle for civil rights and equality in the early 1960's." The recollection is significant, especially for those who lived through the battle (or who at least have a well-grounded historical understanding of it) and who thereby remember the leadership of Dr. Martin Luther King, Jr., who wrote of the time:

> [T]he summer of 1963 was historic because it witnessed the first offensive in history launched by Negroes along a broad front. The heroic but spasmodic and isolated slave revolts of the antebellum South had fused, more than a century later, into a simultaneous, massive assault against segregation. And the virtues so long regarded as the exclusive property of the white South—gallantry, loyalty, and pride—had passed to the Negro demonstrators in the heat of the summer's battles.[39]

In his famous "I Have a Dream" address, delivered in Washington, D.C., in 1963, King put the matter this way:

> Five score years ago, a great American, in whose symbolic shadow we stand today, signed the Emancipation Proclamation. This momentous decree came as a great beacon light of hope to millions of Negro slaves, who had been seared in the flames of withering injustice. It came as a joyous daybreak to end the long night of their captivity.
>
> But one hundred years later, the Negro still is not free. One hundred years later, the life of the Negro is still sadly crippled by the manacles of segregation and the chains of discrimination. One hundred years later, the Negro lives on a lonely island of poverty in the midst of a vast ocean of material prosperity. One hundred years later, the Negro is still languished in the corners of American society and finds himself an exile in his own land.[40]

As Southerners were raising the Confederate battle flag and celebrating the "Centennial of the War Between the States," King was sadly announcing another Centennial—one that marked the occasion of the Negro's continued social death. When, however, he spoke of his "dream," his rhetoric exuded hope for transforming and eliminating this "shameful condition": " . . . when we allow freedom to ring, when we let it ring from every village and every hamlet, from every state and every city, we will be able to speed up that day when all of God's children, black men and white men, Jews and Gentiles, Protestants and Catholics, will be able to join hands and sing in the words of the Old Negro spiritual, 'Free at last, free at last. Thank God Almighty, we are free at last.'"[41]

With these words, King, at least for the moment, transformed the restricted space and time of social death into the openness of a dwelling place where people with differences could acknowledge, caress, and feel at home with each other. It was a time for cultivating conscience, for "knowing together" what was good, right, and just. Recalling the plight of his ancestors and their relationship with the Almighty who answered their prayers, King sounded a call of conscience that was as appropriate then as it is now—a call that, as planned by King and his colleagues, took full advantage of the influential power of the media. As he would later note:

> Normally Negro activities are the object of attention in the press only when they are likely to lead to some dramatic outbreak, or possess some bizarre quality. The march was the first organized Negro operation that was accorded respect and coverage commensurate with its importance. The millions who viewed it on television were seeing an historic event not only because of the subject but because it was being brought into their homes.
>
> Millions of white Americans, for the first time, had a clear, long look at Negroes engaged in a serious occupation. For the first time millions listened to the informed and thoughtful words of Negro spokesmen, from all walks of life. The stereotype of the Negro suffered a heavy blow. This was evident in some of the comments which reflected surprise at the dignity, the organization, and even the wearing apparel and friendly spirit of the participants. If the press has expected something akin to a minstrel show, or a brawl, or a comic display of odd clothes and bad manners, they were disappointed. . . .
>
> As television beamed the image of this extraordinary gathering across the border oceans, everyone who believed in man's capacity to better himself had a moment of inspiration and confidence in the future of the human race. And every dedicated American could be proud that a dynamic experience of democracy in the nation's capital had been made visible to the world.[42]

All that I am saying here about Martin Luther King is brought to mind by a brief reference in the NAACP's resolution to "the battle for civil rights and equality in the early 1960's." The role played by this widely acclaimed "hero" of the movement cannot be overemphasized, for it was King, more than any other African-American leader in the twentieth century, who demonstrated a rhetorical competence that helped to reconstruct the presence, the face, of black Americans beyond the stereotypes that fostered their social death.

We might wonder, then, why the NAACP was not more explicit in recalling some of the story of Dr. King in its boycott resolution. As an organization that was taught by one of its own heroes to be media savvy, and that made much use of "press releases" to inform people about its stance on the matter of the Confederate flag, the NAACP certainly must have known that its resolution would attract the attention of the press. Perhaps the organization felt that it would have been inappropriate to rehearse the social and rhetorical accomplishments of Dr. King once again. When you have to keep reminding people about a certain praiseworthy soul, one runs the risk of giving the impression that this soul is no longer considered to be memorable. Or perhaps the NAACP felt that a rhetorical document announcing a boycott resolution was not the right place to commemorate its hero because, within such a resolution, an "appropriate" recounting of history requires economy in presentation.

Maybe, however, the organization felt that the life and times of Martin Luther King no longer spoke effectively enough to the particular rhetorical situation at hand. Rodger Wilkins, publisher of the NAACP's magazine *The Crisis* (founded by W. E. B. DuBois), lends substance to this possibility when he explains how many young African-Americans today fail to grasp the historical sweep of King's struggle: "It's really hard, because of the generation leap. For those who weren't born in segregation, who didn't live through the civil rights movement, in a culture that was so different, it's almost as if [those of us who stood with King] are a generation who emigrated from the old country." Wilkins goes on to admit that "The NAACP needs to build a new, coherent vision to replace the vision that was present when we were fighting segregation."[43] Chic Smith, the co-chair of Black Youth Vote and founder of Urbanthinktank.org, which focuses on hip-hop culture, agrees: "Young blacks do respect the NAACP but there is a disconnect. They feel like there is no need for that kind of work anymore. They don't know what segregation is."[44]

Whatever the reason, the life and times of Martin Luther King were not a major news component of the NAACP's press releases regarding its resolution and related activities. Defenders of the Confederate flag, however, chose a different strategy as the debate over the removal of the flag continued. Consider, for example, the following words taken from a lengthy document ("Heritage Celebration 2000: Why are We Defending the Flag?") published on the Internet by the Southern Carolina Heritage Coalition (SCHC). This document, I believe, represents the most "well-developed" rhetoric offered publicly by supporters of the Confederate flag:

> Martin Luther King never called for the abolition of Confederate symbols. He never registered any objection to his own state flag. As

a great speaker who understood the power of symbols, Dr. King would certainly have utilized the symbolism of his own native state's banner had he viewed it as a symbol of racism, oppression, white supremacy, the Ku Klux Klan, or of defiance to desegregation. Dr. King never referred to any Confederate symbol provocatively as "an odious blight on the universe . . .[an] ugly symbol of idiotic white supremacy, racism and denigration" nor resolved to commit legal resources to the removal of Confederate symbols from "all public properties" as did the NAACP in 1991.[45]

The rhetorical strategy being used here by the SCHC is as important as it is straightforward: a hero of the opposition is being co-opted to serve the organization's own purposes of discrediting the NAACP. And what do you have when you take away the legitimacy that comes with the name of Dr. King? The answer, according to the SCHC, is simple: "an extremist political and racial organization" whose "true agenda is no secret: the eradication of all Confederate symbols from public view, the outlawing of all celebrations of Confederate memorials which utilize any public funds whatsoever, the renaming of any streets or public buildings which honor Confederate veterans or government officials." In the eyes of the SCHC, the NAACP's ultimate goal is "the 'reeducation' of American youth to believe their ancestors are to be hated, that they should be ashamed of their own heritage" (2). Martin Luther King, Jr., made it possible for the black race to present their genuine face, their humanity and dignity, to the world and to thereby at least begin to put an end to the torment and misery of imposed social death. The NAACP, on the other hand, is allegedly more interested in the activity of de-facing others and in bringing about their social death. "People really need to understand who their political bedfellows are," continued the SCHC. "We South Carolinians also need to fully comprehend that any compromise to appease the NAACP that would involve moving the Memorial flag to a Confederate monument will only move the battle from the dome to the yet-unbuilt monument. History will simply repeat Neville Chamberlain's 'peace in our time' error in negotiating with Hitler" (2).

I think it is fair to say that the comparison being made here between the NAACP and Hitler is, to say the least, outrageous. In making this comparison, however, the SCHC performs a rhetorical maneuver that dissociates itself with "hate groups" such as the Ku Klux Klan who use the Confederate Flag and the Nazi Swastika as symbols of white supremacy. Throughout its document, the SCHC insists that its members are not a bunch of racists and fascists. That people might think otherwise, argues the Coalition, has much to do with the "liberal" media:

Heritage groups like the United Daughters of the Confederacy and the Sons of Confederate Veterans purchase Confederate flags by the thousands to decorate graves, wave in parades, and adorn their property on Confederate Memorial Day. The thousands of honorable displays of the flag are routinely ignored by the media in favor of the handful of Klan or skinhead rallies in which a half dozen members may brandish a Confederate flag. It is rare to find our heritage even covered in *The State* [newspaper] or any other major South Carolina media outlet—but let a dozen Klansmen gather, and there will be television cameras, interviews, articles, and editorials. The flag has not so much been co-opted by racists as it has been adopted as a "whipping boy" by politically biased journalists. (4)

The position of the SCHC is clear: the liberal media, the hate groups, and the "extremist political and racial organization" of the NAACP are the real problems when it comes to gaining a correct understanding of the Confederate flag. In developing this position, the SCHC also makes much of how its stance exemplifies a genuine allegiance to "American" and "Christian" values. The rhetoric here is lengthy but noteworthy:

We live in a pluralistic, multiracial and multiethnic republic. The only way to avoid riots, civil wars, and strife between groups is to adopt a culture of tolerance. Irish Americans have no right to intimidate English Americans into furling the Union Jack. White supremacists have no right to intimidate black Americans from celebrating their heritage and from displaying their symbols. Muslims cannot tear down Stars of David, Protestants cannot demand the removal of Catholic statues of the Virgin Mary. Republicans cannot outlaw the display of Democratic campaign signs. Nor should black Americans be in the business of intolerance of, and intimidation toward, their fellow citizens who are proud of their Confederate heritage.

To capitulate to such hatred is far from Christian. Christians ought not spurn their crosses out of fear of offending unbelievers. The onus is on the unbelievers to be tolerant, not the Christians to be accommodating. Christians are specifically instructed to let their light shine, not to conceal it under a basket. If we South Carolinians—Christians and non-Christians alike—believe the Confederate flag, the crucifix, the Bible, the Star of David, or any other symbol to be honorable and worthy of display, we ought not be deterred by people who mistakenly feel otherwise. We should not cave in even when our attackers appeal to our politeness or devoutness. To do so would be to empower the intolerant and add to a climate of lock-step political correctness that chills free speech and stifles the free exchange of ideas. (5)

The climate being referred to here once again recalls the purported fascist mentality of the NAACP. As can be seen in a press release of his organization where it announced an upcoming demonstration—billed as "[Dr. Martin Luther] King Day at the Dome II: A Day of Dignity"— against the flying of the Confederate flag on state property, the outspoken President and CEO of the NAACP, Kweisi Mfume, typically responded to his opponent's charges by staying focused on the central issue at hand: "The NAACP rejects the *Confederacy-of-the-mind-mentality* of South Carolina's legislators who think that taking the flag from atop the Capitol but placing it on an illuminated, 30-foot flagpole directly in front of the Capitol is acceptable. The new placement is totally unacceptable, equally as offensive and grossly divisive. If people want to fly the Confederate flag, they should fly it on private property and not public grounds."[46]

Is the "*Confederacy-of-the-mind-mentality*" anything like the fascist mentality that supposedly characterizes the world-view of the NAACP? Mr. Mfume did not say; rather he left it to the upcoming demonstration held in the name of Dr. Martin Luther King, Jr., to tell the story. The demonstration coincided with the first official state holiday for Dr. King, a commemoration which was passed in a bill by the state's Senate on May 1, 2000, but only after anti-flag legislators agreed to include a recognition of "Confederate Memorial Day," to be held yearly on the twelfth of May. South Carolina thus became the last state in the nation to officially recognize the King holiday by giving the day off to all state workers.

Compared to the previous year, the attendance at the demonstration was rather small. At 10 a.m., approximately 4,000 people began their march to the Statehouse as they sang the old civil rights hymns "Ain't Gonna Let Nobody Turn Me 'Round" and "This Little Light of Mine" and waved bright colored posters that read "It's Not Our Heritage," "Museum the Flag," and "S.C. Suffers From The 'Confederacy of the Mind.'" Addressing the crowd from the Statehouse steps, speakers complained not only about the flag but also about such issues as racial discrimination in voting, education, and the criminal justice system. Joe Neal, South Carolina Legislative Black Caucus chairman, asked the crowd to turn and look at the flag and chant, "You're coming down!" Nelson Rivers, national field director of the NAACP, referred to the State House monument of a Confederate soldier atop a pedestal (which honors South Carolina's 20,000 Civil War dead) as "that redneck statue." James Gallman, president of the South Carolina Conference of the NAACP, was perhaps the most eloquent as he condemned his state's "Confederacy of the Mind Mentality" with the help of some well-known "redneck" stereotypes:

We come on King Day to celebrate our shared American heritage and shared Southern heritage of freedom, justice, and equality. If that is not your idea of Southern heritage, then you can celebrate it on your car bumper, celebrate it on the back of your pickup truck, celebrate it when you go to the museum, celebrate it when you re-enact battles, celebrate it on your lapel pin and your belt buckle, celebrate it at your house and in your yard, celebrate it in front of your businesses so we'll know where not to spend our money. But don't wave it in our faces here.

Although the crowd that heard and cheered these words was less in number than the 46,000 marchers that attended the rally the previous year, their presence and actions still made a race's revulsion over their continuing social death clear. One elderly protester summed it up nicely when he noted: "I've been on the battlefield since I was a small boy, and I'm a grown man and I'm still on the battlefield. I'm ashamed of South Carolina, but this is my home. I've got nowhere else to go."[47]

A home loses most of its comfort when the dwelling place that it is also encourages the social death of its inhabitants. Not feeling at home in your own home is a sad experience, to be sure. It is not difficult, however, to find a partial remedy for this problem, at least in theory. Supporters of the Confederate flag need only do something that they have not done so far: admit that their heritage is inextricably tied to an evil. Perhaps such an admission would then encourage the NAACP and its supporters, in all fairness, to explicitly state their acknowledgment of how the flag's heritage is not simply reducible to a "bottomless hatred." Although I doubt that these actions would lead to everyone feeling completely satisfied, some progress in the acknowledgment of others, of *both* supporters *and* critics of the flag, would be advanced.

On January 24, 2001, I received an email from a graduate student who was helping me stay in touch with the NAACP and Southern Heritage organizations while I was researching their controversy. He was forwarding an email that he had received a day earlier from a "chairman" of one of these organizations. It read: "I will help if you are going to tell the truth about our people. We have been accused of most everything and really don't trust any person anymore. But the truth about our bloodline will come out when the dumbing down of America is complete. America will fall as Rome did; when the southern Christian is gone." As someone who is committed to the remedy suggested above, I found this message disturbing. Religion was once again being used, as it had been during the Civil War, as a tool for spreading fear about how a supposedly "superior" race of people was in danger of extinction because of "lesser" creatures being allowed to have their own way. My discomfort turned to rage as I thought of how a similar way of thinking had led to the horrible deaths of millions of my Jewish ancestors. Social death. Eugenics. Fascists were present in the controversy between supporters and critics of the Confederate flag, but they stood *not* on the side of the NAACP.

Rage not only produced and fueled this assessment, but it also inspired me to once again head back to Columbia, South Carolina, to witness the first state sanctioned celebration of "Confederate Memorial Day" on May 12, 2001. Around a thousand people were present to cheer the festivities: marchers dressed in Confederate garb, most of them walking, others on horseback; rebel yells; canons firing; a pledge of allegiance to the Flag of the United States of America; a salute to the Flag of South Carolina; another salute to the Confederate Flag; a flyer containing a prayer by Bishop Ellison Capers of South Carolina, 1837–1908:

> Almighty God, our Heavenly Father, we adore Thy Love and providence in the history of our country and especially would like to thank Thee for our Confederate history. We thank Thee for its pure record of virtue, valor and sacrifice. . . .

Pure? "You have got to be kidding," I thought, as the festivities continued: a call to order; the presentation of the colors; roll call of the dead; short addresses by invited speakers; a cannon salute to "*Dixie*"; more rebel yells; taps; retiring of colors; closing remarks.[48]

During the two hours that I spent observing all of these happenings and more, I never saw nor heard, as in the past, any explicitly disparaging remarks about the NAACP (e.g., "The National Association for Retarded People"). Rather, differences were muted and occasionally delivered with eloquence, as was the case when Robert Peeler, Lieutenant Governor of South Carolina, spoke to the crowd: "We denounce those who would rewrite our heritage just as we denounce those who misuse our symbols." Referring to the 27,000 South Carolinians who died during the Civil War, Peeler went on to note "Some died calling their mothers' names. . . . All gave, some gave all. We remember, we will always remember."

Peeler's words were moving. I listened to them while wearing a black ribbon that was tied to my left arm by a middle-aged woman who was dressed in period costume and a widow's black attire. She had asked for permission to tie the ribbon on my arm. I agreed out of respect and a desire not to make a scene by refusing her request. My rage had subsided. My skepticism, however, was still at work. But a ribbon and some words did have me recalling more than once how the saying "Heritage, not a Bottomless Hatred" warranted consideration. In his book *States of Mind*, wherein he has occasion to speak about his skepticism of the "Rebel cause" (although not as it relates to the specific controversy at issue here), Brad Herzog offers an additional yet related reason why such consideration is due:

> I figured that supporting the Rebel soldier meant supporting the Rebel cause. But the more time I spent in the South, the more I began to understand why Confederate descendants strive to maintain

memories that others consider long dead or better forgotten. There are few behaviors more instinctive than protection of a family's honor. There are few nerves more tender than the disparagement of ancestors. Mine were eastern Europeans, and most knowledge of them was lost amid the years and the miles. But southern ties remain fresh and well tended. When you get your hands on an old sepia photograph of your great-great-grandfather in a bushy mustache and a gray uniform, and you see your own eyes staring back at you, it must arouse an instinct to support one who dies fighting for a way of life.[49]

In chapter 1, I discussed how our desire to be acknowledged and remembered after death defines an instinctive, ontological trait of human beings. Herzog is on to something here. Acknowledgment is a life-giving gift. But Herzog is not specific in his use of the phrase "a way of life." If this way was specifically identified with a non-apologetic fervor for the "Providence-based" legitimacy of slavery, would Herzog still have you "see your own eyes staring back at you" as you looked at your kin? And what if the picture in question was that of a Negro slave (perhaps your great-great-grandfather) with scars all over his back from being whipped? Recalling my earlier reference to the Southern aristocrat Mary Boykin Chesnut and her attempted reading of *Uncle Tom's Cabin*, we learned that merely reading about such a tragedy can be too much to bear. This tragedy is brought to mind by an African-American History Monument that was dedicated in January 2001, one that stands to the left and far below the Statehouse dome. No reference was made to this monument by any speaker during the May 2001 celebration of "Confederate Memorial Day." I think it would have been a generous and appropriate thing to do. Perhaps such acknowledgment would have happened if a certain battle flag had also been acknowledged by its critics as being more than a symbol of a "bottomless hatred." Perhaps, however, these critics were waiting for their opponents to acknowledge that, yes, the Confederacy nourished and was nourished by the evil institution of slavery.

Conclusion

The spatial and temporal happening of our own existence sounds a call for acknowledgment: "Where art thou?" This call can also come from others whose existence and well-being are being interrupted by occurrences that place them in jeopardy. The NAACP sounded this call in its stance against the flying of the Confederate flag on public property. Southern Heritage organizations also voiced this call in taking exception to the NAACP's arguments and objectives. Both sides wanted positive acknowledgment in order to stem the tide of social death. Neither side, however, displayed a willingness to return the favor. With their respective rhetorics, both the defenders and critics of the Confederate flag closed themselves off to the "truth": Like it or not, the Confederate flag gives expression to a way of life that thrived in the South in the eighteenth and nineteenth centuries and that was made possible by the evil of slavery justified in the name of God. And like it or not, it is possible that the Confederate flag can mean more than what its detractors claim.

In the struggle to receive the life-giving gift of acknowledgment, people can become rather selfish. Such selfishness, of course, goes against what has been said throughout this book about how the ontological structure and function of human existence calls for a way of being-for-others. Genuine acknowledgment lends itself to the formulation of a specific philosophy of controversy that emphasizes the importance of the rhetorical process of moral deliberation as a way of countering the disease of social death. Moral deliberation can bring about a halt to this ailment. It is a process that, as John Dewey reminds us, involves "doubt" and "hesitation"—time given over to a critical assessment of the "goodness" of courses of action in view of their "consequences for general happiness."[50] In moral deliberation we open ourselves to the related existential questions of whether we are presently doing the right things with our lives and, if not, what must therefore be done to correct the situation. Moral deliberation, in other words, enables us to remain "alert" and "on the lookout" for ways of being good. As Dewey puts it, "The 'good' man who rests on his oars, who permits himself to be propelled simply by the momentum of his attained right habits, loses alertness; he ceases to be on the lookout. With that loss, his goodness drops away from him."[51] Indeed, selfishness is not conducive to the cultivation of goodness in and among beings who are known to cry out "Where art thou?" and who also have an obligation to respond "Here I am!"

That such a relationship has yet to take form between supporters and critics of the Confederate flag is, to say the least, a shame. Race relations in this country are too fragile to be continually disrupted by the lack of positive acknowledgment going on here. The shame of the situation runs deep, to the very heart of the ontological workings of human being.

With the case presented in this chapter we find an illustration of how the thinking and acting of human beings can, owing to their selfishness, lag behind evolutionary progress. Writing about the non-accidental nature of such progress, at least as science sees it, Robert Fripp notes that "To study life's origin [and development] is to collide with one indisputable fact: that, however it came about, life resulted from a falling together of appropriateness."[52] Fripp thus adds another way of thinking about the long history of rhetoric's presence in the cosmos. Remember, a central aspect of rhetorical competence is the capacity to find what is right and fitting (appropriate) for the situation at hand. In the beginning was the Word. Evidence of its presence lies in the "showing/saying" (*Logos*) of our everyday existence and the call for acknowledgment that comes from its heart: "Where art thou?" Religion tells us that this call was first uttered by God. Human beings, be they religious or not, certainly re-call its urgency whenever they find themselves in some state of distress such as being lonely, ill, threatened, or marginalized. We also are known to sound the call in order just to share "good news," as when, for example, we "can't wait" to tell family and friends about some rewarding personal accomplishment. We are creatures who need and desire the gift of acknowledgment.

In the next chapter, I continue to advance my discussion of this fact of life by focusing on a technology—the personal computer—that possesses unprecedented potential in facilitating both the giving and the receiving of this gift but that, as seen in the controversy over the flying of the Confederate flag, can also be employed for selfish purposes. As I hope is clear from what has been said above, such selfishness poses a problem because it contradicts an ethic of being-for-others that is inscribed in the ontological workings of human existence. The evolution of today's ongoing "computer revolution" defines a happening of great ontological significance, especially as its leaders and advocates proclaim its "goodness" for overcoming this problem. The proclamation, related assertions, arguments, and counterarguments define a noteworthy rhetoric of "postmodernity." Zygmunt Bauman tells us that "It remains to be seen whether the time of postmodernity will go down in history as the twilight, or the renaissance, of morality."[53] It is, of course, hard not to root for the later option, which I take to be fundamentally a matter of acknowledgment. My assessment of these related matters opens with a brief discussion of Mary Shelley's classic work of science fiction, *Frankenstein; or, The Modern Prometheus*. This work is well known as a touchstone for cultural critics who would have us realize the possible evils of playing God through science and technology. My use of this work, however, is not limited to this haunting theme. The story of Dr. Frankenstein and his "monster" can also be read as a lesson in acknowledgment.

Chapter Ten

The Computerization of Acknowledgment

Consider these eloquent, albeit desperate, words that were spoken by Dr. Franken-stein's "monster" when he was given the opportunity to reflect on his first moment of self-awareness and share his thoughts with his creator:

> My person was hideous and my stature gigantic. What did this mean? Who was I? What was I? Whence did I come? . . . Hateful day when I received life. . . . Accursed creator! Why did you form a monster so hideous that even *you* turned from me in disgust? God, in pity, made man beautiful and alluring, after his own image; but my form is a filthy type of yours, more horrid even from the very resemblance. Satan had his companions, fellow devils, to admire and encourage him, but I am solitary and abhorred. . . I cherished hope, it is true, but it vanished when I beheld my person reflected in water or my shadow in the moonshine, even as that frail image and that inconstant shade. . . . [S]ometimes I allowed my thoughts, un-checked by reason, to ramble in the fields of Paradise, and dared to fancy amiable and lovely creatures sympathizing with my feelings and cheering my gloom; the angelic countenances breathed smiles of consolation. But it was all a dream; no Eve soothed my sorrows nor shared my thoughts; I was alone. I remembered Adam's suppli-cation to his Creator. But where was mine? He had abandoned me. . . . Oh! My creator, make me happy; let me feel gratitude toward you for one benefit! Let me see that I excite the sympathy of some existing thing; do not deny me my request![1]

Besides being a story about the tragic consequences that can unfold as the result of scientific and technological hubris, Mary Shelley's *Frankenstein* is also about the life-giving gift of acknowledgment and a creature whose call for this gift went unanswered. Dr. Frankenstein constructed this creature as a result of a scientific calling that requires its practitioners to acknowledge and aid others: "Wealth was an inferior object, but what glory would attend the discovery if I could banish disease from the human frame and render man invulnerable to any but a violent death!" (85). Thinking about the "glory" of such a being-for-others was intoxicating: "A new species would bless me as its creator and source; many happy and excellent natures would owe their being to me. No father could claim the gratitude of his child so completely as I should deserve theirs. Pursuing these reflections, I thought that if I could bestow animation upon lifeless matter, I might in the process of time . . . renew life where death had apparently devoted the body to corruption" (97–98).

Driven more by the potential glory than by the altruism of his self-appointed task, however, Frankenstein turned selfish when his creation came to life and showed itself to be a monstrosity: "How can I describe my emotions at this catastrophe, or how delineate the wretch who with such infinite pains and care I have endeavored to form? His limbs were in proportion, and I had selected his features as beautiful. Beautiful! Great God! His yellow skin scarcely covered the work of muscles and arteries beneath" (101). The doctor's success was also a failure. The creature was far from perfect. Frankenstein wanted nothing to do with such a "hideous wretch"—"a thing such as even Dante could not have conceived" (102).

"Where art thou?" There was no one willing to respond "Here I am!" to the creature; no one kind and generous enough to bear his horrific presence, no one able to spend time with a being who had learned to appreciate and employ with eloquence the "godlike science" and technology of language—a technology that he mastered as he secretly listened to the rule-governed speech of others and as he taught himself to read such books as *Paradise Lost* and a volume of Plutarch's *Lives*. The creature sought only acknowledgment and companionship. "[I] hoped to meet with beings who, pardoning my outward form, would love me for the excellent qualities which I was capable of unfolding. I was nourished with high thoughts of honor and devotion" (259). The creature lived for the day that he could offer the life-giving gift to others and receive some degree of appreciation for his efforts. But this never happened. He remained an outcast, a victim of ongoing social death, and his virtues turned evil.

It is important to keep in mind that the creature's fate was sealed as his creator and other human beings continually refused to grant him a dwelling place in their lives that, at least for a moment, would allow him to show the "beauty" of his true self and to feel at home with others. The tragedy here is not without a bit of irony because it was first made possible by one who, *as a scientist*, was obligated to remain open to what is other than himself in order to get at the truth of the specific matter at hand. The creature's physical appearance was ugly, but that fact should not have gotten in the way of the scientist who was devoted to acknowledging the essence of things, the real beauty of their truth.

The creature's imperfection brought out an equally "ugly" imperfection in his creator: extreme selfishness in the face of the other. Coupled with the creature's appearance, this particular imperfection helped to seal Dr. Frankenstein's own fate. His life would unfold as a series of reactions to his creation's presence and doings. Such a sealed fate defines what is commonly referred to today as the phenomenon of "technological determinism": living a life controlled primarily by the operating procedures of our tools and by the cognitive and behavioral habits that take form as we follow technological procedures on a daily basis. This phenomenon is often a source of humor. Consider, for example, some of the entries from the widespread "anonymous" email document "Evidence You Live in the Year 2005": 1) "You just tried to enter your password on the microwave." 2) "You call your son's beeper to let him know it's time to eat. He emails you back from his bedroom 'What's for dinner?'" 3) "You pull up in your own driveway and use your cell phone to see if anyone is home." 4) "You wake up at 2 AM to go to the bathroom and check your email on your way back to bed." 5) "You chat several times a day with a stranger from South Africa, but you haven't spoken with your next-door neighbor yet this year." Clifford Stohl, one of the pioneers of the Internet and also one of its most severe and outlandish critics, also has the phenomenon in mind: "Want a nation of dolts? Just center the [educational] curriculum on technology—teach with videos, computers, and multimedia systems. Aim for the highest possible scores on standardized tests. Push aside such less vocationally applicable subjects as music, art, and history. Dolts are what we'll get."[2]

I will have more to say about Stohl's position in the final section of this chapter. I introduce it here, however, in order to make a point about computer technology that is lost in Stohl's argument, readily revealed in light of Shelley's book, and crucial for my present purposes: The story of Dr. Frankenstein and his creature might have been different if the creature had had a computer connected to the Internet. For then, without having to deal with the problems associated with revealing his face and overall physical presence, he could have joined in an eloquent way the cacophony of "Where art thous?" and "Here I ams!" that are registered in cyberspace everyday as people in need of acknowledgment both receive and give this gift, for example, in emails, chat rooms, and on websites that offer a hospitable dwelling place for individuals experiencing various forms of social death.

The personal computer is a tool capable of advancing ethical behavior in that it is especially attuned to the challenge-response logic that lies at the heart of human existence and that makes itself known in our everyday being-with-and-for-others. No technology in the history of humankind (with the exception of language itself) allows for and facilitates acknowledgment more than the personal computer. Cyberspace offers itself as an awesome transformation of space and time, an immense and easily accessible dwelling place for people to meet, possibly feel at home with others, and thereby know-together what is going on in their lives. People can provide information and, perhaps more importantly, a caring caress to others.

Although I am unaware of any theorist of cyberspace conceiving it as I do— that is, as a dwelling place for the giving and the receiving of the life-giving gift of acknowledgment—the conception certainly underlies the arguments of those who insist that the "virtual communities" found in cyberspace can help revitalize the spirit of civic republicanism.[3] As Robert Bellah and his colleagues remind us, in the civic republican tradition, "community means a solidarity based on a responsibility to care for others because that is essential to living a good life." Moreover, civic republicanism, emphasizing as it does the importance of developing a rhetorically competent citizenry, maintains that the authenticity of

> public life is built upon the . . . languages and practices of commitment that shape character. These languages and practices establish a web of interconnection by creating trust, joining people to families, friends, communities, and churches, and making each individual aware of his reliance on the larger society. They form those habits of the heart that are the matrix of a moral ecology, the connecting tissue of a body politic.[4]

Civic republicanism speaks to the importance of what I have been referring to throughout this book as an ethic of being-for-others. The personal computer is a technology that has the power to advance such an ethic, and thus to facilitate the happening of acknowledgment in that ever-growing transformation of space and time called cyberspace. For creatures like Frankenstein's monster, those who are suffering and dying from a lack of companionship and abject loneliness, cyberspace offers an alternative to their current "hell on earth."

This is not to say that "all will be well" as long as the personal computer is at our fingertips. At its present stage of evolutionary development, this technology not only facilitates the happening of acknowledgment but also transforms the existential occurrence of the phenomenon in specific ways. An obvious example of this transformation, as suggested above, is seen in how the ontological structure of the self's presence in the midst of its being-with-others is afforded greater flexibility in cyberspace. Creatures who suffer social death in "real life" can find sanctuary on the Internet; others are but a few clicks away. But with the transformation of the self's presence in cyberspace, we are faced with an ever important question of interpersonal communication in an especially vivid way: Can we ever "really know" such a *faceless* self? This question gives rise to the much discussed problem of "trust" in computer and cyberspace literature.[5]

With the personal computer come both benefits and burdens exhibiting ontological significance. In the remainder of this chapter, I intend to discuss this twoedged nature of the computer in greater depth, especially as it relates to the existential transformation of the happening of acknowledgment in our lives. Although I do not have any startling revelations to share that can necessarily increase the benefits and decrease the burdens associated with computer use, I do have opinions that make me both an advocate and a critic of what this technology is doing for and to our lives.[6] My discussion of the matter begins "from the ground up" in order to be as fair as possible with both my praise and my blame. I thus continue my practice of grounding the topic in question in the ontology of human existence, discussing how what I term "the call of technology" is embedded in the very texture of our being. In developing the discussion, I will have occasion to recall the major topics that have been considered so far in our examination of acknowledgment: science and religion, the transformation of space and time, the attunement of consciousness, dwelling place, rhetorical competence, home, the caress, appropriateness, teaching, and social death.

Ontology and the Call of Technology

Assessments of computer culture oftentimes make much of the differences that exist between us and our machines. Theodore Roszak's thinking about the human "mind" provides an excellent case in point. He notes:

> The mind, unlike any computer anyone has even imagined building, is gifted with the power of irrepressible self-transcendence. It is the greatest of all escape artists, constantly eluding its own efforts at self-comprehension. It can form ideas about its own ideas, including its ideas about itself. But having done that, it has already occupied new ground; in its next effort to understand its own nature, it will have to reach out still further. This inability of the mind to capture its own nature is precisely what makes it impossible to invent a machine that will be the mind's equal, let alone its successor. The computer can only be one more idea in the imagination of its creator. Our very capacity to make jokes about computers, to spoof and mock them, arises from our intellectual distance from them. If there is anything that frustrates the technician's talent, it is open-ended potentiality.[7]

Indeed, thanks to our ability to "contemplate" and thus be "mindful" of our existence, we can understand that, unlike our machines, we are always more than the functions we perform and identify within the sociopolitical apparatus of modern technological society. We can also understand, however, that, as discussed in chapter 4, we exist as *animalia metaphysica* and that we therefore have a nostalgia for something final and absolute. This passionate longing for order and completeness in our lives makes us the purposive and pragmatic creatures that we are. The everydayness of human existence exhibits an *instrumental* impulse. We put our minds to *use*; they serve as a *means* to any number of *ends*. At its most basic level, a technology is a means to an end. We must therefore face the fact that there is something fundamentally technological about the way that we exist. It might thus be said that a call of technology is embedded in the very ontological structure of our existence.

What I am saying here is not meant to diminish the importance of seeing a difference between human beings and their technological creations. I believe Hannah Arendt is right when, in writing about contemplation and its power of wonder, she notes: "If we had to rely only on men's so-called practical instincts, there would never have been any technology to speak of . . . [Moreover,] it is not likely that our technically conditioned world could survive, let alone develop further, if we ever succeeded in convincing ourselves that man is primarily a practical being."[8] Without the *theoria* of contemplation, practice lacks a major source of vision, and blind behavior can be a dangerous thing indeed. But contemplation that lacks any connection and commitment to the world of practice can also be an affront to the "human condition," especially when circumstances give rise, as they often do, to exigencies that call for a well thought out yet immediate and *practical* response. When offering such a response, we give heed to the instrumental impulse of existence, to the call of technology.

This particular call is as much a fact of life as the call for acknowledgment. In ontological terms, the two are "equiprimordial": there is a "sameness" to them because they are both rooted in the spatial and temporal structure and openness of existence, but they are not identical. A simple example in which both calls make themselves known can help to clarify the matter.

You are sitting at your computer, preoccupied with surfing the net. All of a sudden the computer malfunctions for some unknown reason and you lose your connection. With this particular disruption, you move from a particular involvement with the world of practice (knowing how to surf the net) to the world of theory: contemplating what has gone wrong with your computer so that you can fix the problem and return to being preoccupied with the original task at hand. This desire to return to the world of practice, where all is well and functioning correctly once again, testifies to your hearing and wanting to respond to the call of technology, a call which speaks to the purposive nature of human being. You need some degree of order in your life.

The situation here, however, may not be so simple. A malfunctioning computer might prompt you to not only become more aware of what it takes to complete a given task (surfing the net for some much needed information), but may also cause you to give thought to how a sustained preoccupation with this task is leading to neglect of others (such as family members) who deserve to be treated in a much more caring and respectful way. In this case, the question brought about by the defective tool—"What is going on here, and what can be done about it?"—is no longer restricted to merely knowing how to remedy a technological breakdown. A certain realization has made the situation much more complicated than that.

Another option for action is now apparent—one that, if taken, will further delay your completion of the task as you attend to other pressing concerns. There are people in need of acknowledgment, not just simple recognition. "Where art thou?" The call of technology is still at hand, but now so is the call for acknowledgment. The first call is more concerned with the self; the second call is more concerned with the Other. The call of technology summons the self to act; the call for acknowledgment summons the acting self to remain open to the needs and welfare of others. Not hearing the second call and not being able to fix the breakdown, you might eventually pick up the phone and call some expert for help: "Where art thou?" Desperate to receive a response but not getting one because the expert is too busy to help at the moment, you might find yourself in a situation that is educational. You will know what it feels like when the call for acknowledgment is put on hold by the call of technology.[9]

Both the call of technology and the call for acknowledgment seek our response-ability; they summon us to enact what, as noted in chapter 2, Joan Stambaugh terms "the essential human deed": "Without some kind of response, no poet would write a poem, no composer would write a symphony, nobody would fall in love, no one would find a friend."[10] Stambaugh's examples are more attuned to the call of acknowledgment than simply the call of technology. Genuine and dedicated poets, composers, lovers, and would-be friends struggle to remain open to the truth of something *other* than themselves while engaged in their respective endeavors. But as *animalia metaphysica* and creatures of know-how, we cannot help but respond to the call of technology. Hence the existence of language—that "simple" low tech tool whose basic purpose is to create and maintain meaning and understanding between human beings. The fact that language can be created, used, and, whenever necessary, reformulated in order to display a sensitivity to the specific nature of the otherness of which it speaks testifies to the human ability to hear and to respond to the call of acknowledgment.

A Postmodern Ethos

It is important to remember, however, that these calls that come from our own existence, actually originate in that which is not simply the creation of some self: the *a priori* openness of temporality. Although we can manipulate and order temporality through a variety of measurements (e.g., minutes, hours, days, years), human beings did not create this fundamental (ontological) way of being in the world. There is an otherness to our own existence that begins with the very being of the self, marks our everyday relationships with other things and other people, and works in a deconstructive manner to call "who and how we are" into question. As discussed in chapter 3, this "calling into question" defines a fundamental moral impulse of existence that is always already at work before any particular system of morality is created and that, in opening us to the "not yet" of the future, is forever exposing the "truth" of any human-made system to the uncertainty and the contingency of our existence. Even when conceived in the most all encompassing and "holy" way possible—as God—this call of otherness involves a "surplus of meaning" that transcends the human power of systematization. God's presence is never without absence, without a quality of "Being" that has yet to be captured fully in and by the word. In fact, words and the systems of meaning they sustain as rhetorical economies of language are themselves technologies that operate in accordance with the "logic" of otherness: any system of meaning always enters into an "intertextual" relationship with some *other* system that it is currently transforming. Steeped as we are in its workings, the otherness of existence makes our lives an ongoing "experiment" in the search for goodness, justice, and truth.

I recall these matters because they have come to play an essential role in appreciating what Sherry Turkle terms the "postmodern ethos" of the personal computer. Turkle uses this term to describe how the computer enables us to inhabit a place where it is easier and safer to experiment with our self-identity. Indeed, as discussed above, our online presence in cyberspace is afforded the opportunity to transform itself so that, for example, a "monster" can feel what it is like to be a more attractive person, someone whom others are willing to talk to. According to Turkle, such experiences "help us to develop models of psychological well-being that are in a meaningful sense postmodern" because they accentuate the otherness of existence. In cyberspace, we are "encouraged to think of ourselves as fluid, emergent, decentralized, multiplicitous, flexible, and ever in process."[11] The philosophy of postmodernism emphasizes this point when speaking of the everyday sociopolitical "self" as being, in great part, a technological construction—an effect of language, something that is brought into being by the rhetorical and ideological discourses that are at work in the body politic.

Another illustration of the computer's postmodern ethos is found in the basic dynamics of "hypertext" programs. Such programs are designed to have readers navigate through written material in a non-sequential fashion and to experience how these materials form "a web of relations" with other texts. Hypertext thus calls into question the "modernist" notion of the "self-contained" text that forms the basis of print literacy. As Roland Barthes tells us, no text is a thing unto itself, but instead "consists of multiple writings, proceeding from several cultures and entering into dialogue, into parody, into contestation" with each other as well as with readers who might add to the text's unfolding meaning and destiny.[12] With a "constructive hypertext," readers can direct the text's destination as they become "authors," contributing new material and new links to the document. In the "world of hypertext," writes Jay Bolter, "the reader's attitude toward the text changes. The original text no longer seems inviolate . . . Any text becomes a temporary structure in a changing web of relations with other, past and future, textual structures. In the culture that reads and writes electronically, the original text loses its privileged status."[13]

Moreover, students can become *active* learners with hypertextual reading and writing, rather than *passive* recipients of some author's or teacher's worldview. This experience, according to Richard Lanham, proves to be the fulfillment "not only of the postmodern aesthetic but also of a larger phenomenon that comprehends and explains that aesthetic—the return of the basic traditional patterns of Western education and Western thinking about words and how they are used."[14] Hypertext, in other words, involves its users in the exercise of "rhetorical paideia" and encourages them to think about how they might best contribute to the online text in order to make it as interesting, as persuasive, and as politically and ethically relevant as possible. A well-designed hypertext program thus brings into view an ontological condition of human being: who we are as creatures called by our own existence to interact with our environment and with others in order to survive and who desire acknowledgment of such interactions, especially when we believe them to be praiseworthy. Human existence calls: "Where art thou?" We have an ethical obligation to respond: "Here I am!" The personal computer is especially attuned to the challenge-response phenomenon that is at work here.

A good illustration of the power of a hypertext's postmodern ethos is found in a story that I share with my students about a thirty-five-year-old computer programmer who admitted spending fourteen hours a day at the computer and loving it. The story begins with a bit of personal history concerning the man's vocation or calling: "I was an accounting major, right out of Appalachia, taking statistics class. I'd never seen a computer before. I was stunned. It told me right away if I was right or wrong. I didn't have to wait for a teacher to tell me and make me feel foolish." No negative acknowledgment and social death here. The computer programmer then spoke about a hypertext Bible program on his laptop. "When I sit in church and the minister makes a Bible reference, I call it up, copy it, make notes on what he says, add my own comments, check spelling and save it." Although this story was first published in 1992, it continues to be "ahead of its time." Have you ever seen the majority of a congregation dwelling in the house of the Lord, feeling at home with laptops in hand, clicking and scrolling away?[15]

This question can prompt other ones that bring to mind certain topics that I have related to acknowledgment and that speak of the postmodern ethos of the computer: Did the computer programmer go too far? Where was his sense of decorum or appropriateness? Shouldn't there be a clear boundary marking and respecting the difference between "sacred" space and "cyber" space? In the beginning was "the Word." Today there are sophisticated "hypertext" programs that enable people to keep the authorities (e.g., teachers, ministers) on their toes and accountable. But what is wrong with that? God doesn't like "high" technology? It's debatable, to be sure.

The story of the computer programmer illustrates the much publicized "promise" of technology that, as can be seen in any number of advertisements for personal computers, speaks to us of power, control, speed, and efficiency. The promise also admits something of a "hacker ethic" that is associated with the postmodern ethos of the personal computer: In order to abide by the moral impulse of existence and thereby remain open to otherness, the authority of boundaries should be conceived as limitations to be overcome, not merely accepted.[16] Indeed, Marshall McLuhan's "global village" is now more of a reality than ever before: "Today, after more than a century of electric technology, we have extended our central nervous system itself in a global embrace, abolishing both space and time as far as our planet is concerned."[17] Given the ongoing computer revolution, the promise of technology is often phrased as a warning: We all face the fate of being cast on the "slag heap of technological obsolescence" if we fail to keep up with constant change. "Being unable to work the gadgets through which your world does its business is not funny. It is a dangerous disability."[18] This warning entails a moral imperative, one that would have us behave so as not to be guilty of inflicting injury on ourselves. Remaining low on the learning curve of technological competence is *dis-abling* and thus a self-destructive and unconscionable thing to do. Remember: the call of technology is embedded in the very fabric of human existence. We *are* technological beings.

These last points bring us back to Turkle's argument concerning how life in cyberspace allows for the "psychological well-being" of the self. Notice, however, that since introducing Turkle into the discussion, the emphasis has been more on what the personal computer can do for the self (e.g., the computer programmer) than what the computer and the self can do for others. Turkle's research on computers and identify-formation speaks to us of the importance of what I would term "self- acknowledgment": how cyberspace offers a place where a person can be open to and can experiment with who he or she really is or wants to be. Self-acknowledgment is certainly a practice that informs the process of becoming a mature adult. Hence, Turkle's defense of its occurrence in cyberspace:

> Some are tempted to think of life in cyberspace as insignificant, as escape or meaningless diversion. It is not. Our experiences there are serious play. We belittle them at our risk. ... Without a deep understanding of the many selves that we express in the virtual we cannot use our experiences there to enrich the real. If we cultivate our awareness of what stands behind our screen personae, we are more likely to succeed in using virtual experience for personal transformation.[19]

I think it is fair to say that the jury is still out on whether such personal transformation is all for the good. Moreover, by not paying closer attention to how someone's self-acknowledgment influences and is influenced by others in "real life" (as well as in cyberspace), Turkle fails to give a clear and comprehensive account of a variable that speaks to the postmodern ethos of the computer. I want to bring this variable back into the picture now, although without losing sight of the self and its need for acknowledgment.

Cyborgs

To speak of a self whose well-being is to some extent dependent on the personal computer is to speak of a cyborg: a creature who is part animal and part machine. Cyborgs "interface" with one another as they inhabit "worlds charged with micro-electronic and biotechnological politics," writes Donna Haraway. More now than ever before in our history, "The cyborg is our ontology; it gives us our politics."[20] William Gibson's science fiction classic, *Neuromancer*, offers an example of how this political ontology may someday show itself. Here we read the story of Case, a "cowboy hotshot," who "lived for the bodiless exultation of cyberspace," and who entered this "space" by "jacking in" his nervous system directly to the computer "matrix" by means of special hardware. Maintaining "the elite stance" of the cyberspace expert "involved a certain relaxed contempt for the flesh." Compared to "the consensual hallucination that was the matrix . . . [t]he body was meat." For Case, "it was the Fall" whenever he had to exist within the temporal and spatial constraints of the lived body.[21] In Sherry Turkle's nonfiction work *The Second Self: Computers and the Human Spirit*, we find less extreme examples of what is going on here. There is, for instance, the case of Bert, an MIT sophomore majoring in chemical engineering, who admits he "think[s] of the world as divided between flesh things and machine things. The flesh things have feelings, need you to know how to love them, to take risks, to let yourself go." Bert, however, likes the "perfection" of math, chemistry, and computers. "No risks" here. "I stay away from the flesh things, I think this makes me sort of a nonperson. I often don't feel like a flesh thing myself. I hang around machines, but I hate myself a lot of the time."[22] Bert is a cyborg in distress. Case would probably respond to this by saying, "It's the meat talking, ignore it."[23]

All of us are cyborgs to some degree. It cannot be otherwise. The call of technology lies at the heart of our being. Day in and day out we find ourselves "jacked into" the instrumental matrix of the world of "know-how." When was the last time you spent a day totally unconnected to any piece of technology? And keep in mind also how, as noted above, the "self" you are is in great part a linguistic and therefore technological construction. In this day and age, not being a cyborg is not really an option for us human beings. But we still have options. Owing to our response-ability, we can affirm our "humanity" by making conscientious decisions about how and to what extent we want to connect ourselves to our ever-growing array of technological prostheses. Response-ability and responsibility must go hand in hand. Helen Schwartz has a nice way of telling us why:

> Think for a minute what music Mozart might have written if he'd had the finger length of Meadowlark Lemon, the Harlem Globetrotter who could hold a basketball with one hand. The music of a bionic Mozart might have been better, or maybe worse, but certainly different. This example forces us to consider that a technological extension or prosthesis may not necessarily be a benefit.[24]

Here is another example that does the same thing. Computers and cellular phones enhance the opportunity for people to stay "connected," to "reach out and touch someone." During a discussion of the benefits and burdens of these technologies that took place in a "Communication and Technology" course, a graduate student in rhetoric complained that being "connected" so much was "an assault on her body" and an unwanted disruption of her "private space." She wanted to be "left alone." She wanted more control over her "quality of life." She feared that such technologies made her too susceptible to experiencing "information overload and anxiety." In short, she did not want to be caught up in the suffocating embrace of the caress of existence that is made ever more possible by the hyper-connectivity of the computer revolution. Upon hearing this, an undergraduate, who was doing research in artificial intelligence, responded by telling her that she "would be left behind." He believed that these technologies amplified our "publicness"—who we *are* as social and political beings—and that this amplification was desirable. In the name of community, he argued, "interconnectivity" should be promoted, not thwarted. The grad student maintained that we were becoming too dependent on our technologies and thus "too machine-like" in how we were living our lives. The undergrad disagreed. Both students were noticeably distressed as each continued to oppose the self-declared "humanity" and "responsibility" of the other's position. When all was said and done, the undergrad returned to his AI lab. The grad student went home so she could continue working on her thesis—via her computer, of course.

We are cyborgs. Patients being kept "alive" by life-support technologies are perhaps the best example of this. Oftentimes these patients want to be "disconnected" so that they can die a "humane" and "dignified death." There is no life without death. Moreover, there is no "science" of ethics from which to calculate when, if ever, someone's "good (*eu* . . .) death (. . . *thanatos*)" should be allowed to happen. To what extent are our information technologies keeping us alive? Have you ever wanted to "pull the plug" in the name of your humanity? How many plugs could you pull before you would be "left behind"? At what point would "death" occur? Would that be a "rational" thing for a cyborg to do? What criteria would you use when making the decision?

Questions such as these interrupt the call of technology, for they sound another call: that of "conscience." The call of conscience is rooted in the "meat" side
of our cyborg existence. It summons the lived body to assume the authentic and
ethical task of affirming its freedom through resolute choice. According to Michael Zimmerman, the call of conscience "testifies that human existence has the
power of self-correction. In Aristotelian terms, human beings have their own *telos*
and move toward its full manifestation. Our *telos* is to become open to our possibilities; existence yearns to be truthful.... Conscience is the sign that our temporal
openness is dissatisfied with functioning deficiently."[25]

I sometimes hear the call when I have not been diligent enough in checking
and answering my email. People are waiting. They are lining up in cyberspace. I
am putting them on hold. It's a distressful situation; so many messages and so little time. Email creates a need for time because, as compared to "snail mail," it
dramatically increases our accessibility and accountability. "Now," rather than
"later," is what the speed of email is really about. The other calls. Conscience calls.
Technology calls. All at the same time. I feel like a certain graduate student in
rhetoric. Too much interconnectivity. Not enough private space. Is it worth it? My
body feels the pressure.

Mark Poster tells us that in today's information age "[t]he body is no longer
an effective limit" of the self's "location" in the world. I agree. Because of technological prostheses like email, "I cannot consider myself centered in my rational,
autonomous subjectivity or bordered by a defined ego, but I am disrupted, sub-
verted, and dispersed across social space."[26] With the personal computer comes a
postmodern ethos. A cyborg is as much a "we" as it is an "I," as much an "other" as
it is a "self." But, still, it is I, a self, who hears the call. The other waits for the "essential human deed": a response. Being responsible, I give it (most of the time),
thereby helping to maintain what a student in AI wisely saw as a social and political necessity: the publicness of community.

It is a good feeling to get through all of my email—day in and day out. I have
answered the calls of others. Self-acknowledgment is warranted: I am a responsible teacher, colleague, friend, and citizen. But perhaps I judge too quickly. How
many of my responses were acts of genuine acknowledgment rather than acts of
mere recognition? As first noted in chapter 1, the difference here means a lot. The
ethic of being-for-others depends on recognition becoming acknowledgment.
This process takes time. Email allows us more time to think up "authentic" and
"conscientious" responses to others and to rehearse what we are going to say; it
thus grants us more control over the managing of our personas, our "multiplicitous" selves. A carefully and skillfully worded response can give the impression
that I really care about the other, that I am not merely responding to him or her as
I would to a fly buzzing around my face. How much time in the day do I have to
offer to others genuine acknowledgment (or to come up with a display of fake acknowledgment)? With far too many emails before me, it is good to discover some

that deserve only the quick reflex of recognition. And for those who do not deserve even that, there is the almighty power of the delete key. But all of the other emails give me more pause for thought. Which "self" should take the lead? Yes, indeed, life *is* an experiment. The postmodern ethos of the computer places this fact and the challenge that comes with it right before me. The question raised by the challenge, however, concerns more than *my* psychological well-being. As a computer-using cyborg, the presence and needs of others have never been more apparent.

Community

I was trained to think about computer technology with the following words of John Dewey in mind:

> The highest and most difficult kind of inquiry and a subtle, delicate, vivid and responsive art of communication must take possession of the physical machinery of transmission and circulation and breathe life into it. When the machine age has thus perfected its machinery it will be a means of life and not its despotic master. Democracy will come into its own, for democracy is a name for a life of free and enriching communion.[27]

Such communion presupposes not only a being-for-oneself but also a being-for-others. Observing the postmodern ethos of the personal computer, I suspect Dewey would be hopeful, for this specific "physical machinery of transmission" has had more life breathed into it than any other media technology since Dewey's day.

Taken with all of the life that is going on here, Nicholas Negroponte writes:

> The true value of a network is less about information and more about community. The information superhighway is more than a shortcut to every book in the Library of Congress. It is creating a totally new, global social fabric.

Negroponte emphasizes that his optimism about this phenomenon

> comes from the empowering nature of being digital. The access, the mobility, and the ability to effect change are what will make the future so different from the present. The information superhighway may be mostly hype today, but it is an understatement about tomorrow. It will exist beyond people's wildest predictions. As children appropriate a global information resource, and as they discover that only adults need learner's permits, we are bound to find new hope and dignity in places where very little existed before. . . . We are not waiting on any invention. It is here. It is now. It is almost

genetic in its nature, in that each generation will become more digital than the preceding one.[28]

Negroponte admits that being digital also has its "dark side." The continuing evolution of the computer revolution will bring "cases of intellectual property abuse and invasion of our privacy. We will experience digital vandalism, software piracy, and data thievery. Worst of all, we will witness the loss of many jobs to wholly automated systems."[29] Nevertheless, Negroponte remains optimistic, for he feels certain that with the genetic-like evolution of our digital competencies, we will still be able to better our lives as we continue to learn how to breathe life into our computers. Negroponte makes much of how the quality of our existence will be enhanced as we improve "the interface between people and their computers . . . to the point where talking to your computer is as easy as talking to another human being."[30] And with this improvement will come the sophisticated development of a "digital persona." "One of the reasons that talking cars have been unpopular," writes Negroponte, "is that they've had less personality than a seahorse." For Negroponte, however, the

> Persona of a machine makes it fun, relaxing, usable, friendly, and less "mechanical" in spirit. Breaking in a new personal computer will become more like house-training a puppy. You will be able to purchase personality modules that include the behavior and style of living of fictitious characters. You will be able to buy a Larry King personality for your newspaper interface. Kids might wish to surf the Net with Dr. Seuss. . . . We will see systems with humor, systems that nudge and prod, even ones that are as stern and disciplinarian as a Bavarian nanny.[31]

Although he has nothing specific to say about the life-giving gift of acknowledgment, the world Negroponte is referring to here points to the phenomenon's importance: Computer technology and software should be developed that make the computer more *human*, more *open* to who we are as users who enjoy the company of others, along with the recognition and acknowledgment they have to offer. "The post-information age is about acquaintance over time: machines understanding individuals with the same degree of subtlety (or more than) we can expect from other human beings, including idiosyncrasies (like always wearing a blue striped shirt) and totally random events, good and bad, in the unfolding narrative of our lives."[32] If someone is suffering due to a lack of acknowledgment from others, then she can at least turn on her computer as a way of remedying the problem. The computer as a caring other for a self in need of "heart felt" companionship is a significant part of Negroponte's vision, as well as of those who continue to affirm his claims and speculations.[33]

I am taken with this vision; although Negroponte is back to emphasizing the self over (the human) other. What about the self's obligation of being-for-others, an obligation whose importance is brought into view by the postmodern *ethos* of the personal computer? Is genuine acknowledgment guaranteed by the "fact" that "each generation will become more digital than the preceding one"? Not addressing this issue head on also makes it easy to avoid a related matter that was referred to above: Owing to the hyper-connectivity made possible by the computer revolution, might the world of cyberspace become a dwelling place where the self's caress of the other and the other's caress of the self transform acknowledgment into a suffocating embrace? George Steiner speaks of this existential condition, which he contends is already present, as generating a "pornography of noise" that "sickens the nerve-centers of creativity" and that erodes "both solitude and attendant privacy" with its over-blown claims about "community." Writes Steiner:

> The bias toward the communal, the participatory and the collective is insistent. . . . A dread of solitude, an incapacity to experience it productively, haunts the young. . . . Democracy and mass-consumption, with their ideals of uniformity, of "peer-group" acceptance and approval, condemn solitariness. . . . [I]t is difficult to make out where in cyberspace, under what license, solitude and privacy [, two essential conditions of creativity,] will find breathing space.[34]

Steiner blames the computer for contributing to this loss of the "creative self." Negroponte disagrees as he cheers the technology for its potential to make the self more "self-reliant": "By the year 2020, the largest employer in the developed world will be 'self.' Is this good? You bet."[35] Both, however, lose sight of the other.

Perhaps this concern will have little if any purchase in a future age where the presence of a computer and what it can do for *you, immediately*, becomes more important than what you can do for others. In his critical assessment of how the fast-paced and ever accelerating computer revolution presently lends itself to this anti-communal outcome, Stewart Brand warns: "The worst of destructive selfishness is not *Me!* but *Me! Right now!*"[36] Cultural critics have such selfishness in mind when they argue that life in cyberspace caters to the tendencies of people to be exposed only to the information, opinions, and voices they feel comfortable with and to exclude everything else. Such selective perception promotes the "consumerist" mentality that, with the help of "big business," is known to thrive in cyberspace. Some also believe that this mentality inhibits the online environment's potential to cultivate the climate of civic republicanism that is needed to sustain the "free and enriching communion" of democracy. With this mentality at work, the concern of "Am I satisfied?" is granted priority over the cyber-"citizen's" civic responsibility of being-for-others. Moreover, the problem created by such selfishness is further exacerbated as we realize how, for example, websites that have a specific and identifiable political persuasion tend to provide links to like-minded sites far more than they provide links to "oppositional" sites.[37] Marginalization and social death happen in cyberspace every second of the day. For here is a place where a vast amount of hyperlinks can not only be constructed to help users open themselves to diverse and opposing world-views, but where links can also be employed to instigate the myopic and selfish ways of "groupthink." In this second case, people are conditioned to see the world in "either-or" terms: Either you are with us or you are against us. Either you abide by the party line or you count for nothing.

This "self-consumed" way of thinking goes against the moral impulse of "openness toward otherness" that marks the ontological structure of our temporal existence and that calls on our capacity to enact genuine acknowledgment in order to build community. As discussed in the last chapter, such selfishness is apparent in the way that the NAACP and Southern Heritage Coalitions each made specific use of the computer in telling why the Confederate Battle Flag should or should not be flown over the dome of the State Capital Building in Columbia, South Carolina. There are no links between the websites, nothing that joins the rhetoric of these opposing groups, thereby encouraging users to be open-minded in determining which side really has it right. As neither side has it completely right, linking the sites together might bring to the fore issues that, in order to be adequately addressed, require additional links. This additional information might allow site visitors to realize that the right way to talk about the controversy is in terms of "Heritage, Not A Bottomless Hatred."

With this case in mind, I think it is fair to say that the problem of selfishness has more to do with "human error" than it does with the computer itself. In maintaining this position, however, I do not mean to agree with those like Negroponte who maintain that "Computers are not moral; they cannot resolve complex issues like the rights to life and death."[38] On the contrary, I submit that computers are moral, at least to the extent that their workings reflect the values of the creatures who build and program them; hence the aforementioned "promise" of technology: power, control, speed, efficiency. As facilitated by the computer, these values create both benefits and burdens. We have created this technology along with an awesome space to go with it. Together, they exhibit a postmodern *ethos*—a dwelling place whose character is not unlike the one that we inhabit every second of the day as our temporal existence opens us to the objective uncertainty of the future, to an otherness that extends beyond our finite grasp and that forms the horizon of our everyday way of being with things and with others.

The postmodern *ethos* of the computer provides us with an environment where we can easily and quickly call out to and interact with others who are also calling out to us. Community takes shape in the process, unless selfishness gets in the way. Yet when it does, we, as responsible beings, still have the power to change for the better in the midst of the temporal openness of existence. Such openness allows for change. We did not create this primordial openness. Drawing on our scientific, technological, and artistic capabilities, we did, however, *create its likeness* in the being of cyberspace. Phrased this way, it might seem that there is something "holy" going on here, something whose cosmological history extends at least as far back as a certain singularity's Big Bang happening at the *appropriate* moment, and then even further back to the One who caused this awesome happening to occur *in the first place*. Such speculation brings me to my next set of related topics.

Hyperness, Holiness, and Heroes

We must learn to come to terms with change. Heraclitus said as much well over two thousand years ago. Remember: "You cannot step twice into the same rivers; for fresh waters are ever flowing in upon you."[39] Existence itself offers us the same lesson everyday: Owing to our temporality, we are continually in the "process of becoming" that which we are. "It lies in our nature," writes Karl Jaspers, "to be on-the-way."[40] We constantly find ourselves transcending and thus *moving beyond* the moment at hand. We thus might say that there is something *hyperactive* about our being-in-the-world. This hyperactivity is always at play in our lives; it opens us to the spatial and temporal realm of the "not yet" and thus always speaks to us of the possibility of change, of things being different tomorrow, or one year from now, or fifty thousand years from now. Is there an optimal rate of speed, of progress, for maintaining the good health of our hyperactive being?

In today's information age, change is occurring at an exceptionally rapid rate. The future is more "now" than "later." We find ourselves in an unprecedented state of "hyperness." As *animalia metaphysica*, we might prefer order and stability over this accelerating and sometimes chaotic state of affairs. But let us not forget that, as Søren Kierkegaard once put it, "in existence, the watchword is always forward."[41] We *are* hyperactive beings. Change is a constant made possible by the openness of our existence. Exposed to this openness, we are destined to hear and respond to the call of technology and, as responsible beings, to the call of acknowledgment. Perhaps the quicker we do this the better, especially if we hope to survive in a climate that may just well be another stage in the evolutionary struggle of the "survival of the fittest." But who really knows? Maybe we are moving too quickly with our fast-forward existence. Maybe not.

Although I am unaware of anyone who can provide a definitive response to the issue, it is certainly one that sparks controversy. For there are those, like members of the internationally known "Lead Pencil Club" (LPC), who seek to persuade people that, caught up in the computer revolution, we are indeed moving too quickly and are presently out of control: What computers "are doing to us, our society and our children, is a disaster. We are fed up with the electronic industry's hype of convenience and speed. From the Internet to television to voice mail, to faxes to email to the World Wide Web, we have had it. This nonsense has got to stop."[42] I do not disagree with everything that the LPC has to say about the "downside" of computer technology, but sometimes their logic escapes me.

Consider, for instance, this claim: "Each time you give a machine a job to do you can do yourself, you give away a part of yourself to the machine. That's not practical. If you drive instead of walk, if you use a calculator instead of your mind, you have disabled a portion of yourself. On the other hand, every time you remove a technology from your life, you discover a gift."[43] This claim certainly does not buy into the moral imperative that is associated with how human existence exhibits the call of technology. Rather, the LPC argues that technology is disabling to the self. This argument, at best, is shortsighted. As discussed earlier, a computer that breaks down while you are using it can be a catalyst for the realization that face-to-face communication with your family and friends is a wise and caring alternative to a continuing preoccupation with getting back on the Internet quickly. Technology can get in the way of our acknowledgment of others. But it can also facilitate the accomplishment of this goal.

For example, am I disabling myself if, having just learned that the mother of friend who lives a thousand miles away has just died, I send a caring email rather than walk the distance to express my condolences? Perhaps a less high-tech alternative—a phone call or a hand-written letter—would be more pleasing to the LPC. After all, these options convey a more genuine "presence" (hearing my voice) and a more "personal touch" (my actual hand-writing) than a bunch of electrons structured in "Times New Roman 12 point font" can.

What "portion" of myself am I "disabling" if I choose these less high tech options? And what "gift" do I discover if I choose none of these options and instead decide to walk the thousand miles? Having finally reached my destination (and having explained why it took me so long to respond to the sad circumstances), I might find that in the presence of others I become quite emotional, choked up, and unable to put into words my sincere grief. The best I can offer at that moment are tears and a hug. I suspect that this moment of acknowledgment, especially given all the physical effort that was expended to produce it, would be much appreciated by my friend and his family. Giving and receiving the gift of acknowledgment "in person" makes it all the more meaningful more often than not. But I did not have to be there in person in order to share this gift. A heartfelt and rhetorically competent email could also perform the deed, and in a much more timely manner. The personal computer need not necessarily disable my ability to say "Here I am" to others; in fact, in may improve it, depending on how skilled I am when putting my care and love into words. As we are reminded when reading Shelley's *Frankenstein*, having a way with words can convey more of the depth and genuineness of a person's presence than his or her simply being there in the flesh can.[44]

Life certainly slows down when we turn off our communication technologies, and that can be a very pleasurable, peaceful, and therapeutic way of being at times. But our hyperactive existence and its attendant call of technology remain.

We are purposive creatures who are destined by the openness of our existence to move beyond the moment at hand and toward domains of otherness that call for acknowledgment. The personal computer and the Internet can serve this end. The Internet philosopher Michael Heim puts it this way: "Our fascination with computers is . . . more deeply spiritual than utilitarian," for in "our love affair" with these machines "we are searching for a home for the mind and heart."⁴⁵ Cyberspace is a place where a fundamental aspect of the human spirit—the hyperactive and moral impulse of existence—is allowed to thrive.

Associating computers with the spiritual begs a question that was raised earlier: Is there something "holy" going on here? The question has certainly stimulated the imagination of many writers interested in the nature of cyberspace. For example, in his book *The Talmud and the Internet*, Jonathan Rosen suggests how our searching for a home page in the openness of cyberspace is reminiscent of his Jewish ancestors' wanderings in the openness of the desert and their dependence on the holy and *open-ended* teachings of the Talmud. This holy book, writes Rosen, "offered a virtual home for an uprooted culture." The Jewish people

> became the people of the book because they had no place else to live. That bodily loss is frequently overlooked, but for me it lies at the heart of the Talmud, for all its plenitude. The Internet . . . engenders in me a similar sense of Diaspora, a feeling of being everywhere and nowhere. Where else but in the middle of Diaspora do you *need* a home page?⁴⁶

The postmodern *ethos* of cyberspace lends itself to a "religious" reading. In fact, as Margaret Wertheim makes clear in her comprehensive study of the matter, "The notion of cyberspace as a heavenly space runs rife through the literature. . . . These are not just the imaginings of science fiction writers, more and more they are the real-world dreams of influential members of the techno-scientific elite."⁴⁷ In his equally fascinating study of the matter, Mark Dery adds the following insight: "Ironically, the very scientific worldview and runaway technological acceleration some say have produced the spiritual vacuum and societal fragmentation that are fertile ground for millenarian beliefs are spawning a techno-eschatology of their own—a theology of the ejector seat."⁴⁸ Such a theology presupposes what I have been calling the hyperactive and moral impulse of existence, something that is *other* than a human creation and in whose likeness *we* have constructed the ongoing "home" of cyberspace. Openness is the tie that binds the technological and the religious: "As with Christianity," notes Wertheim,

> cyberspace too is potentially open to everyone: male and female, First World and Third, North and South, East and West. Just as the New Jerusalem is open to all who follow the way of Christ, so cyberspace is open to anyone who can afford a personal computer and a

monthly Internet access fee. Increasingly, libraries and other community centers are also providing access for free. Like the Heavenly City, cyberspace is a place where *in theory* people of all nations can mix together.[49]

In cyberspace people can not only learn to feel at home with others but, in doing so, they can dwell in a place that, although separated from "real life," is nevertheless a step closer to their Maker, to an Otherness whose presence and moral impulse is operating in the openness and hyperactivity of their digital being. Granted, spending too much time in this separated place can pose a danger to their health (recall my earlier comments regarding the life of a cyborg in distress). But according to the story that is told in the Old Testament, the happening of "separation" (*Havdalah*) is an event essential to life. David Gelernter speaks to this point:

> In the beginning, says the book of Genesis, was chaos—*tohu va'vohu*. Chaos is the starting point, and chaos means mixed-togetherness, *un*separation. To banish chaos, you must separate. In the story of creation, God separates light from dark, the waters above from the waters beneath, day from night. To make room for the earth and for man, God forces the chaotic primeval waters open like the Red Sea; the waters are pushed up high and down low.
> Creation and Exodus are a pair. When Israel is born at the Red Sea, God separates the waters once more, just long enough for Israel to emerge, to escape into nationhood. God forces an opening.[50]

It is such a separation that Dery has in mind when, as noted above, he speaks to us of "a theology of the ejector seat" whose "rhetoric of escape velocity" thrusts us up and away toward heaven. For Dery, however, such rhetoric is delusional and dangerous, especially in its Christian transformation, where we find

> the Pentecostal belief in an apocalyptic Rapture, in which history ends and the faithful are gathered up into the heavens. Visions of a cyber-Rapture are a fatal seduction, distracting us from the devastation of nature, the unraveling of the social fabric, and the widening chasm between the technocratic elite and the minimum-wage masses. The weight of social, political, and ecological issues brings the posthuman liftoff from biology, gravity, and the twentieth century crashing down to Earth.[51]

Dery's critical assessment of the computer revolution's "rhetoric of escape velocity" warrants serious consideration, especially because it emphasizes the importance of not allowing such rhetoric to make us forgetful of our finitude and the ethical responsibility that comes with it. We *are* a being-for-others, an identity which entails more than developing a fanatical allegiance to our God and to the home that God allows us to construct and inhabit in cyberspace as we develop what Wertheim disparagingly terms our "cyber-soul."[52] We must keep in mind, however, that the specific rhetoric that directs Wertheim's attention and that informs and instructs this cyber-soul is just an *extreme* brand of discourse meant to encourage only a particular ideological answer to the question: Is there something "holy" going on in cyberspace? In the Judeo-Christian tradition, there is certainly much said about how one's admission into the dwelling place of heaven is dependent on how well we fulfill the earthly obligation of being-for-others.

So *is* there something "holy" going on in cyberspace, something that calls on the human spirit's hyperactivity to continue moving beyond the present? The significance of this question has not escaped the attention of the computer industry, with its constant search for consumers and the capital that comes with them. A full-page magazine advertisement from the computer manufacturer Compaq, provides a case in point.

The words are few; only eight in number. The first three read: "Welcome to Your." The next two that are printed below in big, bold letters running across the entire page: "DIGITAL SANCTUARY." At the bottom right of the page is the word "COMPAQ" with "Inspirational Technology" printed right underneath. On most of the right-hand side of the ad, running approximately two-thirds of the way down the page, is a picture of a casually dressed young man—in his late teens or early twenties—sitting on a portable table, holding a computer keyboard on his leg. The keyboard and a mouse are wired to a computer monitor that sits next to him on the table. The monitor is connected to a hard-drive console that rests underneath the table on a light-colored, wood-stained floor. The young man appears to be in a meditative daze, with his head bowed as he stares down at the floor. Behind him are six vertical windows filled with light, some of which is reflected on the floor.

Do you get the picture? It's quite simple—just what a religious (e.g., monastic) sanctuary should be: a consecrated dwelling place, sparse in furnishings but still blessed by the light of God. Here you are welcome. Here you find refuge, solitude, tranquility. You can feel reverent and at home in this place of worship and inspiration. There is no need to feel rushed, to be overly hyperactive. A personal computer provides the divine link. A medium supplies the message. "Where art thou?" "Here I am!" Although separated from the masses and their frenzied pace of life, you are not alone. Otherness abounds. God does like high technology. Just turn on the computer. Be for others, in peace and quiet. There is a way to find heaven on earth. There is something "holy" going on here. COMPAQ.

A less direct, although I think equally eye-catching, way of exposing the holiness of the personal computer is provided in another full-page magazine advertisement from the computer manufacturer Fujitsu. At the top, right-hand side of the page are the words: "A hero returns." Right below these words, extending one third of the way down the page, is a black and white, full page picture of a crowded office with nine people all staring at you, the reader. Their expressions reflect amazement. Four are seated, the others are standing. Three of them are holding on to pieces of paper. None of them have a computer at hand. Below this picture is another, full-color image of a Fujitsu laptop computer, complete with a pencil-like touch-screen device. The top half of the computer's screen extends into the office photograph. To the left of the computer are the words: "Deal clinching data." To the right the sentence continues: "is just one touch screen tap away." Below and to the left of the picture of the computer is a brief description of the product: "Under 3 lbs., the ultra-portable LifeBook B Series arms the field with everything they need to win over customers. . . . For more on this lean, field-force machine, visit our website." To the left of these words is the website address. Above these words we find the manufacturer's name, "FUJITSU," followed by the words "The Possibilities Are Infinite."

For us mortal beings, the notion of infinite possibilities can have a holy ring to it. With this advertisement, however, such holiness is associated with the Crusade-like, battlefield mentality of big business. In this environment you need to be mobile and quick; thus the importance of "the ultra-portable . . . lean, field-force machine": the "LifeBook B Series" computer that provides ready-access to "deal clinching data." Given the context, this computer is truly a "hero." And you (the viewer), too, can be a hero. Keep in mind that the advertisement is designed so that the people in the picture are looking at you—the one who is walking into their office with a computer in hand that is full of "Life." Indeed, you are serving others by bringing them a life-giving gift of acknowledgment. "A hero returns"— one who embodies the hyperactive and moral impulse of existence and who carries a creation that does the same.

This last point is especially important for my purposes. Heroes are people who act in such a way as to "stand out" from the crowd and who are admired for doing so. Both the act and the admiration are rooted, however, in a more primordial process than they themselves define. The process is that of the ecstatic workings of temporality—the way the no-longer, the not-yet, and the here-and-now interpenetrate each other so that human existence is always in the state of "standing outside and beyond itself" (Gk. *ek-stasis*), at every moment opening out toward the future, toward the world of possibilities. The ontological structure of human being has something heroic about it, and thus we all have the potential to be heroes—those courageous souls who actually act out "human greatness" and thereby illustrate what it takes for a finite being to live on after death in the hearts and minds of others.

Heroes, in other words, speak of the possibility of being immortal and thus "god-like" (hence, their great attraction to humankind). The genuine hero answers the call of others not for egotistical reasons, but rather for the sake of something other than the self, something that is in need of acknowledgment but that is not necessarily expected to return the favor. Certainly a heartfelt thank-you would be nice, but that is not what true heroism is all about. Ernest Becker makes the point this way: "Man will lay down his life for his country, his society, his family. He will choose to throw himself on a grenade to save his comrades; he is capable of the highest generosity and self-sacrifice. But he has to feel and believe that what he is doing is truly heroic, timeless, and supremely meaningful."[53] Like the beings they surpass, heroes need the gift of acknowledgment in order to be remembered beyond the moment of their accomplishments. No heroes, including God, are beyond exception. For even God, as Rabbi Abraham Heschel reminds us, "is in search of man" in order to be acknowledged.[54]

The Fujitsu ad encourages you to envision yourself as the hero, god-like in heart and mind, coming to the aid of others. Like Moses, you have come back to your people with sacred text in hand. You have said nothing so far. Perhaps, like Moses, you know yourself to be "slow of speech" and "slow of tongue" and thus not "eloquent" enough to preach the wonders of your gift. Perhaps, like Moses, you lack the requisite rhetorical competence to spread the word in a moving and truthful way. Overcoming this problem was part of Moses' heroic struggle. With today's computer revolution, however, it is possible to remain silent. The computer's presence says enough; it need only be "touched." You hold something quite special in your hands; something that warrants sharing and that subsequently needs to be caressed by others. Yes, there is something "holy" going on here; something that is open, hyper, and moral, that both grants and welcomes acknowledgment, and that is self and other all at once. And forever more? What finite being can say for sure? Evolution continues.

God, as they say, works in mysterious ways. Is the personal computer an evolutionary sign of God's presence, a creation of a creation who, for the time being, is destined to remain open to otherness and to the numerous questions it poses?[55] Computer companies address this question with advertisements that must display some degree of artistic and rhetorical competence if, as it is said in the business world, they are to become "invited guests in people's homes."[56] As noted throughout this book so far, such competence plays an essential role in opening people to what others believe to be good, just, and truthful. The art of rhetorical competence is thus also called for in cyberspace. I mentioned this fact earlier when, during my critique of one of the major arguments made by the Lead Pencil Club, I emphasized how a rhetorically competent email could be more effective interpersonally than the mere presence of a self before others. I will have more to say about this matter in the next and final section of this chapter as I take a closer look at the relationship that exists between the personal computer, acknowledgment, and rhetorical competence. I will also discuss how this relationship shows itself in what I take to be one of its most important contexts: the existential milieu of teaching and education.

Teaching and the Spirited Education

Right around the time that the personal computer revolution was taking off (1982), the philosopher Calvin Schrag had this to say to his fellow educators about the changing times:

> A university that does not respond to the technological develop-
> ments of the current age can be said to be both nonresponsive in
> the behavioral sense and irresponsible in the moral sense. It might
> seriously be questioned whether a stance of nonresponse is indeed
> possible. Technology is an inescapable fact of our contemporary
> cultural existence. We are reminded of the disarming reply of Tho-
> mas Carlyle to Margaret Fuller's stoic affirmation, "I accept the uni-
> verse!" Responded Carlyle, "Gad, she'd better!" . . . The more diffi-
> cult requirement that we face, however, is that of responding
> responsibly to this cultural fact.[57]

Like Schrag, I believe that universities must constantly position themselves to respond responsibly to the moral challenge posed by the computer revolution. I also agree with Schrag's contention that such a response requires the questioning and critical reflection of collaborative moral deliberation, for only through such rhetorical and conscientious behavior can the members of a given community genuinely acknowledge one another as they try to coexist with technology, making a place for it in their lives without becoming its mere servants.[58] Such "servant-hood" portends the possibility of an extremely rigid and unforgiving type of tech-nological determinism. We find this in Shelley's *Frankenstein*, especially when the creature, overwhelmed by his creator's selfish ways, feels compelled to say to the scientist: "Slave, I before reasoned with you, but you have proven yourself unwor-thy of my condescension. Remember that I have power, you believe yourself mis-erable, but I can make you so wretched that the light of day will be hateful to you. You are my creator, but I am your master; obey!" (208). The deadly consequences that resulted when this command was ignored could have been avoided if Dr. Frankenstein had assumed the ethical responsibility of being a devoted teacher to a creation who was in desperate need of acknowledgment.

Let us take a moment to recall how acknowledgment defines the essence of teaching: The tasks before the dedicated teacher always include finding a way to transform space and time into a dwelling place where people can open themselves to and feel at home with each other, take an interest in whatever is being said, and come to know together its reasonableness, worth, and perhaps how to make it more enlightening, revealing, truthful, accurate, and applicable to people's lives. Teaching, in other words, is an ethical activity requiring rhetorical competence. Dedicated teachers help others cultivate their conscience and, in so doing, serve as models for learning how to say "Here I am" to those in need of acknowledgment, guidance, and friendship. Dedicated teachers welcome the challenge of authenticity that comes with their calling: the challenge of putting themselves on the line in front of others and running the risk of learning that they have yet to get things right. The whole experience admits a "religious" quality that can be, and to a certain extent should be, entertaining for the students as well as for the teacher. The genuine teaching experience defines a being-for-others that is reciprocal; its spirited ways live and die on how well acknowledgment is cultivated in the classroom *between* people, their topics, and their texts. There is something heroic about being a good teacher and a good student.

Technology can facilitate this honorable way of being. Consider how email serves the student-teacher relationship. Owing to this communication technology, a teacher's office hours have been extended to twenty-four hours a day. With this transformation of time and space, the dwelling place of the educational setting has expanded, making it easier for both students and teachers to make their presence known to each other. The personal computer is certainly a tool for enhancing acknowledgment, for opening the self to others and others to the self. Engaging in and regulating this interpersonal exchange is part of the teaching experience. And it takes rhetorical skill, especially if the exchange is not to become a suffocating embrace. The inappropriateness of being in someone's face too frequently and for too long can try their patience to the point that the desire to give and to receive acknowledgment gives way to the more expedient act of simply offering some form of recognition. The genuine teaching experience, however, cannot thrive on this offering alone. There is, if you will, no "Tuesdays with Morrie" if teacher and student only take the time to recognize one another because they are satisfied with this rather noncommittal way of being-with-and-for-others.

Although it can be used as a "crutch" by students who, for one reason or another, opt not to develop their conversational and rhetorical skills in the classroom or in face-to-face sessions with their teachers, email still makes a freedom of expression possible, allowing students who suffer from the anxiety of "communication apprehension" to give and receive acknowledgment. Indeed, this electronic mode of communication has saved more than a few students in my classes whose reticence was not only incorrectly interpreted by me in an uncomplimentary way, but also broke the rule of mandatory class participation. This rule adheres to the age-old Socratic argument that such participation, and the "risk" that goes with it, allow for and encourage the development of the students' moral character by involving them in a dialogical process whereby interlocutors are open to each other's potentially conflicting positions.[59] The process is thus attuned to what I have described throughout this book as the moral impulse of human existence, an impulse that calls on us to assume the ethical responsibility of our freedom of choice while at the same time remaining open to what others have to say about the matter at hand.

With the rule of mandatory class participation, students are free to not speak their minds in every class session, but they are not free to remain silent throughout the semester. Sooner or later they must put themselves on the line, speak up, share their ideas and criticism, acknowledge and be acknowledged by others. I try to facilitate this process by way of instruction and behavior that make clear to one and all that the classroom is a dwelling place where people can feel at home with each other, and where a student need not be afraid of being ridiculed for "saying something stupid." The process, of course, is one of those things that is easier said than done, especially when dealing with students who suffer from communication apprehension.

Reading what these students are sometimes willing to share when their presence is routed through cyberspace can be instructive. Consider, for example, the case of "Anna," a senior undergraduate who was enrolled in my special seminar, "Communication Ethics and Acknowledgment." She did not say a word in class for the first three weeks of the semester because, despite my encouragement, she was fearful of "saying something stupid" in front of her peers. Her communication apprehension also prevented her from contacting me by email or making an appointment to see me to discuss her problem in more detail.

Finally, in the evening after a class discussion about how the "instant messenger" (IM) service available to students, faculty, and staff through the university was affecting the culture and communication climate on campus, Anna sent me the following email:

> Dr. Hyde: I thought I'd share this with you: "Don't worry, IM is working again . . . life can return to normal" and "My computer is always scared when IM doesn't work because I want to throw it out the window." These are current "away messages" of two of my friends on Instant Messenger. The Internet was down last night, and you would have loved to see the reactions. People were obsessively checking to see if the Internet was working, and when it wasn't, they'd curse it for 5 minutes afterwards. "We pay enough money at this school for them to keep the Internet working. . . ." I just thought it proves how dependent we are [on our computers]—some more than others—and how many can't handle being disconnected for any period of time. Very interesting. . . . Have a good weekend.

I was surprised by this sudden change in behavior and admitted as much in my return email. But I thanked her for this new information and once again encouraged her to be more vocal in class. During the next meeting of the class, Anna had an opportunity to share with her peers what she had shared with me via email. When she once again chose not to take advantage of this opportunity, I ad-libbed a transition in the discussion in order to tell the class about the email and who sent it. Although she remained silent, Anna had a smile on her face as the class enjoyed sharing some additional stories about the Internet going down.[60]

The ice had finally broken. Another Internet transaction between Anna and me occurred shortly after dinner. We talked more about the workings of IM on campus, prompting her to share the following observation about technology and its relationship to acknowledgment: "It's pretty fascinating. People leave messages like 'Someone leave a message to cheer me up' or 'Today is my birthday, send me some lovin.' Indeed, cyberspace is filled with "Where art thous?" and "Here I ams!" I asked her if she had minded my acknowledgment of her in class that day. "I was a little embarrassed," she said, "just because it's always a little nerve-wracking to have the spotlight on you in class. But I admit I was happy when you mentioned my thoughts. . . . I also told my friend Chris that you might use his quote about throwing the computer out the window in your book, and he was very excited."

Helping students to become, among other things, happy and excited about their education is certainly a goal of the committed teacher. Acknowledgment serves this goal. The personal computer is a tool for acknowledgment. Negroponte tells us that "Brevity is the soul of e-mail."[61] Not necessarily! Students who have important things on their mind can reach out for help by writing long emails. Given the particular student involved, responses sometimes require a rhetorical competence that is not confined to the "short and sweet." The personal computer enables us to save a lot of time when getting in touch with others. Cyberspace admits a fast-paced rhythm. But once in touch, the process of bringing about genuine acknowledgment can certainly slow things down a bit.

Cyberspace, of course, allows for this process, too.

Taking the time to visit and explore students' websites and web diaries ("blogs") is another way that teachers can learn about who their students *are*. Constructing an informative, friendly, welcoming, and entertaining website and web diary that keeps the attention and interest of others, so that they remain open to and feel at home in the creator's dwelling place, also requires rhetorical competence. The architecture of any website or web diary is made to sound both a call and a response: "Where art thou?" "Here I am!" Students are known to put a lot of themselves into this architecture for, like their teachers, they, too, need acknowledgment and are happy and excited when they receive this life-giving gift.

Of course, the use of the computer in the classroom also can facilitate the process of acknowledgment. As anyone who has tried it successfully knows, incorporating material found on the Web into courses and presentations can add a creative dimension to teaching. This creativity, which was not possible before the computer revolution, can be used to inspire the attention of students. For example, when teaching students about the relationship between acknowledgment and cosmology (chapter 2), I make use of an interactive website, "Molecular Expressions: Science, Optics, and You."[62] With the help of computer animation, this site allows visitors to view the Milky Way at a distance of 10 million light years (10^{23}

meters) from the Earth. You can then continue to move through space toward the Earth in successive orders of magnitude of ten—until you reach a tall oak tree just outside the buildings of the National High Magnetic Field Laboratory in Tallahassee, Florida. After that, you can move from the actual size of a leaf into a microscopic world that reveals leaf cell walls, the cell nucleus, chromatin, DNA, and finally into the subatomic universe of electrons, protons, and quarks (10^{-16} meters). The demonstration allows me to illustrate in an exceptionally vivid way what I term the "significant insignificance" of humankind's home in the universe.[63] Students find the demonstration to be not only "dazzling," "awesome," "entertaining," and "quite humbling," but also a stunning "epideictic display" of some truth. The creators of the website warrant praise for their rhetorical competence. I try to enhance an understanding and appreciation of their revelation with my use of a PowerPoint presentation that complements my prepared lecture material. When all goes right, the class typically proves to be intellectually stimulating and entertaining. Acknowledgment is known to serve such ends.

What I am saying here about computers, rhetorical competence, and acknowledgment has not gone unchallenged in the literature of education. For there are those, like the computer analyst Clifford Stohl, who maintain that

> good schools need no computers. And a bad school won't be much improved by even the fastest Internet links. . . . [A] good teacher can handle her subject without any multimedia support. . . . [T]he enjoyment of scholarship has nothing to do with making learning fun. . . . With or without a computer, a mediocre instructor will never kindle a love for learning. And a good teacher doesn't need the Internet to inspire her students to excellence.[64]

Indeed, there are times when too much dependence on email, downloaded material from the Web, and PowerPoint demonstrations can get in the way of the acknowledgment and learning that should be going on in the classroom. Stohl's book is a joy to read, provided you keep this one-sided account in mind. I consider him rhetorically competent when it comes to poking fun at the limitations and misuse of computers. For example, here is Stohl discussing what he terms "the plague of PowerPoint":

> Imagine a boring slide show. Now add lots of generic, irrelevant, and pyrotechnic graphics. What have you got? A boring slide show, complete with irrelevant whiz-bang graphics. . . .
>
> Once, foibles, yarns, and a few jokes sympathetically linked speaker to audience. Now, everyone's . . . staring at the video screen or reading their handouts. The speaker becomes an incidental accessory behind the lectern.

Not that the speaker cares. He's too busy fiddling with buttons and watching the screen. With his back to the audience, the orator knows what the next slide will say, as does the audience [with handouts in hand]. Should he forget a line or head off on a tangent, the program prompts him back to the prepared talk.[65]

When it comes to the educational means and ends of rhetorical competence, acknowledgment, and learning, computers can too easily become an impairment:

What motivates an audience? Emotion. Passion. Fire. A sense of warmth, excitement, shared adventure. A PowerPoint-driven meeting delivers chilly, pre-programmed video graphics. You see graphs, numbers, bullet charts. But dancing sprites and flashing logos can't inspire zeal, loyalty, outrage, or a clarion call to action. . . .

I can imagine Abraham Lincoln at Gettysburg, sporting a video projector and PowerPoint. He'd show a graphic of eighty-seven calendars flipping by, fading into an animation of Washington crossing the Delaware. Highlighted on his bullet chart would be the phrases "A new nation," "Conceived in liberty," and "All men are created equal."[66]

My students enjoy reading Stohl's observations about PowerPoint, especially this last paragraph. He has a good take on the absurd, which makes his writing entertaining and fun—the very things that he objects to when they are facilitated by computers inside the classroom. This contradiction is not missed by my students. Throughout their education, they have experienced both boring and interesting electronic presentations. They thereby know that Stohl is, at best, telling a half-truth and, at worst, using his rhetorical competence to manipulate and dupe the reader.

The study of the computerization of acknowledgment, especially in the educational setting, requires that we develop a much more comprehensive understanding and appreciation of rhetorical competence than what Stohl provides. The personal computer need not take total control of this artistic capacity, one that is needed by teachers and students in order to share the life-giving gift of acknowledgment with each other. The dwelling place found in education flourishes or decays as teachers and students attend to a moral challenge that is rooted in the existence of human being—a challenge that sounds both the call of technology and the call for acknowledgment. In closing this chapter, allow me to offer one final example that speaks to the importance and the difficulty of this challenge.

Members of the Information Systems staff at my university (Wake Forest) are currently at work trying to extend the university's technological learning curve. They are designing and testing a hand-held computer that they maintain will increase the quality and character of communication between students and faculty—without anyone uttering a word. The new technology, christened PocketClassroom (PCL) by its designers, enables students to view web pages and check and send emails using a wireless card. More importantly, the technology allows students to increase their participation in the classroom by providing better feedback to the teacher. Students can use their PCL to anonymously ask questions during class about material that they may not understand, and teachers can conduct impromptu quizzes and get immediate results in order to gauge the effectiveness of their lecture. The software also features its own web server, allowing the instructor to launch class-specific websites and PowerPoint presentations while walking around the classroom and conversing with individual students. Multiple choice questions can be asked, with responses sent to the teacher through the PCL. Answers can be recorded and organized in a bar graph on the teacher's computer and projected on a classroom screen for the whole class to see in real time. An on-screen bar graph (ranging from "+10 to–10") recording student responses to the teacher's classroom presentation is also possible.[67]

The PCL certainly serves the need for student/teacher interaction, especially in larger lecture courses where such interaction—and the acknowledgment that can arise from it—are, practically speaking, quite difficult (if not impossible) to sustain. The PCL caters to acknowledgment as it provides a new opening for students to reach out to their teachers. Always on the mind of the conscientious classroom teacher is the question "Where art thou?" Are students understanding and appreciating all that he or she is saying? The PCL offers students a way to produce an ongoing response to this question, and the teacher need never know who, exactly, made their presence known with a specific response, a specific "Here I am!" The PCL thus lessens the risk that comes with the seeking of acknowledgment, the chance that opening yourself to another might, depending on his or her specific response to you, incite hurt feelings and social death.

As noted earlier in this chapter, such risk not only adds to the existential robustness of being acknowledged, but also represents an important ingredient in the development of moral character. For students suffering from communication apprehension, the lessening of this risk, at least for the time being, makes good sense. Sooner or later, though, students have a responsibility to open themselves as much as possible to this risk. The ontological structure of human being demands as much. The PCL, at the very least, facilitates the beginning of a response to this demand. It is a tool for acknowledgment; it provides an opening to teachers by allowing for instantaneous feedback on their work in the classroom. Such feedback is only limited by the student's willingness to type a message on his or her PCL and send it to the teacher.

Of course, not having the speed and memory of a state-of-the-art computer, teachers have a limit to how much feedback they can process and respond to effectively. Preliminary testing of the PCL in an introductory lecture course in physics at Wake Forest has demonstrated that "too much feedback" can become anti-productive because it hampers the flow and coherency of the teacher's lecture. But exactly how much feedback properly warrants the description of "too much" feedback? The question forces us to consider the variable of "individual differences" with respect to both teachers and students. These differences are influenced by at least two related things: the social and cultural conditioning that comes with everyday existence and the physiology of cognitive functioning.

There are teachers and students who are better than other teachers and students because they have received more caring, stimulating, and effective training in their social and educational schooling and because they are better at processing what they perceive and then doing something creative with it. The PCL can help to *perfect* these social and physiologically based skills. For example, a teacher who is open and responsive to negative feedback certainly displays a more caring attitude in the classroom than a teacher who dismisses the educational value of this feedback does. Such moral responsibility also rests on the shoulders of the students who, with PCL in hand, should refrain from sending "bogus" answers to the teacher, responses that are not a true reflection of their undivided attention and their understanding of the material. Unfortunately, students are known to sometimes do to teachers what teachers are known to sometimes do to students: mess with their heads and hearts.

Still, the PCL provides a way to enhance the openness and honesty that informs the process of acknowledgment. Recall, for example, how a bar graph recording real time responses to the teacher's lecture can be projected onto a classroom screen. What more could dedicated and morally responsible teachers and students ask for than an educational experience whose technologically enhanced transparency now reveals more about the "truth" of the dynamics that are going on during the teacher/student interaction than ever before? Standing in front of dedicated and morally responsible students, the truly outstanding (if not perfect) teacher would be easy to see: a constantly unfolding bar graph projected on a screen would remain between a level of, let's say, +8 to +10. With more practice, perhaps an even higher state of perfection could be achieved as the teacher learned to deal *more* efficiently with *more* feedback at a quicker rate. The bar graph would be like an electrocardiogram that helps one understand something about "the heart" of the matter. The PCL could thus play a role in the "design of excellence" that all worthwhile educational institutions struggle to achieve.

This struggle corresponds to what Kenneth Burke describes as the "principle of perfection" that motivates a good deal of human behavior. Burke points to the nature of a specific "low" technology—language—to illustrate this tendency:

> The principle of perfection is central to the nature of language as motive. The mere desire to name something by its "proper" name, or to speak a language in its distinctive ways is intrinsically "perfec-

tionist." What is more "perfectionist" in essence than the impulse, when one is in dire need of something, to so state this need that one in effect "defines" the situation? And even a poet who works out cunning ways of distorting language does so with perfectionist principles in mind, though his ideas of improvement involve recondite stylistic twists that may not disclose their true nature as judged by less perverse tests.[68]

The designers of the PCL are certainly driven by the perfectionist principle. At the present state of human evolution, however, the practical employment of this principle is usually far from perfect. For, despite our capacity to raise ourselves above the other creatures of the earth with our ability to speak of "the good," our sense of this specific "God term"—as demonstrated, for example, in religious debates and wars—has yet to obtain universal acceptance. We are finite beings caught up in the muck and mire of our spatial and temporal existence. Different people, living in different circumstances, with different needs, often make "the good" a disputable term. Thus the potential problem with the PCL: Although this technology values acknowledgment and the quick response, its functional design is not precisely attuned to the essential spirit of education, especially as this spirit involves the complex dynamics of acknowledgment. When it comes to assessing all that is going on with these dynamics—a specific setting (time and place) of an interaction and the capacities (attunement of consciousness, ethical responsibility, rhetorical competence) of the characters involved in the setting—the PCL's bar graph is too simplistic.

To expand on this last point: What *exactly* is being measured as students use the PCL to respond to their teacher's presentation? In the best case scenario it would be the "learning" made possible by acknowledgment and the dwelling place it creates. Such learning, however, involves more than the mere transmission of information between teacher and student. Learning presupposes a certain way or style of presenting the information in order to attune it to the student's consciousness and make it interesting enough for him or her to pay attention to it. Learning, in other words, presupposes the enactment of what I have been describing throughout this book as rhetorical competence.

Georges Gusdorf comments on the importance of this competence for the "great educator" when he discusses how such a person seeks to help others find their "own voice" and to stimulate them to discover their "innermost need[s]." "Such is the task of the teacher, if, going beyond the monologue of instruction, he knows how to carry the pedagogical task into authentic dialogue where personality is developed. The great educator is he who spreads around himself the meaning of the honor of language as a concern for integrity in the relations with others and oneself."[69]

As a technology that can at least help to initiate the process of acknowledgment in the classroom, the PCL has a role to play in developing the "pedagogical task" being noted here. Yet, like an electrocardiogram, the PCL's bar graph at best tells only part of the story of the condition at hand. A teacher whose pedagogical performance in class fluctuates between a +8 and a +10 throughout the semester may indeed be a person of great rhetorical competence. He or she may display intelligence, wit, sensitivity, and other capacities that help students to appreciate the relevance of the lessons of the day, find these lessons entertaining, and feel at home in the dwelling place of the classroom. With regard to the PCL, however, the problem comes when we reduce these capacities to the quantifications of a bar graph. Appreciating the dynamics of acknowledgment requires more than a numerical response, which may or may not be an indication of the capacities and complexities at work.

The PCL is, at best, a tool for cultivating acknowledgment; it offers no guarantee that this life-giving gift and all that must be at work to give and receive it are present and permanent. Theory and research in education have a long way to go before we are good enough to develop a technology that can offer a definitive assessment of the workings of acknowledgment in the classroom environment, especially given the differences that exist in these environments due to such things as course topics, requirements, and the extant biases and capacities of teachers and students. As the ancient Greeks long ago told us, different situations require different rhetorical competencies on the part of those who seek to improve the educational quality of the specific situation at hand.

It would be a serious mistake at the present time to see the PCL as a technology that can provide "some really solid data" on the quality of teachers and whether they should be rewarded (e.g., granted tenure, promotion, and a salary raise) or released. Such a mistake would be an example of how the short-sightedness, impatience, and ignorance of human beings can influence their metaphysical longing for something final and absolute, turning it into the condition of being "rotten with perfection." The character of Beth in the film *Ordinary People* (discussed in chapter 7), exhibited this way of being, along with its tendency to be closed-minded to any viewpoint that would call its habits and attitudes into question. The potential of the condition manifesting itself in our lives is ever-present as we attend to the challenge of being as open-minded as possible when answering both the call of technology and the call for acknowledgment.

Chapter Eleven

The Rhetor as Hero

The ontological nature of this specific challenge to be open-minded has been emphasized throughout this book. The challenge originates in the disclosing of the fundamental spatial and temporal character of existence, in the way we are open to the future, to the continual uncertainty of what is not yet in our lives, an uncertainty that calls into question what at the time we hold to be "the truth" of any number of matters of interest. This "call of conscience," however, does not work in just an interruptive and deconstructive way; our openness to what is not yet also calls on us to assume the ethical responsibility of affirming our freedom through resolute choice. Along with others, we can think and act in a constructive way in order to make the world a more meaningful and moral place to be. Confronting us with its deconstructive dynamics, existence challenges us to engage in reconstructive tasks, over and over again. It calls: "Where art thou?" And for the benefit of others and ourselves we must respond: "Here I am!" The life-giving gift of acknowledgment is born of this entire process.

As detailed in chapter 2, religion relates this process back to God, to One who not only called everything into being through an act of acknowledgment but who is also in need of this gift from all of those who can give it. Religion makes no sense without the workings of acknowledgment. The same can be said of science, its journey back to the beginning goes only as far as the Big Bang and the evolutionary process that was initiated. Sometime during this process, creatures evolved who, in a moment of acknowledgment, were able to reflect on the awesomeness of their own existence. They wondered about where they came from and pondered what it means to be. Scientists are still working hard to address these and related questions: Why does the universe go to all the bother of existing? Why does it allow for creatures who can be awed by and acknowledge its wonders? Does the universe itself really call for such acknowledgment? Is that truly part of its logic and laws? Is there an Intelligent Designer behind all the chaos and order that appears before us, or is it all merely chance and accident? Religion is ever-ready to chime in as science puzzles over these matters. Religion would have science broaden the range and flexibility of its attunement of consciousness, its way of being open to and acknowledging all that there is. Science, on the other hand, argues that it is not being true to itself when *its* procedure of acknowledging the dynamics of the cosmos is made "less rigorous" by engaging in metaphysical gymnastics—"God-of-the-gaps" thinking.

The debate between religion and science over the origins of our earthly dwelling place (and how we are "at home in the universe") is bound to continue for some time. Remember the words of Nobel Laureate, Richard Feynman: "We are not smart. We are dumb. We are ignorant. We must maintain an open channel" to whatever the essential truth shows itself to be.[1] I have made much of how the human capacity for rhetorical competence has an important role to play in this endeavor of acknowledgment. As discussed throughout chapters 4 through 7, the art of rhetoric helps to open people to the possible truth of matters. Rhetoric facilitates acknowledgment by transforming space and time into dwelling places where people can feel at home with each other, engage in collaborative deliberation, and know together ways of resolving disputed concerns. The rhetor initiates and directs this process as he or she exhibits competence in the related activities of the showing-forth (epideictic display) of some intended object of consciousness and in the appropriate and stylistic use of language: saying the right thing at the right time and in the right way in the struggle for consciousness. The rhetor is an architect, a builder of dwelling places, homes, habitats where the caress of others is a welcoming occurrence.

The rhetor brings to language what science finds in its study of the cosmos: structure, order, harmony, and beauty. Rhetoric and science both have an appreciation of aesthetics (e.g., the eloquently arranged public address, the beautiful mathematical equation). Religion is not surprised. Aesthetics aids acknowledgment, and acknowledgment was supposedly at work in the very beginning with the uttering of the first words: "Let there be!" Religion sees God as the true scientist, rhetor, and artist. God first shares the life-giving gift of acknowledgment, setting forth a principle of perfection to guide the evolution of all that there is.

This book is not concerned with whether religion is right or wrong in advancing this contention. I am open to religion for the same reason that I am open to science: both provide clues for developing a phenomenological understanding of the ontological workings of acknowledgment. The presence of acknowledgment is crucial in the teaching environment (chapter 8); its absence promotes social death (chapter 9); its computerization (chapter 10) shows promise but still falls short of perfection—that god-like quality that first showed itself with a Big Bang and that informs and is informed by the human capacity for rhetorical competence. In the last three chapters, I had occasion to relate this capacity briefly to the notion of heroism. The present chapter expands on this relationship as I make a case for the importance of what I term the rhetor as hero. Admittedly, the literature of rhetorical theory and criticism is filled with studies that, at least implicitly, encourage such a praiseworthy view of the rhetor. I know of none, however, where the phenomenon of acknowledgment is used as a basis for examining the topic. To do so is to realize how the genuine rhetorical hero is committed to the pursuit of truth.

Rhetorical Heroism and Truth

Among their many attributes, heroes are people who exhibit greatness in some achievement and are admired for doing so. With their extraordinary actions and praiseworthy character, heroes thus "stand out" from the crowd. Ralph Waldo Emerson saw fit to make mention of such outstanding souls when writing about the nature and importance of "eloquence": "Certainly there is no true orator who is not a hero. . . . The orator must ever stand with forward foot, in the attitude of advancing. . . . His speech is not to be distinguished from action. It is action, as the general's word of command or shout of battle is action."[2] This claim calls into question a well-known maxim of our culture—"Actions speak louder than words"—that is famous for its "put-down" of the practice of rhetoric. And the metaphor that informs the eloquence of Emerson's claim lends it further force, for, indeed, heroes and war are readily related. When speaking of the true orator's heroism, however, Emerson's understanding of "war" emphasizes what he terms "a military attitude of the soul" that is not directed toward the actual killing of others. Instead, this attitude is needed by the orator who would "dare the gibbet and the mob," the rage and retribution of a misinformed and closed-minded public, when attempting to move its members beyond the blinders of their "common sense" beliefs and toward a genuine understanding of what, for the orator, is arguably the truth of some immediate matter of concern. For Emerson, the heroism of the true orator is made possible not only by one's "power to connect his thought with its proper symbol, and so to utter it," but also, and primarily, by one's "love of truth and . . . [the] desire to communicate it without loss."[3]

Eloquence is born of such power, love, and desire. As Kenneth Burke succinctly puts it: "The primary purpose of eloquence is not to enable us to live our lives on paper—it is to convert life into its most thorough verbal equivalent" in order to better understand, appreciate, and deal with the reality of which we are a part.[4] The true orator, the rhetor as hero, is a person committed to this task of eloquence. In working out the moral grounds of "civic republicanism" as he countered Plato's critique of the orator's art, Cicero made clear the value and necessity of such rhetorical action: For "what function is so kingly, so worthy of the free, so generous, as to bring help to the suppliant, to raise up those who are cast down, to bestow security, to set free from peril, to maintain men in their civil rights? . . . The wise control of the complete orator is that which chiefly upholds not only his own dignity, but the safety of countless individuals and of the entire State."[5] Indeed, the rhetor as hero, which Cicero certainly aspired to be, is the embodiment of dignity. His or her presence and action allow for an epideictic display of what, as Leon Kass reminds us, "*dignitas*" is all about: "worthiness, elevation, honor, nobility, height—in short, excellence or virtue."[6] In his assessment of the political style that characterizes Cicero's republican theory of rhetoric and that Cicero practiced in public forums with the hope of gaining the fame that he believed was warranted given his heroic endeavors, Robert Hariman is thus correct to emphasize that "The republican community understands heroism not as the conquest of an alien warrior, but as the individual's triumphing over personal limitation to become the exemplar of civic virtue. . . . The republican politician achieves greatest glory as the heroic individual seizing the moment by voicing immortal words at the height of great events."[7]

To credit the rhetor as hero with the ability to express "immortal words" is certainly to bestow on such a person a "god-like" quality: the capacity to be inventive, to arrange materials in an appropriate, orderly, and beautiful way, to favor the good and the just, and, of course, to speak "the truth" of what *is*. Focusing as he does on political style—which he defines as "*a coherent repertoire of rhetorical conventions depending on aesthetic reactions for political effect*"[8]—Hariman omits any explicit discussion of how this last matter has anything to do with the rhetor's heroic endeavors. This omission is warranted to the extent that readers know how Cicero's understanding of political style and civic virtue encompasses philosophical instruction for appreciating whatever truth can be established about any given topic of discussion. "Philosophy," Cicero insists, "is essential to a full, copious and impressive discussion and exposition of the subjects which so often come up in speeches and are usually treated meagerly, whether they concern religion, death, piety, patriotism, good and evil, virtues and vices, duty, pain, pleasure, or mental disturbances and errors."[9] In his phenomenological study of the functions of speech, Georges Gusdorf expands on and further clarifies the matter by associating the rhetorical artistry needed to cultivate civic virtue with what he terms "the ceaseless heroism necessary in pursuing the struggle for style"—a struggle where "Concern for the right expression is bound up with the concern for true reality: accuracy (*justesse*) and integrity (*justice*) are two related virtues."[10] Cicero makes the point this way: ". . . if we bestow fluency of speech on persons devoid of . . . [the] virtues of [integrity and supreme wisdom], we shall not have made orators of them but shall have put weapons into the hands of madmen."[11]

In the remainder of this chapter, I discuss in further phenomenological detail and assess critically by way of a case study the specific relationship that binds the rhetor as hero with "the concern for true reality"—that is, with the concern for being open to the disclosing, the "showing-forth," of what *is*. Phenomenologically speaking, truth happens, first and foremost, as an act of disclosure, a revealing or epideictic display of something that presents itself to us and that we appreciate by way of an act of acknowledgment. Both the assertion and the validity of any "truth claim" presuppose the occurrence of this process.[12] I make an issue of the relationship between the rhetor as hero and the concern for true reality because, as is the case with Hariman, rhetorical scholars too often sidestep the issue when arguing for the heroic relevance of a given orator. As a result, the notion of heroism—which as far as I know has yet to be carefully investigated by rhetorical scholars—ends up being conceived more as what Michael McGee disparagingly terms an "ideograph" than as a carefully understood phenomenon that is necessarily related to a concern for true reality and that, like it or not, thus requires rhetoricians, in any given case, to deal with a specific issue that Plato, in his critique of the orator's art, made forever lasting.[13]

The presence of rhetoric, be it heroic or not, presupposes the question of truth. Abraham Lincoln, for example, becomes less of a rhetorical hero than he is typically acknowledged to be if we do not buy into the truths that he is famous for advocating, or if we question Lincoln's sincerity regarding these truths by pointing to certain controversial (e.g., "racist") statements he made in his career. Rhetorical analyses of Lincoln are warranted because of what is perceived to be his consistent and instructive display of rhetorical virtuosity in making these "necessary" truths known to others and because analysts, in agreeing or disagreeing with this perception, feel compelled to make sure that their audiences "have it right" when it comes to appreciating the truth of the matter. As with Cicero, we can point to Lincoln's "republican" style when making a case for his rhetorical brilliance, but it is the truth (or true opinion) of which this style speaks that should also be considered when crediting Lincoln with being a genuine rhetorical hero.[14]

The specific case study of concern here is the terrorist attack on the World Trade Center and the Pentagon on September 11, 2001 ("9/11"). This horrific situation, which continues to unfold today with the reality and consequences of the Iraq war, brought to light in vivid detail just how important heroes can be to those caught up in immense tragedy.[15] The extensive literature on 9/11 is filled with narratives detailing the courageous acts of all sorts of people: firefighters, police officers, physicians and nurses, clergy, construction workers, airline personnel and passengers (especially those on Flight 93, which crashed in Pennsylvania before it reached its target). The list could go on. In adding the rhetor to this list, I subscribe to the argument that the events of 9/11 defined a monumental occasion for would-be rhetorical heroes to display their talents as they sought to disclose the truth, make sense of the horror and chaos at hand, and thereby help in the treatment and guidance of an anxious and terrified American public.[16]

The various rhetorical artifacts that direct my attention span the political spectrum. Special attention is given, however, to certain discourses of President George W. Bush. The order of presentation of the artifacts is the result of my attempt to construct a coherent narrative about the relationship between rhetoric, heroism, and truth. This narrative allows me to clarify further and thus expand on what has been said so far about the relationship and to ground my assessment of the artifacts in terms of what I take to be the ontological basis of the relationship, or what is described as the heroic structure of human existence that presents itself as a primordial form of epideictic discourse and that speaks a moral directive heard as a call of conscience. This call, we have seen, summons us to be open to and to articulate with rhetorical competence—that is, to acknowledge—the truth of what *is*. The circumstances of 9/11 worked to disclose the ever present happening of this evocative event.

The Call of 9/11

The rhetorical landscape of 9/11 came into being as soon as the planes struck the towers of the World Trade Center. What was witnessed then was at one and the same time a gut-wrenching spectacle and an awesome symbolic act. A marvel of modern architecture that embodied such American values as freedom, human dignity, democracy, the thriving marketplace of capitalism and its good life, was disintegrating. The scene was a vivid epideictic display of American vulnerability, and of a long-cultivated loathing of the ascendancy of a too popular American lifestyle. A terrifying rhetoric was uttered without a word as terrorists staged for the world to see with the help of massive media coverage a stunning exhibition of hatred and truth, at least as they would have it. The rhetorical landscape further materialized as the towers burned and collapsed, as police, firefighters, and other rescue workers did their heroic duty, and as people from all walks of life struggled to find words that made some sense of these events and subsequent happenings.

In his essay "Simile," Richard Powers assumes the challenge of this struggle and, in so doing, provides an insight on 9/11 that is especially instructive for my purposes. Powers reports that he was preparing to meet his undergraduate writing class at the University of Illinois when he heard the news. "The day's topic was to have been figurative speech: metaphor and simile in fiction." On the way out of his office, he "saw the first headlines. Then the images and the repeating, unreal film. And every possible class lesson disappeared in that plume."[17] Powers goes on to admit that like "the rest of the world," he found himself "losing ground against the real" and "helpless to say what had happened." He writes:

> And when the first, stunted descriptions came, they came in a flood of simile. The shock of the attack was like Pearl Harbor. The gutted financial district was like Nagasaki. Lower Manhattan was like a city after an earthquake. The gray people streaming northward up the island covered in an inch of ash were like the buried at Pompeii.[18]

Powers describes what he heard as an "outpouring of anemic simile" that "with startlingly little variation . . . resorted to the most chilling refrain: like a movie. Like 'Independence Day.' Like 'The Towering Inferno.' Like 'The Siege.' Like bad science fiction. Like a Tom Clancy novel." Indeed, remarks Powers, "The magnitude of this day could not be made real except through comparison to fiction. Nothing but the outsize scale of the imaginary was big enough to measure by." Powers thus maintains that "No simile will ever serve. In its size and devastation and suddenness, the destruction of Sept. 11 is, in fact, like nothing, unless it is like the terrors experienced in those parts of the world that seemed so distant on Sept. 10."[19] The truth that showed itself on 9/11 at the World Trade Center and the Pentagon was "unspeakable" for the time being because, unlike other countries, this truth had yet to be conveyed to Americans with such shock and awe. Powers's remarks on the consequences of this truth are noteworthy: "The America [we] woke to on Tuesday morning was, like the skyline of New York, changed forever. The always-thereness of here was gone."[20] A very fitting and truthful simile, especially as Powers clarifies it with another suggestive phrase. Powers has a way with words—a talent that he continues to share with readers as he concludes his essay with the following instructive observation:

> The final lesson of my writing class came too soon. There are no words. But there are only words. To say what the inconceivable resembles is all that we have by way of learning how it might be outlived. No comparison can say what happened to us. But we can start with the ruins of our similes, and let "like" move us toward something larger, some understanding of what "is."[21]

Powers wants to understand the truth of a sudden and devastating event whose magnitude seems beyond measure. His rhetoric directs our consciousness to the presence of a time and place that is strange and terrifying. Powers refers to this presence when he speaks of "losing ground against the real." When "the always-thereness of here" vanishes, something still remains. "The real" is one way to describe what this something is. For my present purposes, however, we need a more nuanced description of the matter.

The specific presence at issue here defines what I have described throughout this book as the "ecstatic" temporal process of "the openness of Being": the way in which the *no-longer* (the past), the *not yet* (the future), and the *here and now* (the present) interpenetrate each other so that human existence is always in the state of "standing outside and beyond itself" (Gk. *ek-stasis*), at every moment opening toward the future, toward the world of possibilities, and thus toward the realm of objective uncertainty where the finality of death will eventually take place, though we don't know when.[22] Commenting on the fundamental and truthful nature of this process—how it serves as a basis for understanding, knowing, and making the truth of anything else public—Martin Heidegger writes: "To be certain of an entity means to *hold* it for true as something true. But 'truth' signifies the uncoveredness of some entity, and all uncoveredness is grounded ontologically in the most primordial truth, the disclosedness of [human existence]." Heidegger thus emphasizes that, with the relationship that we hold with this disclosedness, we are constantly and "essentially 'in the truth.'" In other words, we are necessarily involved with a revelatory process that defines a "good" (an essential ingredient of life), sustains everyday existence, and can be thought of and spoken about by the human creatures who are living it.[23]

Recall that this specific ontological structure of existence is itself not a human creation. The openness of Being is a happening that is always already at work disclosing itself before we decide to notice and to calculate its presence. Human existence, in other words, has something about its nature—a primordial dimension of time and space—that, in truth, is *more* and thus *other* than its own making. Crises and their breakdowns (e.g., a serious and incapacitating illness; the events of 9/11) expose us to this otherness ("the real") as they disrupt our everyday, taken-for-granted habits and routines ("the always-thereness of here") and thereby bring us face-to-face with the ecstatic temporality of the openness of Being.[24] As discussed in chapter 3, from this encounter originates the primordial "saying" of the world, a revealing or uncovering of the "givenness" of human being, a showing-forth of how we fundamentally exist as those beings who are always already situated in the truth. Regarding the genre of rhetoric most steeped in this primordial discursive event (epideictic), Quintilian has said: "Indeed I am not sure that this is not the most important department of rhetoric in actual practice."[25] A phenomenology of the ecstatic temporality of human existence lends ontological support to this claim. The "saying" or disclosing of our temporal existence defines the most primordial form of epideictic speech and "public address."[26] Moreover, this saying speaks to us of the heroic nature of our existence and its call of conscience—a call that is most apparent when some crisis causes "the always-thereness of here" to disintegrate, leaving us exposed to the truth, the objective uncertainty, of the openness of Being.

With the call of conscience comes a call for moral judgment and decisive action, a call that emanates from out of the ecstatic temporality of our existence. Owing to the suddenness and severity of the crisis that exposes us to this call, the situation is likely to inspire anxiety—the state of *not feeling at home* with our surroundings—as we must now face the primordial truth of our Being and, with it, the possibility of our own demise.[27] The call of conscience allows for the possibility of being courageous in adverse circumstances. The heroic acts of individuals testify to this fact. Any act of heroism presupposes the answering of the call of conscience. Heroes and conscience go hand in hand. Heroes provide the material that directs a society's moral compass, offer instructions for understanding what human greatness is, and inform members of society about what it takes for a finite being to live on after death in the hearts and minds of others. Indeed, as Ernest Becker points out in his discussion of the matter, a given culture's symbolic "hero system" speaks of the possibility of being immortal and thus "god-like" (hence, its great metaphysical attraction to humankind).[28]

Let us keep in mind, however, that this attraction to "outstanding" achievements is rooted in a more primordial event than the achievement itself. Heroes emerge by responding to a call of conscience that is, itself, made possible by the *out-standing* ecstatic function of our temporal existence. We *are* creatures whose truth is situated in the openness of Being, in an event of disclosure that is other than a human creation and that calls on us to be standout souls. The ontological structure of human existence has something fundamentally heroic ("god-like") about it. Is this to suggest that the heroic structure of existence is *meant* to have us think about and remember the work of God? No one can say for sure. I simply take the matter of heroism as a given, something that a phenomenological appreciation of existence reveals: we *are* beings of heroic potential who must face the fact that our fate is to be open and to listen to a constant calling that challenges us with the ethical and moral struggle of coming to know and to speak the truth.

The Rhetor as Hero

Powers speaks to us of a moment when Americans were abruptly exposed to this challenge. The horror of 9/11 reached down to our very Being. Powers' rhetoric is directed toward our heroic nature, our ability to *stand out* from a specific situation—where "There are no words. But there are only words"—in order to assume the responsibility of producing some rhetorical action that moves us beyond the "ruins of our similes" so that we can gain a more accurate "understanding of what 'is." Powers responds to the call of conscience by calling on the heroic potential of readers to speak the truth. In assuming this task, as William Barrett reminds us, we demonstrate an appreciation of how "the primary function of language, if we have something to say and are not merely babbling, is to uncover something within the world, to bring it into the open; and it can do this only because it itself transpires within the open world."[29] The would-be rhetorical hero (e.g., Powers) assumes the responsibility of using discourse to disclose a phenomenon's own disclosure, *its* being and truth. The call of conscience calls for nothing less than this: a most genuine and truthful act of publicity. With such inventive and descriptive phrases as "the always-thereness of here was gone," Powers also reminds us of how the rhetor answering this call must find an appropriate way to express the truth so that it can assume a publicly accessible form and function effectively in the social and political arena.

The rhetor as hero is involved in a struggle for consciousness. People in a state of crisis and anxiety are in need of discourse that can help them make sense of the horror and chaos at hand and that can also lessen the trauma of their not feeling at home with their environment. We might say that the rhetor as hero becomes a "home-maker," the builder of a "dwelling place" that affords protection, as he or she responds to this need.[30] A strong example of the type of discourse that should inform this response was heard as the events of 9/11 exposed people to the openness of Being and evoked an economical but quite meaningful response: "Oh my God!"[31] With this specific plea/prayer to the "One" who many consider to be the greatest hero of all time, Being took on a name. In the presence of horror, human beings, without giving it a second thought, screamed for help from One who, when everyone else is gone, incapacitated, or doesn't care, is supposedly always there to acknowledge and aid the neediest of souls.

Calling on the saving grace of the Almighty is the most common way that human beings give expression to who they are as metaphysical creatures. In dealing with the uncertainty of our temporal existence and the anxiety that such uncertainty inspires, we have developed a passionate longing for some degree of completeness in our lives, "a nostalgia for something final and absolute."[32] The term "nostalgia" speaks of that state of being where we are "homesick" and thus in need of a dwelling place that can help us regain the feeling of being at home with others. The discourse of the Judaic-Christian tradition pays special attention to the treatment of this sickness; the metaphor of "home" plays a crucial therapeutic role in this tradition. Recall that the Hebrew word for "dwelling place"— *makom*—is also a name for God, the ground and the source of everything that exists, the very place of Being itself. The Bible teaches people how to be at home with God here on earth so that, when the time comes, they can return home to their Maker in heaven. The act of prayer opens our earthly home to God and God's heavenly home to us.[33]

President Bush designated September 14, 2001, as a "National Day of Prayer" for those who lost their lives on 9/11, their family and friends, and all mourning Americans. The dwelling place where he and others gathered was The National Cathedral in Washington, D.C. Here, in this "house of God," Bush made it clear that "Our purpose as a nation is firm. Yet our wounds as a people are recent and unhealed, and lead us to pray." Admitting that "God's signs are not always the ones we look for," and that "We learn in tragedy that his purposes are not always our own," the president reassured his audience that "the prayers of private suffering, whether in our homes or in this great cathedral, are known and heard, and understood." The president made a truth-claim here, which he expanded on in the conclusion of his speech: "As we have been assured, neither death nor life, nor angels nor principalities nor powers, nor things present nor things to come, nor height nor depth, can separate us from God's love."

This truth-claim certainly contributed to the task of making heart-sick and anxious people feel more at home with the crisis situation. They dwelled together in the face of death, yet they were in a place that was built, as they say, "for the love of God." The president was doing what the rhetor as hero is supposed to do: answering the call of conscience and being an honest-to-goodness "home-maker" to a people whose home was attacked. The "enemies of human freedom," Bush noted, "have attacked America, because we are freedom's home and defender." Bush reminded us that this home is rooted in "the commitment of our [founding] fathers."[34] From a religious perspective, the roots run deeper than that, for freedom is a gift from God—one that is supposed to be respected and used wisely, as when, for example, a person acts heroically in order to be a "good Samaritan" or the "keeper" of his or her "brothers and sisters."

President Bush is an evangelical Christian who is known to seek truthful guidance more from his "Holy Father" than from his political forefathers.[35] While guiding Americans in praying to this greatest of heroes, Bush wisely and respectfully made much of the related earthly heroics of Americans who, on 9/11, displayed their national and moral character as they answered a certain call and began the reconstructive task of administering to the ruins of a massive deconstructive act of terror. In his National Cathedral address, Bush emphasized that "We have seen our national character in rescuers working past exhaustion; in long lines of blood donors; in thousands of citizens who have asked to work and serve in any way possible." Moreover, he noted, "we have seen our national character in eloquent acts of sacrifice. Inside the World Trade Center, one man who could have saved himself stayed until the end at the side of his quadriplegic friend. A beloved priest died giving the last rites to a firefighter." He then offered additional examples in order to illustrate further how "Americans showed a deep commitment to one another, and an abiding love for our country." In short, they acted in a god-like way.

Notice that, in telling this story about heroes, Bush associated their endeavors with "eloquent acts of sacrifice" that would help to guide America's response to the terrorist attacks. Eloquence is a term that is first and foremost associated with the art of rhetoric. The actions of heroes mark out epideictic events as they show-forth the noble and virtuous qualities of human beings, speaking to us of our potential for being better than we typically are. "To praise a [person]," writes Aristotle, "is in one respect akin to urging a course of action."[36] Bush took advantage of how the heroic admits a fundamental rhetorical and spiritual quality. As someone who is supposed to be heroic when addressing the American people about crises in their lives, President Bush became the rhetor as hero talking about the hero as rhetor. Rhetorical heroism was in full force that day.

The hero as rhetor takes on special significance in the literature dealing with the events of 9/11. Stories and pictures of heroes appeared in the media coverage of these events on a daily basis. These pictures put more of a "face" on the lessons offered by these stories. The heroic and rhetorical (epideictic) nature of the stories are compelling to creatures whose ecstatic existence displays an essential ingredient of heroism.[37] The American Red Cross made use of this rhetorical climate when sounding its specific call for help. In a nationally distributed letter that was mailed to previous donors immediately after the events of 9/11 (and that pictured a military "Silver Cross" as part of its letter head), the Red Cross talks about heroism:

> If you rescued a child from a burning building, you'd be featured on the evening news. If you saved a life in combat, you'd receive the Silver Star and come home to a ticker-tape parade. And although your

recent donation of blood didn't make the local news, or even
prompt a parade, it's every bit as heroic. Maybe more so.

Think about it. Most people go through their entire lives without
saving one life. You may have saved three lives with *every* pint you
donated. Heroic? No question about it....

You are an integral part of the [Red Cross] tradition of dedication and compassion....

It's people like you who helped us earn that reputation. Your selfless act helps us carry out our mission.

On a flyer accompanying the letter are the words: "When something feels
this *good*, why not make it a habit?" Another accompanying flyer contained a
"Special Designation" sticker that read: "Active Hero." Giving blood is giving life;
thus it certainly qualifies as a gift of acknowledgment, and a heroic one at that.
"Where art thou?" "Here I am!" In this situation we are told that the "I" is "selfless,"
without ego. Indeed, heroes sacrifice *for others* and feel good about it. As more and
more people made the sacrifice of giving blood, their heroic actions gained rhetorical significance. Giving blood became an epideictic event, a showing-forth of
patriotism capable of moving others to action.

In his September 20, 2001, "Address to a Joint Session of Congress and the
American People," President Bush contined to be the rhetor as hero talking about
the hero as rhetor. This strategy took form as Bush emphasized how his fellow
Americans "will remember what happened that day, and to whom it happened. . .
. Some will remember an image of fire, or a story of rescue. Some will carry
memories of a face and a voice gone forever."[38] Bush's memories, however, would
be associated with a certain object that he held in his hand: "the police shield of a
man named George Howard, who died at the World Trade Center trying to save
others. It was given to me by his mom, Arlene, as a proud memorial to her son.
This is my reminder of lives that ended, and a task that does not end." Bush continued by emphasizing that he would "not forget this wound to our country, or
those who inflicted it." He would "not yield." He would "not rest." And he would
"not relent in waging this struggle for the freedom and security of the American
people."

These words initially attuned the audience's consciousness to the recent past,
to memories of a specific place and time when chaos, suffering, and death reigned.
Bush, however, transformed this place and time by displaying (showing-forth) a
badge of courage and by naming both the hero who once wore it and the hero's
mother who gave it to the president in memory of her son. The suffocating influence of misery was not without the life-affirming influences of honor and pride.
Epideictic discourse and the good feeling it can inspire was used once again to
counter an earlier and "murderous" form of epideictic discourse (the symbolic destruction of the World Trade Center and the damage to the Pentagon). The inspi-

ration helped to make clear a "task that does not end." This task is the democratic "struggle for the freedom and security of the American people." The president's words created a dwelling place where these people could begin to feel at home with one another once again, know-together what needed to be said and done, and be hopeful of a better future. The president offered himself as a leader and a hero who would "not rest" until his job was completed with as much perfection as possible. As he put it when concluding his address, "God is not neutral" on matters of "freedom and fear, justice and cruelty."

Political pundits praised the rhetorical competence that the president displayed in his September 20 address. They thought he offered a resolute and eloquent response to the call of conscience as he spoke of the brave and the free, the spirit of democracy that they embodied, and how he, too, would sustain this spirit. Bush was the rhetorical hero, truth-teller and home-maker that he had to be in countering the act of terrorists who, as the president made clear in his address, would not deceive us with their "pretenses to piety." An example of the pretenses that Bush had in mind is found in the words of Osama bin Laden, the mastermind of the terrorist attacks, as he defended the actions of his al-Qaeda followers:

> America has been hit by Allah at its most vulnerable point, destroying, thank God, its most prestigious buildings. . . . What America is suffering today does not constitute even a negligible part of what we [Muslims] have suffered for decades. Our nation has undergone more than 80 years of this humiliation, its sons are killed, its blood flows, its holy places are attacked without reason—but no one hears or answers. God guided the path of a group of vanguard Muslims who destroyed America and we implore Allah to raise them up and admit them to paradise.[39]

For Bush, such rhetoric was just another product "of all the murderous ideologies of the twentieth century." The terrorists who spouted it were destined to "follow in the path" of these ideologies "to where it ends: in history's unmarked grave of discarded lies." The president's exposing of such ideology took place throughout his September 20 address: The members of al-Qaeda "are the same murderers indicted for bombing American embassies in Tanzania and Kenya, and responsible for the bombing of the U.S.S. Cole." The terrorists "practice a fringe form of Islamic extremism that has been rejected by Muslim scholars and the vast majority of Muslim clerics." The terrorists seek "to kill Christians and Jews, to kill all Americans, and make no distinction among military and civilians, including women and children." The terrorists support, and are supported by, the Taliban regime that rules Afghanistan, a country where "many are starving and many have fled," where "women are not allowed to attend school," and where "you can be jailed for owning a television." The terrorists "hate" our "democratically elected government . . . our freedom of religion, our freedom of speech. . . . With every atrocity, they hope that America grows fearful, retreating from the world and forsaking our friends. They stand against us, because we stand in their way."

The rhetor as hero is obligated to seek and to tell the truth. This obligation is rooted (at least empirically) in what was defined above as the ontological and heroic structure of existence. More than any other form of government, democracy prides itself on being true to this structure, its call of conscience, and the freedom provided by its openness—which makes all the other freedoms (e.g, freedom of speech, freedom of religion) possible. Sissela Bok reminds us how democracy further emphasizes the importance of this ontological feature of openness by stressing how the moral justification of actions "cannot be exclusive or hidden" but, instead, must "be capable of being made public." Such publicity "is connected more directly to veracity than to other moral principles" and the "principle of veracity" is essential to the livelihood of democratic institutions.[40] There are, of course, occasions when the deceitful practice of covering up the truth is morally justifiable. As Bok notes, "There would be no difficulty in defending openly the policy that persecutors searching for their innocent victims can be answered dishonestly."[41] But such a case is more the exception than the rule when it comes to maintaining the proper function of democracy and the principle of veracity that informs this function. Bok thus stresses that "in any situation where a lie is a possible choice, one must first seek truthful alternatives. And only where a lie is a *last resort* can one even begin to consider whether or not it is morally justified."[42]

I make these points with Bush still in mind. Although his September 20 address displayed the work of a rhetorical hero, there remained more truth to tell about the terrorists than he admitted—truth that complicates Bush's simple black-and-white depiction of the matter and, in so doing, calls the authenticity of his heroism into question (to the point that we might accuse him of being purposely deceitful). Examining how other would-be rhetorical heroes made clear what Bush did not is necessary in order to judge the worthiness of the accusation.

More Truth to Tell

In his response to 9/11, "In the Ruins of the Future: Reflections on Terror and Loss in the Shadow of September," Don DeLillo begins by noting that

> In the past decade the surge of capital markets has dominated discourse and shaped global consciousness. Multinational corporations have come to seem more vital and influential than governments. The dramatic climb of the Dow and the speed of the Internet summoned us all to live permanently in the future, in the utopian glow of cyber-capital, because there is no memory there and this is where markets are uncontrolled and investment potential has no limit.

On September 11, however, this way of being changed.

> Today . . . the world narrative belongs to terrorists. But the primary
> target of the men who attacked the Pentagon and the World Trade
> Center was not the global economy. It is America that drew their
> fury. It is the high gloss of our modernity. It is the thrust of our
> technology. It is our perceived godlessness. It is the blunt force of
> our foreign policy. It is the power of American culture to penetrate
> every wall, home, life, and mind.[43]

The contrast offered here by DeLillo establishs a truth that gives direction
to the rest of his essay and that Bush only introduces through his negative acknowledgment: Yes, the terrorists hate what America stands for, but their hatred
is not without reasons that are worth at least some consideration. DeLillo's word
choice when describing what "drew [the terrorists'] fury" makes the point.
America is seen not only as a show-off ("high gloss of our modernity"), but a
show-off that is pushy ("thrust") with its wares, domineering ("blunt force")
with its ideology, unethical ("perceived godlessness"), and invasive ("the power
. . . to penetrate"). DeLillo does not side with this viewpoint, but he nevertheless
sees it as being real. It is a "counter narrative" whose truth is presently at work—
without a doubt—and it must be respected for what it is and for what it can do.
Attending more closely to the matter, DeLillo's rhetoric is as eloquent and
thought-provoking as it is frightening:

> Our tradition of free expression and our justice system's provisions
> for the rights of the accused can only seem an offense to men bent
> on suicidal terror.
>
> We are rich, privileged, and strong, but they are willing to die. This
> is the edge they have, the fire of aggrieved belief. . . . Plots reduce the
> world. [The terrorist] builds a plot around his anger and our indiffer-
> ence. He lives a certain kind of apartness, hard and right. . . .
>
> Does the sight of a woman pushing a stroller soften the man to
> her humanity and vulnerability, and her child's as well, and all the
> people he is here to kill?
>
> This is his edge, that he does not see her. . . . [T]here is no de-
> fenseless human at the end of his gaze. . . .
>
> We can tell ourselves that whatever we've done to inspire bitter-
> ness, distrust, and rancor, it was not so damnable as to bring this
> day down on our heads. But there is no logic in apocalypse. They
> have gone beyond the bounds of passionate payback. This is heaven
> and hell, a sense of armed martyrdom as the surpassing drama of
> human experience.

[The terrorist] pledges his submission to God and meditates on the blood to come.[44]

The rhetorical power of DeLillo's description unfolds as he acknowledges the terrorist's mindset and way of being with a more nuanced reading of the topic than what Bush has to offer. His rhetoric brings to life the outlook of death held by the terrorist—an outlook that both inspires and blinds those who share its ideology and follow its instructions about such matters as heroism and cowardness. With DeLillo, we are encouraged to be more understanding and less immediately dismissive of an enemy who will not let the charge of coward make him feel less than the hero he was trained to be. Such understanding does not simply translate into positive acknowledgment, although it does slow down the unhesitating embrace of simple negative acknowledgment. Compared to Bush's discourse, DeLillo's *halting* rhetoric provides readers with a perspective that is more conducive to encouraging robust deliberation about the matter at hand, especially because it was expressed at a later and thus more appropriate time than earlier and highly criticized remarks made by such political commentators as Susan Sontag and Bill Maher regarding the "non-cowardly" actions of the terrorists.[45]

DeLillo's rhetorical strategy and timing work to keep readers open and attuned to the immense complexity of a tragedy and, as he makes clear, to the irony that accompanied it:

> For those who may want what we've got, there are all those who do not. These are the men who have fashioned a morality of destruction. They want what they used to have before the waves of Western influence. . . .
>
> The World Trade towers were not only an emblem of advanced technology, but a justification, in a sense, for technology's irresistible will to realize in solid form whatever becomes theoretically allowable. . . .
>
> Now a small group of men have literally altered our skyline. We have fallen back in time and space. It is their technology that marks our moments, the small lethal devices, the remote-control detonators they fashion out of radios, or the larger technology they borrow from us, passenger jets that become manned missiles.
>
> Maybe this is a grim subtext of their enterprise. They see something innately destructive in the nature of technology. It brings death to their customs and beliefs. Use it as what it is, a thing that kills.[46]

With observations like this last one in mind, I read DeLillo as being horrified by what the terrorists did but at the same time trying to appreciate the full scope and function, the "truth," of their existence. Certain words of Rabbi Abraham Heschel come to mind once again: "The greatest hindrance to knowledge is our adjustment to conventional notions, to mental clichés. Wonder or radical amaze-ment, the state of maladjustment to words and notions, is, therefore, a prerequisite for an authentic awareness of that which is."[47] DeLillo takes us beyond various con-ventional notions and mental clichés regarding terrorists that we find in Bush's dis-course. With what it shows-forth and acknowledges, DeLillo's rhetoric calls the sim-plicity of the truth-claims contained in that discourse into question. The stylistic presentation of his rhetoric thus has something of a deconstructive ring to it—a ring that makes readers pause to wonder about the matter at hand and may even en-courage them to acquire an even more authentic awareness of the truth of this mat-ter. By encouraging such wonder, deconstructive rhetoric also plays a role in the he-roic process of home-making, although this role is primarily one of "breaking ground" for whatever dwelling place will eventually be rhetorically reconstructed.

Unlike Bush, DeLillo does not explicitly say how we should react to the ter-rorists. Rather, maintaining his deconstructive style, he leaves us to continue won-dering about the wound that the terrorists inflicted on the *ethos* of America, an in-jury that needs to be tended to with determination and resolve. I sense that retaliation is certainly not out of the question for this rhetor; on the contrary, the truth he offers with his rhetoric might very well move readers to advance the ac-knowledgment that he inspires and thereby to spread the word about the necessity of resolute reaction and reconstruction. Democracy must not be made to live on its knees. But the deconstructive ring of DeLillo's rhetoric and the wonder it in-spires are also capable of keeping readers open to his topic. Without such open-ness, democracy mutates into something less than it is supposed to be.

Allan Gurganus maintained this openness and found a similarity between the truth of the terrorists and a truth of his history as a born and bred Southerner: General Sherman's burning of mansions and plantations in Gurganus' home state of North Carolina during the Civil War. "Sherman left these as a lesson," writes Gurganus. "The biggest, grandest structures ever built got leveled. This was pay-back to our arrogant country that'd forgot its kindnesses, its professed gentility, its obligations to all other nations (especially a certain big one to the north)." Gur-ganus enhances the eloquence of the analogy by detailing how "Stern fire-masters on fast horses trotted through here one hot, Biblical afternoon. These strangers, dispassionate as surgeons, willing to give their lives for another system of law, speaking a strange dialect, torched the very emblems of our enterprise and grace. . . . [These emblems] were savaged without warning, at real human costs, all just to make a moral point."[48]

Gurganus goes on to clarify *his* moral point as he relates the past to the pre-sent, to the flame and smoke engulfing the World Trade Center. He speaks of a certain "arrogance" that he believes informs the character of his country, an arro-gance that had a role to play in the nightmare of 9/11:

Deprived of another great competitive world power, we rarely use our solo authority for beneficence. Instead, we treat our signed treaties as some salad bar; our sacred world, we pick and choose. We honor those agreements that will turn a profit for our donor-friends. We hold all other nations to the letter of the law. And we can't imagine why we aren't beloved abroad.

Today . . . what I fear most is not just a religion that anneals its believers into sacrificing everything for a hate-based God. I'm scared of our having become a law-unto-itself nation so entitled and self-referential. . . . This amazing invention lately seems so cut off, so arrogant, we did not even *know* we could still be hurt.[49]

Gurganus's rhetoric reminds, indicts, and makes matters ever so personal. He critiques his country for the benefit of his country. Like DeLillo, he acts heroically, putting a deconstructive impulse to work in order to tell a truth that many others would later confirm and repeat in the media when talking and writing about a certain arrogance that opened the door to 9/11. This truth was even powerful enough to gain the attention of President Bush and his speechwriters, although their way of telling it was less deconstructive and more reconstructive in nature. Reflecting one year later on the truth of 9/11 as he addressed a GOP gathering in South Carolina, President Bush remarked: "I believe that out of the evil done to America, the culture of our country is changing from one which has said if it feels good, go ahead and do it . . . if you've got a problem, blame somebody else, to a culture which says each of us are responsible for the decisions we make in life."[50]

I do not know if those like DeLillo and Gurganus would be satisfied with this reconstructive rephrasing of the truth. An act of self-acknowledgment that leads to the realization that you have become too selfish and arrogant when dealing with others is certainly a necessary step for remedying the problem. In the case of America's involvement in events leading up to 9/11, however, this realization also opens us to additional truths regarding the terrorists, truths that took shape in the later years of the "Cold War" and that, once acknowledged, further call into question President Bush's "straight-forward" explanation of why the terrorists hate freedom-loving Americans. A brief summary of these truths will be helpful, especially because, as far as I know, they were never detailed in any official public statements from the Bush administration following the events of 9/11.

Before they became terrorists, bin Laden and his fellow "holy warriors" (mujahideen) in Afghanistan were "rebels" supported by the United States in its ongoing confrontation with the Soviet Union, which in 1978 ruled Afghanistan with a Communist puppet regime (the People's Democratic Republic of Afghanistan). The United States, via the CIA, began arming and training the mujahideen in June 1979.[51] In a 1998 interview for the French newspaper *Le Nouvel Observateur*,

Zbigniew Brezinski, who in 1979 was President Jimmy Carter's national security adviser, admitted that this aid was initiated to inspire Soviet military intervention, thereby producing the "Afghan trap" that would give "the USSR its Vietnam War." Asked if he ever regretted having supported the Islamic fundamentalists, having given arms and advice to future terrorists, Brezinski replied: "Regret what? . . . What is most important to the history of the world? Some stirred-up Muslims or the liberation of Central Europe and the end of the Cold War?"[52]

Aid to the mujahideen continued throughout the Reagan administration. President Reagan praised them as "freedom fighters." But with the withdrawal of Soviet troops from Afghanistan in early 1989, the country collapsed into virtual anarchy as different factions of the mujahideen and their warlord leaders struggled for power. Content with the success of its "Afghan trap," the United States now chose to be only a witness to the carnage resulting from this struggle.

In 1994, the Taliban movement came into being, promising a restoration of order, peace, and much needed reform. The Taliban captured Kabul in September 1996, thereby beginning their rule in Afghanistan. The order promised by the movement was instituted, but it came with a great cost. The Taliban's brand of extreme Islamic fundamentalism led to the brutal repression of minorities, strict sanctions against public demonstrations and expression, and the denial of education, health care, and employment possibilities for women. The United States was well aware of such costs but still chose to support the Taliban's reactionary program and individuals such as Osama bin Laden, who sought refuge in its operations. Despite the suffering it fostered in Afghanistan, the movement's achievement of order, stability, and power in the country was a welcomed development for the United States. After all, America was an "ally" who helped make this development possible and who might now persuade Taliban leaders to allow American oil companies to use Afghanistan as a "friendly" route for gaining access to Caspian sea oil.[53]

As the United States should have realized all along, bargaining with the Taliban proved impossible. The ideologies at work here were, to say the least, incommensurate. The United States recognized the Taliban as a means to an end. The Taliban not only knew this, but also regarded the moral, political, and economic workings of the United States as an ongoing insult and threat to the Islamic faith which, as interpreted by those like bin Laden, commanded retaliation, not positive acknowledgment, for "the love of Allah." We might think of the overall situation as being somewhat analogous to the story of Dr. Frankenstein and his creature: The United States had a hand in the creation of a "monster" that took serious exception to the way its "master" ended up treating it.

This analogy receives support from writers such as Rahul Mahajan, who reminds us that when Madeleine Albright, then Ambassador to the United Nations and soon to be Secretary of State, appeared on *60 Minutes* on May 12, 1996, she did not contest the claim that, owing in great part to the sanctions on Iraq initiated after the Gulf War, a half million Iraqi children had died—more than all the children who died in Hiroshima. When asked if she thought that the price was worth it, Albright replied: "I think this is a very hard choice, but the price—we think the price is worth it." Mahajan then writes:

> That is the philosophy of terrorism. The people who crashed planes into the World Trade Center killed almost four thousand people because they resented U.S. domination of the Middle East. The U.S. government helped to kill a half million children in Iraq in order to preserve that domination.

Mahajan goes on to emphasize that "This does not mean efforts should not be made to stop terrorists of the ilk of Osama bin Laden. It simply means that terrorist efforts to stop them should not be made." Mahajan ends his remarks with the following recommendation: "If Albright appears on *60 Minutes* again, this time she should be asked whether she thinks U.S. policy goals in the Middle East were also worth the deaths of thousands of Americans."[54]

Mahajan intends to make Americans feel much less at home with the rhetoric of the Bush administration and with those like William Bennett, who insist that "We are a target not because of anything we have done, but because of who we are, what we stand for, what we believe, and what our nation was founded upon: the twin principles of liberty and equality."[55] On the contrary, *the United States had a role to play in events leading up to the horror of 9/11!* Obviously, being true to the temporal and heroic structure of human existence that calls for a disclosing of truth can have its costs. You can end up discovering more than you really want to know and admit. But democracy is supposed to allow this to happen. While not condoning the acts of the terrorists, Mahajan takes full advantage of this liberty. More than the discourses of DeLillo and Gurganus, his rhetoric moves readers along a path of deconstruction with little effort given to reconstruction, beyond emphasizing that "citizens of the United States have an obligation to oppose its crimes even before they would oppose the crimes of others over whom they have less control."[56] As was the case with both Susan Sontag and Bill Maher (referred to above; see note 45), you risk being seen as "un-American" if you start on this path at an inappropriate time or stay on it for too long without offering a "fair amount" of reconstructive (positive) rhetoric. Telling the truth without a sense of decorum can be problematic.

The rhetoric surrounding the events of 9/11 contains various attempts to deal with this issue of propriety. Consider, for example, the discourse offered by Rabbi David Wolpe in an address given to his congregation in the United States before America retaliated against the Taliban and the terrorists. Early in the address, Wolpe admits:

> I am trying to focus on my own sins, but it is hard. I know that the magnitude of others' sins does not wipe out my own, but it is hard.

The United States has wreaked a good deal of havoc in the world. In this time of repentance, we have much to repent for as a country, as individuals. We are not guiltless. We should not let the horror cut off our self-examination.

We are sinners, but we are not deserving of this cruelty. We are imperfect, but we are not evil. This is the face of radical evil.

And it must be fought.[57]

Wolpe is more truthful (heroic) than Bush is when it comes to dealing with an important matter of self-acknowledgment. He is not without sin. His country is not without sin. Confessing your sins in a place of worship is not only an appropriate thing to do, it also defines a "heroic act," forcing you to *stand out* from the habits, routines, and the shelter of conformity of everyday existence in order to assume *personal responsibility* for unjust thoughts and actions. "Where art thou?" "Here I am!" The stories and teachings of the Old Testament would not be what they are without this often occurring "exchange" between God and mere mortals, whereby these mortals acknowledge their responsibility to the "most Holiest" of others.[58] Such self-acknowledgment also defines a maneuver that has long been recognized by the rhetorical tradition as an invaluable aid for enhancing a speaker's credibility. Admitting your sins right from the start helps to guard against the charge of appearing overly self-righteous and deceitful.

Might there be a way of further reducing the chances that this charge could be made? Could a more detailed account of the truth of America's historical relationship with the terrorists be offered? Beyond noting that "Yes, it is obscene to see the plane go into the [World Trade Center]" and that "America's [media fed] obsession with the vivid image is not our best feature," Wolpe does not specify the sins in question.[59] So what exactly is Wolpe referring to when he speaks of how our country "has wreaked a good deal of havoc in the world"? Perhaps he has our country's historical relationship with the terrorists in mind. Indeed, "self-examination" must continue in the face of horror. But what exactly should we be examining and acknowledging for ourselves and to the world? Wolpe opts for ambiguity over precision when dealing with this question, at least until he tells his audience that "we should feel gratitude" that we still have "the power" of resolute response and retaliation.

To be powerless is not moral, it is merely powerless. Jews remember too vividly the days we had no power. The millions who perished in Stalin's camps without a word, whisked away at night. The millions who died in concentration camps, and the world turned away because the Jews were expendable.

After the carnage of the 20th century, the Jew who is not grateful for power is unforgivably naïve. Do not lament our power. We know too much history. It is the only bulwark blocking the abyss. Powerlessness in the face of evil leads to Auschwitz.[60]

Instead of remaining focused and elaborating on his country's sins, Wolpe reverses his confessional, deconstructive strategy and returns to the sins of others, recalling in more detail than did Bush in his September 20 address one of the "murderous ideologies of the twentieth century." This past is ever so painful to the Jewish people. "Never forget!" is the well-known promise and demand that these people make to each other in light of the atrocities done to them in the name of Nazi ideology and other ones (e.g., Islamic fundamentalism) that also advocate the annihilation of the "children of Israel." Wolpe keeps this promise as he demands that the 9/11 atrocities be remembered, thereby serving as a warrant for retaliation against terrorists whose presence and actions, like the Nazis before them, register "the face of radical evil." The Jewish people "have seen this face" for too long a time, writes Wolpe. "We are the world's canary in the coal mine, and though we do not wish to be the first to know, we are."[61]

Indeed, Wolpe and his people "know too much history"; it thus makes sense for him to recommend for certain others what these others recommend for Wolpe and all those who support his position. The recommendation is the same one that Bush made when he, too, recalled some of this history to justify his actions. In both cases, however, the history that is remembered is quite selective. The historical relationship between the terrorists and the United States is omitted. Granting that this omission is not simply the result of being ignorant or forgetful of history, it is reasonable to conclude that it is part of an intended rhetorical strategy for encouraging specific judgments and actions. The potential effectiveness of this strategy is dependent on, among other things, audiences *not knowing* or *not fully appreciating* enough about the history and consequences of the relationship in question. In a country that prides itself on its democratic *ethos*, its being a place that is genuinely attuned to the heroic structure of human existence and what this structure calls for (an openness to and a disclosing of the truth), Wolpe's and Bush's omissions invite the charge of being deceptions, a covering-up of the truth. Deception is not the action of a genuine rhetorical hero unless, as Bok points out, "the hero" in question represents a community that encourages "deceit to survive and conquer."[62]

Jewish culture has been caught up in a struggle for survival for over two thousand years. Its ongoing bloody conflict with the Palestinians continues to threaten the land, the original dwelling place, where the children of Israel worship God and practice democracy. Of course, Israel's expansion of this homeland since winning its independence from the British over fifty years ago also threatens the original dwelling place where Palestinians worship Allah. I suspect that Wolpe's decision to cover up the truth when calling for retaliation against the terrorists is not unrelated to this conflict and his fear of losing. "Powerlessness in the face of evil leads to Auschwitz." This claim speaks more to Wolpe's being a devout member of the Jewish faith than it does to his being a patriotic American. In the specific context that it was made, the claim is powerfully appropriate: it expresses a truth that Wolpe's audience deserves to hear and that trumps another truth that remains ambiguous. But we can only go so far down the path of deconstruction before a need for reconstruction, for feeling at home in the world, is felt in our hearts. Remember, the call of conscience calls for both of these rhetorical activities.

Wolpe's claim initiates his reconstructive response to this call. But isn't there still an obligation to say more about how the "United States has wreaked a good deal of havoc in the world"?[63] I consider this question with President Bush in mind once again.

The Ongoing Call for Heroic Rhetoric

In a recent critical assessment of Bush's September 20 address, David Zarefsky maintains that, "given the contemporary American culture," it would have been politically and rhetorically unwise for Bush to acknowledge any related historical matter that might call the country's resolve into question. "The options were not even imagined," claims Zarefsky, "and to have pursued them would have been suicidal." Zarefsky's rationale for this claim emphasizes how crises like 9/11 "do not invite deliberation"; rather, "their urgency forestalls it" and encourages instead a "rhetoric of war." Such rhetoric "constructs an enemy unworthy of international deliberation and assumes a unity of purpose that does not require deliberation at home. Rather than setting forth claims and arguments, it constitutes a kind of argument by definition, setting forth partial discourses as if they were the complete picture and uncontestable." Although Zarefsky concedes that the "dwelling place" constructed by this rhetoric of "the closed fist" can and does serve "a positive social purpose" in wartime, he worries about its potential to condition the American public to become too mindless and thus unappreciative of the full democratic scope and function of rhetoric.[64] Expressing such concern is as close as Zarefsky comes, however, to considering the issue of President Bush's deceit. Zarefsky therefore leaves us to ponder whether this deceit was justifiable in a discourse that served "a positive social purpose."[65]

George Harper addressed the issue head-on after listening to President Bush's March 17, 2003 explanation of why he was going to order the United States armed forces to invade Iraq and end the regime of Saddam Hussein.[66] In this speech, Bush continued to use his well-rehearsed and generally accepted conception of the terrorists to justify his decision: "The terrorist threat to America and the world will be diminished the moment that Saddam Hussein is disarmed. . . . We are a peaceful people—yet we're not a fragile people, and we will not be intimidated by thugs and killers." No mention was made of the historical relationship that the United States had with the terrorists. Rather, the president stressed how "Terrorists and terror states do not reveal [their] threats with fair notice, in formal declarations—and responding to such enemies only after they have struck first is not self-defense, it is suicide."[67] In his critique of this particular claim, Harper notes: "Bush here alluded to the supposed surprise nature of the 9/11 attacks. The American people were indeed surprised, but only because we had been lulled into complacency by our government, anxious to distract us from the dangers to which it was exposing us with its aggressive foreign policy." Continuing to expose the president's deceit, Harper further emphasizes that "Had the American people been informed, from the beginning, that terrorism upon our citizens would be the price paid for military adventures in the Middle East, perhaps our politicians would have received a different message from the voters."[68]

Perhaps. But this suggestion presupposes an attempt on the part of the president to engage in an all-out heroic and rhetorical action that facilitates acknowledgment of the truth of the matter in question. The president would thus have to expand his role as a "stand-out" teacher in order to inform us about our country's historical relationship with the terrorists, enhance the intelligence of "contemporary American culture," and thereby help to remedy what Robert Hariman describes as the American public's tendency to be "dumb as a stump, way short of a load, stupid" when it comes to being knowledgeable about matters of foreign policy.[69] On an issue of great importance to our country and many others, the president would be taking a big step toward meeting a specific moral obligation that calls the rhetoric of the closed fist into question.

Such an obligation, we must remember, is not utopian—something that has no (*u*) place (*topos*) on earth. On the contrary, the source of this obligation, although not a human creation, is no further away than our own existence, our most fundamental "dwelling place." With its openness, our existence calls for acts of deconstruction and reconstruction so that an understanding of the truth of what is can take form and progress. While reflecting on the horror of 9/11, Jacques Derrida makes much of this specific evocative and epideictic event: It is something that "is not privative. It is not inaccessible, and it is not what I can indefinitely defer: it is announced to me, sweeps down upon me, precedes me, and seizes me *here now*, in a nonvirtualizable way, in actuality and not potentiality. It . . . never leaves me in peace and will not let me put it off until later. . . . It is what is most undeniably *real*."[70] At every moment of our lives—before, on, and after 9/11—we are faced with the challenge of being remarkably competent, heroic, and rhetorical souls. Derrida associates this ongoing challenge with what he terms the "invincible promise" of democracy to maintain the integrity of our openness to Being; for "the inherited concept of democracy is the only one that welcomes the possibility of being contested, of contesting itself, of criticizing and indefinitely improving itself."[71] With the case of 9/11 in mind, however, it makes good sense to ask: Should we attempt to keep this promise even with people who think the world would be a "better place" without the promise and those who are willing to make it?

Not living in a perfect world, we need heroes to express and encourage us to keep the promise of democracy, a promise that respects the truth of who we *are*: creatures whose fundamental way of being on earth *is* heroic. Owing to the onto-logical structure of human existence, we are fated to be open to what is other than the self—be this other the ecstatic temporality of existence that is not a human creation and that speaks to us of metaphysical and spiritual matters or be it other mortal creatures whose presence is there to behold in the openness of Being. Our destiny entails the constant challenge of coming to terms with the truth of what-ever this otherness may be. Meeting this challenge is especially important when our ability to live in peace is at issue. The horrible events of 9/11 might not have happened if the rhetorical strategy of deception had been questioned more seri-ously by the Bush administration. Although still finding the heroic ways of de-mocracy offensive, bin Laden and his followers perhaps might then have heard expressions and admissions that worked to temper their hatred for and actions against others whose heroism is currently still tainted by the practice of deception. As I write, the Bush Administration shows no signs of engaging in acts of genuine, rhetorical heroism regarding our country's historical relationship with the terror-ists. The truth is still covered up even as staunch supporters of the administration, like well-known conservative journalist George Will, call for a change in rhetorical tactics: "Since Sept. 11, Americans have been told that they are at war. They have not been told what sacrifices, material and emotional, they must make to sustain multiple regime changes and nation building projects. Telling such truths is part of the job description of a war president"—especially if he seeks to perform his job in a genuinely heroic way.[72]

But what if the people do not want to hear the whole truth about matters of importance? Or what if, for whatever reason, they are not prepared to deal with the truth and the anxiety and homesickness that can accompany it? In such rhe-torical situations, the moral obligation announced by the "otherness" of the heroic structure of human existence is still at work, and still demanding of a response. Granted, meeting this demand may seem impossible at the time—"suicidal," to repeat Zarefsky's remark. Nevertheless, the demand persists, for it is who we are: an openness that, by way of a primordial form of public address (epideictic dis-course), calls for the disclosing of the truth of what is. Reflecting on the events and consequences of 9/11, Francis A. Beer asks: "How do we remain true to ourselves and our long-term vision of our open society?"[73] A moral directive that calls from the heart of human existence supplies direction for answering this question.

The case of 9/11 forces the issue of how the rhetor, being true to the essence of democracy, is obligated to perform this heroic act. With its emphasis on "the concern for true reality," the ontological and phenomenological approach empha-sized here suggests a rigorous standard for assessing the authenticity of rhetorical heroism. The relationship identified between truth and heroism allows for the op-tion of political suicide. When it comes to being a genuine hero, there is no guarantee of surviving the task at hand. All the heroes that risked their lives and died on 9/11 attest to this fact of life. If only some heroic rhetor could have found a way to save us from the horror of that day. I think it is fair to say that no patriotic American would deny the importance of such wishful thinking. Genuine rhetorical heroes who dwell sincerely, thankfully, and honestly in the land of democracy are obligated to risk sacrificing their (s)elected livelihood for the "good" of those who voted (and did not vote) them into power and who, by way of deliberation, are right to demand the truth from *their* officials. Dana L. Cloud is correct when she insists that "without a normative ideal of deliberation we cannot have democracy."[74] Let us keep in mind, however, that this "normative ideal" is grounded in and thereby made possible by the ontological and heroic structure of human existence, the openness of Being that is the basis for all critical endeavors directed toward uncovering the good and the bad of humankind's rhetorical practices.

The call of conscience that comes to us from out of this openness is forever demanding of acknowledgment. It may also be interpreted as "comforting" by those who associate its presence with God, the One who supposedly always has in mind our perfection, or who, at least, respects our freedom and is always wishing us well. Even then, however, the call's demand can be hard to take. The cosmos came into being approximately fifteen billion years ago. We, however, have yet to evolve as a species that has outgrown its selfish tendencies. As Burke puts it, our striving for perfection is known to turn "rotten."[75] The existence of extreme fundamentalism is a case in point, as is what Jürgen Habermas, speaking about the tragedy of 9/11, describes as a "materialist West" that "encounters other cultures—which owe their profile to the imprint of one of the great world religions—only through the provocative and trivializing irresistibility of a leveling consumerist culture."[76]

Habermas's criticism of the "materialist West" is evident in some of the artifacts that have been examined in this chapter so far. Recall, for example, DeLillo's observation of how "the high gloss of [America's] modernity" and "the thrust of our technology" is seen as "invasive" to and "destructive" of Muslim culture. The scope and function of consumerism all too easily impedes the genuine acknowledgment of "the other." For writers like Judith Shulevitz and Thomas de Zengotita, however, our consumerist mentality is also damaging to the American public. Reflecting on the events of 9/11, Shulevitz found it necessary to admit:

> Somewhere deep in my heart, I have always longed for a catastrophe like the present one. Such wishes may seem appalling once they have come true, but we harbor them nonetheless. . . . There's nothing like being under attack to clarify what's important and to sweep away the nonsense on which we tend to squander our public attention: petty political squabbling, the enervating celebrity gossip. Never again to have to think about Gary Condit or Britney Spears!

To focus as a nation on our future and that of our children! These are instinctively attractive and ennobling ideas. Only once those other topics disappear, if they disappear, do we begin to appreciate how lucky we had been to be obsessed by them.[77]

Shulevitz's admission returns us to the first rhetorical artifact that was discussed in the present case study: Richard Power's essay that attunes our consciousness to the presence of a time and place where has vanished "the always-thereness of here" and thus where, in a moment of anxiety and awe, we are forced to stand face-to-face with the truth of Being and its call of conscience, its call for responsible thought and action. The call awakens us to our authenticity. We are more than "the nonsense on which we tend to squander our public attention." The moment is at hand where the question of "our future" must be taken seriously, without distraction: "Where art thou?" A response is needed: "Here I am!" This response of personal responsibility defines an event of acknowledgment, a happening that speaks to the issue of what it means to be a human being. We *are* creatures who are open to the future and who must thus assume the burden of affirming our freedom through resolute choice for the benefit of ourselves and others. Indeed, human existence is so structured as to admit an "instinct" for freedom. This instinct informs our heroic potential, our ability to "stand out" from the crowd in order to do exceptional things for the good of all. Of course, the challenge here can be daunting. Shulevitz admits as much when commenting on how "lucky" we are to be creatures whose authenticity can become lost in our obsessions with "petty political squabbling" and "enervating celebrity gossip." We are creatures whose love of distracting "entertainment" encourages escape from the more serious form of the activity, the form that is essential for the happening of acknowledgment: entertaining or "giving careful thought to" how we might better construct the moral nature of our dwelling places.

The events of 9/11 called us to wonder about the value of our consumerist passion for entertainment, a passion that can lead us to be forgetful and take other important and necessary concerns for granted. In his essay "The Numbing of the American Mind: Culture as Anesthetic,"[78] De Zengotita points out that this thoughtlessness is a product of a culture whose rhythm has taken on the tempo of our high tech times; like the cursor on our computers, we are being programmed to always "move on" with our lives:

> When you . . . see your 947th picture of a weeping fireman, you can't help but become fundamentally indifferent because [in our high tech, consumerist culture] you are exposed to things like this all the time, just as you are to the rest of your options. Over breakfast. In the waiting room. Driving to work. At the checkout counter. *All the time.* I know you know this already. I'm just reminding you.[79]

De Zengotita wants us to remember what the media of corporate America encourages us to forget as it "overloads" us in a "profitable" and entertaining way with things to remember. The more we tune in, the more we tune out. For the purpose of survival and in order to maintain our well-being, we permit ourselves to become comfortably numb in our everyday existence.

> So, if we were spared a gaping wound in the flesh and blood of personal life, we inevitably moved on after September 11. We were carried off by endlessly proliferating representations of the event, and by an ever expanding horizon of associated stories and characters, all of them, in their turn, represented endlessly, and the whole sweep of it driven by the rhythms of The Show—anthrax, postal workers, the Bronx lady, the Saddam connection, Osama tapes, al Jazeera's commentary on Osama tapes, Christiane Amanpour's commentary on al Jazeera's commentary on Osama tapes, a magazine story about Christiane Amanpour . . . . Conditioned thus relentlessly to move from representation to representation, we got past the thing itself as well, or rather, the thing itself was transformed into a series of signs and upon it we were borne away from every shore, moving on, moving on.[80]

We live in a culture where it *pays* to produce distractions, short attention spans, and mindlessness. Such an environment is more conducive to cultivating recognition than the life-giving gift of acknowledgment. Developing our "concern for true reality" is thereby placed at a disadvantage. Yet we dare not give up the struggle of trying to improve ourselves, for the heroic structure of existence and its call of conscience are ever present, and this fact of life, made clear by the horror of 9/11, must not be taken for granted and forgotten.

Conclusion

Long ago there evolved a creature capable of wondering about itself, its place in the cosmos, and what it all means. Acknowledgment was at work in that moment of awe and wonder as our prehistoric ancestors found themselves opened to the openness of Being—and its challenging call of conscience—like never before. The moment marked a place in time and space where the evolving universe became aware of itself. The story of Adam and Eve speaks of this monumental moment of self-awareness, as does the story of the Big Bang and its evolution. Acknowledgment is crucial for the sayings and doings of both religion and science.

I emphasized this last point throughout this book while attending to a specific question concerned with the well-being of humankind: What would life be like if no one cared enough to take the time to acknowledge your existence and thereby make a place for you in their life? The question typically comes to mind only when our lives, for whatever reason, are not being nourished enough by this life-giving gift. We are beings that need to receive acknowledgment *and* that also need to give it to others. Being capable of self-awareness, we know how much it can hurt when our need to be needed is ignored or deemed to be worthless by others.

Acknowledgment is recognition evolving into a more receptive and morally attuned state of consciousness. According to the scientist Paul Davies, this process not only "represents a *fundamental* rather than an *incidental* feature of existence," it also offers itself as "a deep and satisfying basis for human dignity." Davies makes this claim as an advocate of the "science of self-organization and complexity," which emphasizes "the fact that the universe *is* creative" and that its scientifically discernible "laws have permitted complex structures to emerge and develop to the point of consciousness—in other words, that the universe has organized its own self-awareness." For Davies, this fact provides "powerful evidence that there is 'something going on' behind it all. The impression of design is overwhelming. Science may explain all the processes whereby the universe evolves its own destiny, but that still leaves room for there to be a meaning behind existence."[1]

Davies leaves open the door to "God-in-the-gaps" thinking. The well-known and respected science writer, Timothy Ferris, is not someone who favors such thinking. He nevertheless has a nice way of accommodating its presence:

> [I]n a creative universe God would betray no trace of his presence, since to do so would be to rob the creative forces of their independence, to turn them from the active pursuit of answers to mere supplication of God. And so it is: God's language is silence. . . . God ceases speaking with the book of Job, and soon stops intervening in human affairs generally, leading Gideon to ask, "If the Lord be with us, why then . . . where be all his miracles which our fathers told us of?" The author of the Twenty-second Psalm cries ruefully, "My God, my God, why hast thou forsaken me?"
>
> Whether he left or was ever here I do not know, and don't believe we ever shall know. But one can learn to live with ambiguity—that much is requisite to the seeking spirit—and with the silence of the stars. All who genuinely seek to learn, whether atheist or believer, scientist or mystic, are united in having not *a* faith but faith itself. Its token is reverence, its habit to respect the eloquence of silence. For God's hand may be a human hand, if you reach out in loving kindness, and God's voice your voice, if you speak the truth.[2]

Reverence, the eloquence of silence, loving kindness, the truth: these are some of the things that were taken into account in the ontological and phenomenological story of acknowledgment offered here. A fundamental aspect of the story concerned how the openness of existence makes itself known and can thereby be acknowledged in that dwelling place offered it by human being, a place where the call of conscience challenges our moral capacity. Perceiving and responding to this challenge entails certain other fundamental phenomena associated with the happening of acknowledgment: the emotional attunement of consciousness, the transformation of time and space, and the creation of dwelling places where we can experience an appropriate caress and feel at home with others while deliberating about and knowing together the truth of matters of importance.

I have argued that this entire process, from beginning to end, has something rhetorical about it. The showing-forth of what *is* marks a primordial moment of epideictic rhetoric—a moment that can be traced back to the first light of the Big Bang and perhaps even further than that. Moreover, the art of rhetoric has a seminal role to play in promoting whatever good judgment can be produced as we engage in collaborative deliberation with others in the search for truth. The production of such judgment, especially in times of crisis, should be acknowledged as a heroic endeavor. The rhetor as hero abides by an ethic that is not utopian; on the contrary, it is no further away than the rhetor's own existence, his or her most fundamental dwelling place. With its openness, existence calls for acts of deconstruction and reconstruction so that a genuine understanding of what is can take form and progress.

Although the topic of the rhetor as hero was not discussed in detail until the final chapter of my story, such a character, to various degrees, appears throughout this book: Annie Dillard, Richard Feynman, Abraham Heschel, Robert Frost, Mitch Albom, Morrie Schwartz, Judith Guest, Martin Luther King, Jr., and a host of people who dwell in cyberspace. The rhetoric offered by all of these individuals speaks of the importance of being open to "otherness." Salvation from loneliness and escape from social and biological death are possible when the happening of acknowledgment is encouraged by some rhetorically competent and heroic individual who is willing to take the time to construct a dwelling place for others where some degree of peace of mind, happiness, and hope is possible. The moral imperative at work here finds expression, for example, in Christ's teaching to turn the other cheek so as not to close off our relationship with others. The extreme difficulty of performing this task is well known. The moral imperative that is always already at work, remains, however (as it did before and after Christ put it into words.) Its presence is *other* than a human creation, although it makes itself known in the primordial temporal and spatial workings of the openness of this being's existence. From where, or what, or whom did this imperative originate? Perhaps it is all just one big accident.

The universe is expanding, creating openness as it does. Our sun has reached its half-life; it has approximately four and a half billion years before it burns out, thus ending the existence of the solar system. The first simple organisms, bacteria and blue-green algae, came to life on earth about three billion years ago. Human civilization has a recorded history of no more than five to six thousand years. The rise of modern science began just a few centuries ago. Modern medical science is less than a century old. The computer revolution is less than thirty years old.

Humanity has advanced much in a very short amount of time. If we do not end up destroying ourselves beforehand, where do you think we will be one thousand years from now? One million years from now? Ten million years from now? In the great cosmological and evolutionary scheme of things, this last figure is but a blink of the eye. The blink happens on a small planet in a galaxy that shares space and time with approximately 10^{11} (1,000,000,000,000) other galaxies in the observable universe. Each galaxy contains about as many stars and each is typically one hundred thousand light years across.[3] Our presence in the universe, I think it is fair to say, is rather insignificant. How dare we be as selfish and self-centered—as rotten with perfection—as we sometimes are? Egotism and closed-mindedness are not our best features. Indeed, they get in the way of our acknowledging a *very* big truth.

Still, there remains something significant about our insignificance: we are open to and are thus able to acknowledge, wonder, and speak about the call of Being. We are creatures whose existence marks out a place where the truth of things can happen, be appreciated, and be put to good use. We are home-makers. This essential vocation, unfortunately, has yet to produce perfect results, for we have yet to figure out how to employ the full potential of our capacity for acknowledgment on a consistent basis. Hope remains, however. The openness of existence allows us to keep trying to meet this challenge as we continue to evolve.

How long it will take to successfully complete the endeavor is anybody's guess. The longer the struggle takes, the more we will learn about just how imperfect we have been up until that time. I suspect it will be a very humbling moment. Self-awareness has its costs. But these costs are worth it as long as we are determined to understand and correct what it is about ourselves that inhibits our ability to share with others the very gift that we are presently using in an effort to stay open to ourselves.

What would it be like to live in a world where sharing and receiving the life-giving gift of acknowledgment was the accepted rule of the day—an obligation that we loved to fulfill, any time, any place, and with anybody? In such a "perfect" world, acknowledgment would have evolved into something else: a sort of Oneness with Otherness. Does that sound too "religious"? How about calling it a "singularity" of humankind? Maybe such a state exists beyond (behind) one of the Universe's many black holes. Scientists have not ruled out this possibility.[4] Before we get there, however, we need a lot of practice in doing whatever it takes to share with others, and with all that stands before us, the life-giving gift of acknowledgment.

Notes

Notes to Preface

1. University of South Carolina Press, 2001.

2. George Steiner, *Grammars of Creation* (New Haven, Conn.: Yale University Press, 2001).

3. See, for example, Gregory Bateson, Don D. Jackson, Jay Haley, and Janet H. Weakland, "Toward a Theory of Schizophrenia," *Behavioral Science* 1(1956): 251–264; Gregory Bateson, *Steps to an Ecology of Mind* (New York: Ballantine, 1972).

4. Martin Buber, *The Knowledge of Man: Selected Essays*, ed. M. Friedman, trans. M. Friedman and R. G. Smith (Amherst, N.Y.: Humanity Books, 1998): 57–58.

5. R. D. Laing, *Self and Others* (2nd ed.) (New York: Penguin, 1969): 98–107; Paul Watzlawick, Janet H. Beavin, and Don D. Jackson, *Pragmatics of Human Communication* (New York: Norton, 1967): 82–90; Evelyn Sieburg, *Family Communication: An Integrated Systems Approach* (New York: Gardner, 1985): 183–189.

6. See, for example, Kenneth N. Cissna and Ron Anderson, "Communication and the Ground of Dialogue," in *The Reach of Dialogue: Confirmation, Voice, and Community*, ed. Ron Anderson, Kenneth N. Cissna, and Ronald C. Arnett (Cresskill, N.J.: Hampton Press, 1994): 9–30; Kenneth N. Cissna and Ron Anderson, *Moments of Meeting: Buber, Rogers, and the Potential for Public Dialogue* (Albany: State University of New York Press, 2002); Ronald C. Arnett, *Dialogic Education: Conversation About Ideas and Between Persons* (Carbondale: Southern Illinois University Press, 1992); Ronald C. Arnett, "A Dialogic Ethic 'Between' Buber and Levinas: A Responsive Ethical 'I'," in *Dialogue: Theorizing Difference in Communication Studies*, ed. Rob Anderson, Leslie A. Baxter, and Kenneth N. Cissna (Thousand Oaks, Calif.: Sage Publications, 2004): 75–90.

7. "Confirmation," "affirmation," "validation," and "acknowledgment" are terms that also find purchase in the literature of "social support." See, for example, Teresa L. Albrecht and Mara B. Adelman (eds.), *Communicating Social Support* (Newbury Park, Calif.: Sage, 1987); Brenda Penninx, "Social Support in Elderly People with Chronic Diseases: Does It Really Help?" (Doctoral Dissertation, Institute for Research in Extramural Medicine of The Vrije Universiteit, 1996); Brant R. Burleson

and Erina L. MacGeorge, "Supportive Communication," in *Handbook of Interpersonal Communication*, ed. Mark L. Knapp and John A. Daly (Thousand Oaks, Calif.: Sage, 2002), 374–424. "Social support" is defined as the "verbal and nonverbal communication between recipients and providers that reduces uncertainty about the situation, the self, the other, or the relationship, and functions to enhance a perception of personal control in one's life experiences" (Albrecht and Adelman, 19). Although they can be related to each other, social support and acknowledgment are distinct constructs. For example, a healthcare provider can offer support to a patient by taking the time to converse with him or her. But such conversation can happen without genuine acknowledgment being achieved; for not all "supportive" conversations are intended to produce openness, respect, a climate of comfort, trust, and hence an interpersonal dynamic intended to enhance the good health and well-being of others. These and related aspects of acknowledgment will be covered in greater detail throughout this book. Moreover, within the social support literature one finds little appreciation of two related topics that are crucial to the present project: (1) the ontological workings of acknowledgment and (2) how the *rhetorical competence* of subjects plays a role in these workings and thereby facilitates the acknowledgment of other people and other things. Regarding this last point, also see Dilip Parameshwar Gaonkar's "Introduction" to "The Forum: Publics and Counterpublics," *Quarterly Journal of Speech* 88 (2002): 410–412. Although he does not specifically mention "acknowledgment," Gaonkar makes the argument, particularly with the rhetorical tradition in mind, that the existence and good standing of any academic discipline presupposes, among other things, a rich and specialized vocabulary of "key terms" that speak to the scope and function of the discipline's specified areas of expertise and that thereby help to "credential" the discipline's claimed worthiness and status. A related prerequisite for maintaining the discipline's good health involves its members in the process of "building theory from the ground up" whereby the meaning of their specialized vocabulary is refined and clarified in order to ensure that, as time goes on, its significance and applicability are better understood and appreciated by people both "inside" and "outside" the discipline. The present project certainly is an attempt to build theory from the ground up by centering on the key term of acknowledgment.

Notes to Chapter 1

1. Ernest Becker, *The Denial of Death* (New York: The Free Press, 1973), 152–153.

2. This is not to suggest, of course, that all negative acknowledgment is harmful. For example, being shown by a student in a caring way that I have done something "wrong" in class can be beneficial to all concerned.

3. As Calvin O. Schrag notes, "the blurring of the grammar of acknowledgment with the grammar of recognition is one of the most glaring misdirections of modern epistemology." See his *God as Otherwise than Being: Toward a Semantics of the Gift* (Evanston, Ill.: Northwestern University Press, 2002), 117–118.

4. Considering the definition of "recognition" found in the *Oxford English Dictionary* (OED)—"The action or fact of perceiving that some thing, person, etc., is the same

as one previously known; the mental process of identifying what has been known before; the fact of being thus known or identified"—can also help to distinguish this phenomenon from acknowledgment as I have just defined it. The phenomenon of acknowledgment entails more than the mental process of identifying what has been known before. Thanks is owed to Lisbeth Lipari for this insight. In his *The Struggle of Recognition: The Moral Grammar of Social Conflicts*, trans. Joel Anderson (Cambridge, Mass.: MIT Press, 1996), Axel Honneth offers a comparative analysis of the role of recognition in the philosophies and social theories of G. W. F. Hegel and George Herbert Mead. He also makes mention of the work of Immanuel Kant, Karl Marx, Georges Sorel, and Jean-Paul Sartre. From my perspective, what Honneth has to say about these individuals' respective assessments of "recognition" (*Anerkennung*: to ascribe to individuals "some *positive* status") would be more accurately expressed with the term "acknowledgment" (cf. "Translator's Note," viii–ix). Throughout the book, Honneth's discussion of his central topic remains on an abstract philosophical level. No case studies are presented to clarify the practical application of his assessments. This omission, too, adds to the confusion of how acknowledgment and recognition differ in scope and function. A host of case studies are presented throughout the present work as a way of avoiding this problem. A systematic study of acknowledgment requires that one integrate theory and practice as carefully as possible.

5. Stanley Cavell, *The Claim of Reason: Wittgenstein, Skepticism, Morality, and Tragedy* (New York: Oxford University Press, 1979), 389, 435.

6. Stanley Cavell, *Must We Mean What We Say?* (New York: Cambridge University Press, 1976), 255.

7. Ludwig Wittgenstein, *On Certainty*, ed. G. E. M. Anscombe and G. H. von Wright, trans. Denis Paul and G. E. M. Anscombe (New York: Harper and Row, 1969), #378.

8. In all fairness to Cavell, I suspect that he might contend that his assessment of acknowledgment in light of his readings of such Shakespearean plays as *King Lear* (in *Must We Mean What We Say?* 267–354), as well as *Antony and Cleopatra, As You Like It, Hamlet, Othello*, and others (in *The Claim of Reason*, 329–496), does have something to say about the life-giving capacity of acknowledgment. I would not disagree. Indeed, the genius of Shakespeare is far-reaching and Cavell's painstaking reading of the Bard is, to say the least, quite fine. Still, as I hope to make clear, the life-giving capacity of acknowledgment is considerably more complex and extensive than Cavell admits.

9. Brant R. Burleson and Erina L. MacGeorge, "Supportive Communication," in *Handbook of Interpersonal Communication*, ed. Mark L. Knapp and John A. Daly (Thousand Oaks, Calif.: Sage, 2002), 374–424.

10. My use of the term "evolution" here reflects my appropriation of various arguments set forth in the literature of evolutionary psychology. See, for example, Robert Wright, *The Moral Animal: Evolutionary Psychology and Everyday Life* (New York: Vintage Books, 1994), esp. 327–344.

11. Kenneth Burke, *Permanence and Change*, 2nd rev. ed. (New York: Bobbs-Merrill, 1954), 37.

12. Plato, *Gorgias*, trans. W. D. Woodhead, in *The Collected Dialogues of Plato*, ed. Edith Hamilton and Huntington Cairns (Princeton, N.J.: Princeton University Press, 1961), 456b–c. For a discussion that takes exception to Plato's unflattering representation of Gorgias, see Bruce McComiskey, *Gorgias and the New Sophistic Rhetoric* (Carbondale: Southern Illinois University Press, 2002).

13. See Garry Wills, *Lincoln at Gettysburg: The Words That Remade America* (New York: Simon & Schuster, 1992).

14. Richard M. Weaver, *The Ethics of Rhetoric* (Chicago: Henry Regnery, 1965), 175, 178.

15. Ibid., 175; also see Richard M. Weaver, *Visions of Order: The Cultural Crisis of Our Time* (Baton Rouge: Louisiana State University Press, 1964), 7. Praising Lincoln in this way can be called into question by certain "racist" claims that he made during his famous debates with Stephen A. Douglas during the summer and fall of 1858. I deal with this matter in greater detail in chapter nine when analyzing the present day controversy regarding the flying of the Confederate Battle Flag over the Statehouse dome in South Carolina.

16. George Steiner, *Grammars of Creation* (New Haven, Conn.: Yale University Press, 2001), 9–11. Hereafter cited in the text as *GC*. As is the case with a host of books that have been published in various fields over the last fifty years and that reflect disillusion with where "progress" has taken us in the twentieth century, Steiner's contention here serves as a major warrant for the writing of his book which, as will be discussed shortly in the text, offers itself as a remedy for the condition he bemoans. This remedy, especially as it involves developing a reappreciation of theological and literary matters, also has much precedent in literatures pertaining to these fields. Commenting on what he sees to be the uniqueness of his book, Steiner notes that his book is "an *in memoriam* for lost futures and a stab at understanding their transmutation into something 'rich and strange' (though the 'richness' is, perhaps, in doubt). In another sense, I want to consider the word and concept 'creation' at a moment when Western culture and argument are so fascinated by origins" (15–16).

17. Steiner, in my humble estimation, offers a "too quick" assessment of science and deconstruction. Although I, too, at times will be critical of these enterprises, I also will have more positive things to say about them throughout the book.

18. This discussion will draw heavily from the writings of both Heidegger and Levinas. Although Steiner turns to Heidegger throughout his book as a way of emphasizing the importance of creativity in the arts and in philosophy, he avoids any specific assessment of Heidegger's understanding of acknowledgment and the role it plays in his philosophy. Chapters 2 and 3 of the present book deal with this matter in great detail. Levinas is briefly mentioned by Steiner, who credits the French philosopher with offering a "noble doctrine" of "altruism" that, in the end, fails to go "to the heart of the question": "Is there in creation an enormity of irrelevance so far as human life is concerned?" (40). With Levinas, too, however, Steiner avoids the topic of acknowledgment, which, as will be indicated in chapter 6, plays a crucial role in

Levinas's theory of "the caress." In this theory, the Judaic appreciation of "acknowledgment" as a "primordial" communicative act and response ("Where art thou?" "Here I am!") receives much attention. Hence, it is interesting to note that although Steiner draws from his Judaic heritage to support his thesis about creation, he has nothing explicit to say about how acknowledgment figures in to this central question /answer narrative structure of the Old Testament. I attend to this matter throughout the chapters of this book.

Notes to Chapter 2

1. Annie Dillard, *Teaching a Stone to Talk: Expeditions and Encounters* (New York: HarperPerennial, 1983), 95. The story here is entitled "On a Hill Far Away." Further references to this work will be cited in the text.

2. Joan Stambaugh, *The Finitude of Being* (Albany: State University of New York Press, 1992), 56.

3. Edward S. Casey, *Getting Back into Place: Toward a Renewed Understanding of the Place-World* (Bloomington: Indiana University Press, 1993), ix.

4. For a much more detailed discussion of the meaning and significance of the Word (*Logos*) in the New Testament, see Rudolf Bultmann, *Theology of the New Testament*, vol. 2, trans. Kendrick Grobel (New York: Charles Scribner's Sons, 1955), 40–69. Also see Susan Wells, "Logos," in *Encyclopedia of Rhetoric*, ed. Thomas O. Sloane (New York: Oxford University Press, 2001), 456–468. I will have more to say about *epideixis* and *kairos* in chapter 4.

5. Martin Rees, *Before the Beginning: Our Universe and Others* (Reading, Mass.: Perseus Books, 1997), 1. Also see Martin Rees, *Our Cosmic Habitat* (Princeton, N.J.: Princeton University Press, 2001), where he continues to evaluate how a "universe hospitable to life—what we might call a *bio-philic* universe—has to be very special in many ways" (xvi).

6. My discussion of religion throughout this book is rooted primarily in the Judeo-Christian tradition. I realize, of course, that what is said about religion from this "Western" perspective is not necessarily the case with other religions, most notably Eastern religions.

7. Warren Zev Harvey, "Grace or Loving-Kindness," in *Contemporary Jewish Religious Thought: Original Essays on Critical Concepts, Movements, and Beliefs*, ed. Arthur A. Cohen and Paul Mendes-Flohr (New York: The Free Press, 1987), 302.

8. Abraham Joshua Heschel, *God in Search of Man: A Philosophy of Judaism* (New York: Noonday Press, 1955), 136.

9. See his *The Guide for the Perplexed*, tr. S. Pines (Chicago: University of Chicago Press, 1974).

10. Hugh Ross, "Astronomical Evidences for a Personal Transcendent God," in *The Creation Hypothesis: Scientific Evidence for an Intelligent Designer*, ed. J. P. Moreland (Downers Grove, Ill.: InterVarsity Press, 1994), 141.

11. With "the sociology of science literature" in mind, one anonymous reviewer of my original manuscript argued that "'Science' as a noun creates a hypostatization that

tends to deny just how human and historically situated scientists are." The term "Science," continues the reviewer, "is a misleading abstraction in the sense that its use tends to evade how incredibly varied the activity covered by the term is, and that it is human beings acting as scientists that produce what we call *post hoc* 'science'." I am well aware of the literature referred to by the reviewer and thus the argument that he or she recalls. That said, I hope that readers who are also familiar with this literature will excuse what may be considered a "rather simplistic" treatment of the scientific enterprise. I submit, however, that the argument I intend to make about how acknowledgment plays a central role in this enterprise is still valid even if it is not presented in the context of a more thorough evaluation of the "varied activities" of scientists.

12. See Max Weber, "Science as a Vocation," in *From Max Weber: Essays in Sociology*, trans. and ed. H. H. Gerth and C. Wright Mills (New York: Oxford University Press, 1946), 129–156.

13. See, for example, Hugh Ross, *The Creator and the Cosmos: How the Greatest Scientific Discoveries of the Century Reveal God*, rev. ed. (Colorado Springs: NavPress, 1995); John Polkinghorne, *The Faith of a Physicist: Reflections of a Bottom-Up Thinker* (Minneapolis: Fortress Press, 1996); Gerald L. Schroeder, *The Science of God: The Convergence of Scientific and Biblical Wisdom* (New York: Broadway Books, 1997); Gerald L. Schroeder, *The Hidden Face of God: Science Reveals the Ultimate Truth* (New York: Simon & Schuster, 2001).

14. Martin Rees, *Before the Beginning*, 177.

15. Ibid., 8.

16. Paul Davies, *God & the New Physics* (New York: Simon & Schuster, 1983), 55–56.

17. Stephen Hawking, "Foreword," in Martin Rees, *Before the Beginning*; also see his *A Brief History of Time* (the updated and expanded tenth anniversary edition), (New York: Bantam, 1998), 187–191.

18. Davies, *God & the New Physics*, 70, 209. Also see Paul Davies, *The 5th Miracle: The Search for the Origin and Meaning of Life* (New York: Simon & Schuster, 2000). The latter half of this book "is devoted to a radical new theory of the origin of life" (biogenesis) that does not retreat to "the God-of-the-gaps" in emphasizing how "life began *inside* the Earth."

19. Hawking, *A Brief History of Time*, 83–117.

20. On July 21, 2004, Hawking presented a paper in Dublin, Ireland at the 17th International Conference on General Relativity and Gravitation where he argued—using more sophisticated mathematical calculations than he had used in the past—that black holes *are* able to expel their contents back into the universe, albeit "in a mangled form." If these calculations are eventually judged by the scientific community to be accurate, Hawking's new received theory would call into question the possibility that the singularity of a black hole can be a "source" of another "baby universe" that exists parallel to ours. Even if the theory proves to be correct, however, what I am saying about acknowledgment and its role in scientific inquiry would still hold true.

21. Gerald L. Schroeder, *Genesis and the Big Bang: The Discovery of Harmony Between Modern Science and the Bible* (New York: Bantam, 1990), 149–150. Also see his *The Science of God* and *The Hidden Face of God*. In this later work, Schroeder offers a wonderful discussion of the immensely complex biological and chemical structure of the human body as a way of suggesting how life speaks of the "reality" of intelligent design.

22. Rees, *Before the Beginning*, 246.

23. Hawking, *A Brief History of Time*, 190.

24. See William A. Dembski, *Intelligent Design: The Bridge Between Science and Theology* (Downers Grove, Ill.: InterVarsity Press, 1999); Daniel C. Matt, *God & the Big Bang: Discovering Harmony Between Science & Spirituality* (Woodstock, Vt.: Jewish Lights Publishing, 1996); John Angus Campbell and Stephen C. Meyer (ed.), *Darwinism, Design, and Public Education* (East Lansing: Michigan State University Press, 2003).

25. John A. Wheeler, *A Journey into Gravity and Spacetime* (New York: W. H. Freeman), quoted in Rees, *Before the Beginning*, 245. Wheeler's theory is identified with what he terms the "participatory anthropic principle," which emphasizes a conception of the universe as observer dependent. That is, observers are necessary to bring the universe into being. For the most thorough discussion of the history and development of this principle, see John D. Barrow and Frank J. Tipler, *The Anthropic Cosmological Principle* (New York: Oxford University Press, 1986). Also see Timothy Ferris, *The Whole Shebang: A State-Of-The-Universe(s) Report* (New York: Simon & Schuster, 1998). In discussing Wheeler's theory, Ferris maintains that "the anthropic principle is the [intelligent] design argument in scientific costume" (304).

26. Rees, *Before the Beginning*, 245.

27. Ibid., 6.

28. Regarding this argument, also see Brian Greene, *The Elegant Universe: Superstrings, Hidden Dimensions, and the Quest for the Ultimate Theory* (New York: Vintage Books, 2000), and his *The Fabric of the Cosmos: Space, Time, and the Texture of Reality* (New York: Alfred A. Knopf, 2004).

29. For a fuller discussion of the Hippocratic Oath and medicine's treatment of patients, see my *The Call of Conscience: Heidegger and Levinas, Rhetoric and the Euthanasia Debate* (Columbia: University of South Carolina Press, 2001), esp. 124–150.

30. Heschel, *God in Search of Man*, 76–78.

31. Ibid., 78.

32. See, for example, Steven S. Schwarzschild, "Conscience," in *Contemporary Jewish Religious Thought*, ed. Arthur A. Cohen and Paul Mendes-Flohr (New York: Free Press, 1987), 87–90.

33. For two well-argued yet opposing views on the (un)necessary conflict that exists between science and religion, see Stephen Jay Gould, *Rocks of Ages: Science and Religion in the Fullness of Life* (New York: Ballantine, 1999); and Huston Smith, *Why Religion Matters: The Fate of the Human Spirit in an Age of Disbelief* (New York: HarperCollins, 2001).

34. Stuart Kauffman, *At Home in the Universe: The Search for Laws of Self-Organization and Complexity* (New York: Oxford University Press, 1995).

35. Ibid., 23. Also see Stuart Kauffman, *Investigations* (New York: Oxford University Press, 2000).

36. Kauffman, *At Home in the Universe*, 4–5.

37. Ibid., 302, 304.

Notes to Chapter 3

1. Arthur Conan Doyle, "A Scandal in Bohemia," in *The Complete Original Illustrated Sherlock Holmes* (Secaucus, N.J.: Castle Books, 1976), 11. Further references to this story will be cited in the text.

2. See, for example, Edmund Husserl, *Ideas Pertaining to a Pure Phenomenology and to a Phenomenological Philosophy* (The Hague: Martinus Nijhoff, 1982).

3. Martin Heidegger, "Letter on Humanism," trans. Frank A. Capuzzi and J. Glenn Gray, in *Basic Writings*, ed. David Farrell Krell (New York: Harper & Row, 1977), 237.

4. Martin Heidegger, *Parmenides*, trans. Andre Schuwer and Richard Jojcewicz (Bloomington: Indiana University Press, 1992), 7.

5. Heidegger, "Letter on Humanism," 210.

6. Ibid., 230.

7. Martin Heidegger, *Being and Time*, trans. Edward Robinson and John MacQuarrie (New York: Harper & Row, 1962), 32.

8. Martin Heidegger, *An Introduction to Metaphysics*, trans. Ralph Mannheim (New Haven, Conn.: Yale University Press, 1959), 205.

9. Martin Heidegger, *Identity and Difference*, trans. Joan Stambaugh (New York: Harper and Row, 1969), 31.

10. Heidegger, *Being and Time*, 312–348.

11. For a detailed account of the Massacre and its consequences, see the "special issue" of *Time* magazine, December 20, 1999: 6, 40–59.

12. S. C. Gwynne, "An Act of God?" *Time* (December 20, 1999): 58–59. The student who testified to this killing, however, later denied telling the story. The matter is thus still open to debate.

13. Heidegger, *Being and Time*, 228–235.

14. See Francis X. Clines, "Columbine Spurs Pilot Computer Program to Spot Potentially Violent Students," *New York Times* (October 24, 1999): 16; Nancy Gibbs, "The Columbine Effect," *Time* (March 19, 2001): 22–28; John Cloud, "The Legacy of Columbine," *Time* (March 19, 2001): 33–35.

15. Nancy Gibbs and Timothy Roche, "The Columbine Tapes," *Time* (December 20, 1999): 40–51.

16. Lisa Belkin, "Parents Blaming Parents," *The New York Times Magazine* (October 31, 1999): 60–67, 78, 94, 100.

17. Adrian Nicole LeBlanc, "The Outsiders: How the Picked-on Cope—or Don't," *The New York Times Magazine* (August 22, 1999): 38.

18. This point is particularly well-developed in Robert Wright's *The Moral Animal: Evolutionary Psychology and Everyday Life* (New York: Vintage, 1994).

19. Heidegger, "Letter on Humanism," 193.

20. Heidegger, *An Introduction to Metaphysics*, 62, 191–192.

21. Of course, like any human endeavor, phenomenological discourse is "always already" value laden; it thus carries with it something of a "prescriptive" nature.

22. Heidegger, *Being and Time*, 342–348, 358; also see 296–298.

23. Ibid., 395.

24. See, however, my *The Call of Conscience* (74–78, 217n.22), where I do critique Heidegger for his "inauthenticity."

25. Martin Heidegger, *Existence and Being*, trans. Douglas Scott, R. F. C. Hull, and Alan Crick (South Bend, Ind.: Henry Regnery, 1949), 355.

26. William Barrett, *Irrational Man: A Study in Existential Philosophy* (New York: Doubleday/Anchor Books, 1958), 154.

27. Heidegger, *Existence and Being*, 338, 343.

28. Anatole Broyard, *Intoxicated by My Illness and Other Writings on Life and Death* (New York: Ballantine, 1992), 50.

29. Heidegger, *Being and Time*, 358.

30. Heidegger, *Existence and Being*, 357; also see Martin Heidegger, *Discourse on Thinking*, trans. John M. Anderson and E. Hans Freud (New York: Harper and Row, 1966), 46.

31. Martin Heidegger, *What Is Called Thinking?* trans. J. Glenn Gray (New York: Harper and Row, 1968), 121.

32. Heidegger, "Letter on Humanism," 210.

33. Heidegger, *What Is Called Thinking?* 140, 202–228.

34. Heidegger, *Existence and Being*, 306, 355, 358; *Discourse on Thinking*, 90.

35. Heidegger, *What Is Called Thinking?*, 142.

36. For a discussion of how "natural theology" is also committed to an empirically based assessment of its subject matter, or what the author terms "bottom-up" thinking, see John Polkinghorne, *The Faith of a Physicist: Reflections of a Bottom-Up Thinker* (Minneapolis: Fortress Press, 1996).

37. Heidegger, *Existence and Being*, 358.

38. Heidegger, "Letter on Humanism," 236.

39. Heidegger, *Existence and Being*, 359.

40. Heidegger, "Letter on Humanism," 233–235.

41. Heidegger, *Parmenides*, 135–136.

42. David A. Cooper, *God Is a Verb: Kabbalah and the Practice of Mystical Judaism* (New York: Riverhead Books, 1997), 66–67.

43. Ibid., 67.

Notes to Chapter 4

1. Martin Heidegger, "Letter on Humanism," trans. Frank A. Capuzzi and J. Glenn Gray, in *Basic Writings*, ed. David Farrell Krell (New York: Harper and Row, 1975), 235.

2. Ibid., 239–242.

3. Heidegger reminds us that the oldest word for "saying" is *logos*: "Saying which, in showing, lets beings appear in their 'it is'." The saying power of language is what enables any discourse to give expression to things that call for attention. Heidegger further reminds us that the word for "saying" (*logos*) is also the word for Being. Indeed, Being is constantly disclosing and showing itself in how things are, in the presencing of all that lies before us, in the circumstances of life that call for thought. The truth of Being is a saying, a showing, a phenomenon that presents itself for understanding. This is what Heidegger is referring to when he speaks of the "call of Being": the primordial "saying" whose showing is thought provoking. And this is why Heidegger tells us that if we are to listen attentively to this call, we must "follow the movement of showing" so as to let whatever concerns us speak for itself. Heidegger insists that this is the one true way of phenomenology; its discourse must be responsive to a most fundamental calling. See Martin Heidegger, *On the Way to Language*, trans. Peter D. Hertz (New York: Harper and Row, 1971), 155; *Being and Time*, trans. Edward Robinson and John MacQuarrie (New York: Harper and Row, 1962), 56; *On Time and Being*, trans. Joan Stambaugh (New York: Harper and Row, 1972), 25, 44–45, 65–67, 82.

4. See Martin Heidegger, *The Question Concerning Technology and Other Essays*, trans. William Lovitt (New York: Harper and Row, 1977), 10; *Existence and Being*, trans. Douglas Scott, R. F. C. Hull, and Alan Crick (South Bend, IN: Henry Regnery, 1949), 282–284; *Poetry, Language, Thought*, trans. Albert Hofstadter (New York: Harper and Row, 1971), 213–229.

5. Heidegger, *Poetry, Language, Thought*, 152.

6. Ibid., 216.

7. Heidegger, *Existence and Being*, 276.

8. Ibid., 283–284.

9. Heidegger, "Letter on Humanism," 241–242.

10. Ibid., 241.

11. See Martin Heidegger, *Plato's Sophist*, trans. Richard Rojcewicz and André Schuwer (Bloomington: Indiana University Press, 1997), and *Grundbegriffe der Aristotelischen Philosophie* (an unpublished transcript of Heidegger's 1924 Summer Semester lecture course at Marburg, in the Marcuse Archive in the Stadtsbibliotek in Frankfurt am Main).

12. Hans-Georg Gadamer, *Truth and Method*, 2nd rev. ed., trans Joel Weinsheimer and Donald G. Marshall (New York: Crossroad, 1991), xxxviii.

13. Richard J. Bernstein, *Philosophical Profiles* (Philadelphia: University of Pennsylvania Press, 1986), 219.

14. For an excellent work on the topic, see Karsten Harries, *The Ethical Function of Architecture* (Cambridge, Mass.: MIT Press, 1997).

15. Hans Blumenberg, "An Anthropological Approach to the Contemporary Significance of Rhetoric," trans. Robert M. Wallace, in *After Philosophy: End or Transformation?* ed. Kenneth Baynes, James Bohman, and Thomas McCarthy (Cambridge, Mass.: MIT Press, 1987), 441.

16. Isocrates, *Antidosis*, trans. G. Norlin (Cambridge, Mass.: Harvard University Press, 1982), 253–56.

17. For a historical treatment of these matters, see Brian Vickers, *In Defense of Rhetoric* (New York: Oxford University Press, 1989).

18. John Poulakos, *Sophistical Rhetoric in Classical Greece* (Columbia: University of South Carolina Press, 1995).

19. See Aristotle's *Rhetoric: A Theory of Civic Discourse*, trans. George A. Kennedy (New York: Oxford University Press, 1991), bk. I, 1354a, 1355a–b; bk. II, 1381a. Also see Aristotle, *The Politics of Aristotle*, trans. Ernest Barker (New York: Oxford University Press, 1979), 1252b, 1253a, 1281b.

20. Calvin O. Schrag, *Communicative Praxis and the Space of Subjectivity* (Bloomington: Indiana University Press, 1986; rpt. West Lafeytte, Ind.: Purdue University Press, 2003), 198–99.

21. Heidegger, *Being and Time*, 178. The bracketed phrase here corresponds to the original German: "in der rechten Weise." See Martin Heidegger, *Sein und Zeit* (Tübingen: Max Niemeyer, 1979), 138–39.

22. Martin Heidegger, *The Basic Problems of Phenomenology*, trans. Albert Hofstadter (Bloomington: Indiana University Press, 1982), 171–72.

23. See Thomas H. Huxley, "Evolution and Ethics," in *Evolutionary Ethics*, ed. Matthew H. Nitecki and Doris V. Nitecki (Albany: State University of New York Press, 1993), 29–80; and John Dewey, "Evolution and Ethics," in *Evolutionary Ethics*, 95–110.

24. See, for example, Paul R. Falzer, "On Behalf of Skeptical Rhetoric," *Philosophy and Rhetoric* 24 (1991): 238–54.

25. This position is most commonly associated with Cicero's rhetorical and moral theory of "civic republicanism," which I discuss in my *The Call of Conscience: Heidegger and Levinas, Rhetoric and the Euthanasia Debate* (Columbia: University of South Carolina Press, 2001), 10–13.

26. Heidegger, *Poetry, Language, Thought*, 66.

27. Ibid., 74–75.

28. Maurice Natanson, *Literature, Philosophy, and the Social Sciences: Essays in Existentialism and Phenomenology* (The Hague: Martinus Nijhoff, 1968), 135–36.

29. Ibid., 139–40.

30. Walter Jost and Michael J. Hyde, "Rhetoric and Hermeneutics: Places Along the Way," in *Rhetoric and Hermeneutics in Our Time*, ed. Walter Jost and Michael J. Hyde (New Haven, Conn.: Yale University Press, 1997), 1–42.

31. John Bridges, *How to Be a Gentleman: A Contemporary Guide to Common Courtesy* (Nashville, Tenn.: Rutledge Hall Press, 1998), 97.

32. Cicero, *De officiis* (I. 11–14), trans. Walter Miller (Cambridge, Mass.: Harvard University Press, 1913).

33. Coluccio Salutati (fourteenth-century humanist), as quoted in Brian Vickers, *In Defense of Rhetoric* (New York: Oxford University Press, 1989), 272.

34. Cicero, *De officiis*, I. 103.

35. See Mario Untersteiner, *The Sophists*, trans. Kathleen Freeman (New York: Philosophical Library, 1954), esp. his discussion of Gorgias, 92–205.

36. Cicero, *Orator* (71–74), trans. H. M. Hubbell (Cambridge, Mass.: Harvard University Press, 1962).

37. Georges Gusdorf, *Speaking (La Parole)*, trans. Paul T. Brockelman (Evanston, Ill.: Northwestern University Press, 1965), 74–75.

38. Ibid., 75–76.

39. Ibid., 75.

40. See Alfred North Whitehead, *Process and Reality* (New York: The Free Press, 1978), who does equate God's creative work with the process of "persuasion."

41. Friedrich Nietzsche, "Description of Ancient Rhetoric," in *Friedrich Nietzsche on Rhetoric and Language*, ed. and trans. Sander L. Gilman, Carole Blair, and David J. Parent (New York: Oxford University Press, 1989), 21–23.

42. See, for example, Paul de Man, "The Rhetoric of Temporality," in *Blindness and Insight* (Minneapolis: University of Minnesota Press, 1983), 187–191; "The Rhetoric of Tropes (Nietzsche)" and "The Rhetoric of Persuasion (Nietzsche)" in de Man, *Allegories of Reading: Figural Language in Rousseau, Nietzsche, Rilke, and Proust* (New Haven, Conn.: Yale University Press, 1979), 103–18, 119–31.

43. See, for example, Kenneth Burke, *A Rhetoric of Motives* (Berkeley: University of California Press, 1969); also see Jost and Hyde, "Rhetoric and Hermeneutics: Places Along the Way," 17–19.

44. Quintilian, *Institutio Oratoria*, trans. H. E. Butler, 4 vols. (Cambridge, Mass.: Harvard University Press, 1985), 2.1.10.

45. E. M. Cope, *An Introduction to Aristotle's Rhetoric* (London: Macmillan, 1867), p. 121.

46. Lawrence W. Rosenfield, "The Practical Celebration of Epideictic," in *Rhetoric in Transition: Studies in the Nature and Uses of Rhetoric*, ed. Eugene E. White (University Park: The Pennsylvania State University Press, 1980), 133.

47. Ibid., 145.

48. Ibid., 143, 145–146, 150. This same take on epideictic is also the basis of Rosenfield's thinking in "Central Park and the Celebration of Civic Virtue," in *American Rhetoric: Context and Criticism*, ed. Thomas W. Benson (Carbondale: Southern Illinois University Press, 1989), 221–66.

49. The little that Heidegger does have to say about the topic is offered in his *Grundbegriffe der Aristotelischen Philosophie*, 5.6.24.

50. Rosenfield, 148.

51. As Aristotle notes, for example, "To praise a man is in one respect akin to urging a course of action." (*Rhetoric* 1, 9, 1367b35).

52. For a discussion of how definitions are themselves arguments, see Edward Schiappa, "Arguing About Definitions," *Argumentation* 7 (1993): 403–17.

53. Ludwig Wittgenstein, *On Certainty*, ed. G. E. M. Anscombe and G. H. von Wright, trans. Denis Paul and G. E. M. Anscombe (New York: Harper and Row, 1969), secs. 611, 612.

54. Raphael Demos, "On Persuasion," *The Journal of Philosophy* 29 (April 1932): 226.

55. Ibid., 228.

56. Ibid., 229.

57. Wittgenstein, *On Certainty*, 141–142.

58. Charles Taylor, *Sources of the Self: The Making of the Modern Identity* (Cambridge: Harvard University Press, 1989), 72.

59. Jacques Derrida, "Violence and Metaphysics: An Essay on the Thought of Emmanual Levinas," in *Writing and Difference*, trans. Alan Bass (Chicago: University of Chicago Press, 1978), 138.

60. Jacques Derrida, "Deconstruction and the Other," interview with Richard Kearney, in Richard Kearney, *Dialogues with Contemporary Continental Thinkers: The Phenomenological Heritage* (Manchester: Manchester University Press, 1984), 118.

61. Ibid., 116, 120.

62. Jacques Derrida, *Limited Inc.*, trans. Samuel Weber and Jeffrey Mehlman (Evanston, Ill.: Northwestern University Press, 1988), 147.

63. Derrida's use of the word "différance" (as opposed to "difference") is meant to capture this simultaneous "differing" and "deferring" economy of language.

64. *Journal of the American Medical Association*, 259 (1988): 272. For a detailed discussion and critical assessment of the essay, see my *The Call of Conscience*, 124–50.

65. Emmanuel Levinas, *Outside the Subject*, trans. Michael B. Smith (Stanford, Calif.: Stanford University Press, 1994), pp. 135–43.

66. Levinas's philosophy is discussed in much greater detail throughout chapter 6.

67. Derrida, "Deconstruction and the Other," 116–26.

68. For an excellent and even-handed elaboration of this point, see Eugene Goodheart, *The Skeptic Disposition in Contemporary Criticism* (Princeton, N.J.: Princeton University Press, 1984).

69. Garry Wills, *Lincoln at Gettysburg: The Words That Remade America* (New York: Simon & Schuster, 1992).

70. Emmanuel Levinas, *Alterity & Transcendence*, trans. Michael B. Smith (New York: Columbia University Press, 1999), 96, 163.

71. Ibid., 5.

72. Ibid., 175.

73. Steven Weinberg, *Dreams of a Final Theory: The Scientist's Search for the Ultimate Laws of Nature* (New York: Vintage Books, 1992), 247.

74. Weinberg, 245.

75. Ibid., 250–251.

76. Ibid., 250.

77. Ibid., 261.

78. Ibid., 132–165, 259.

79. David Bohm, *On Dialogue*, ed. Lee Nichol (New York: Routledge, 1996), 27.

80. See, for example, Steve Fuller, "Science," in *Encyclopedia of Rhetoric*, ed. Thomas O. Sloane (New York: Oxford University Press, 2001), 703–713.

81. Richard P. Feynman, *The Meaning of It All: Thoughts of a Citizen-Scientist* (Reading, Mass.: Perseus Books, 1998), 25–28.

82. Ibid., 28.

83. Ibid., 49–50.

84. Ibid., 56–57.

85. Ibid., 39.

86. Ibid., 12.

87. Lee Smolin, *The Life of the Cosmos* (New York: Oxford University Press, 1997), 163.

88. Ibid., 176.

89. Ibid., 299–300.

90. Ibid., 177. Smolin is not interested in discovering the ultimate laws of nature that would lead to a "final theory" of the universe, for he posits that the laws of physics are "time-bound," not "timeless" (201–10).

91. Weinberg, *Dreams of a Final Theory*, 165.

92. Ibid., 243–246, 255.

93. Steven Weinberg, *The First Three Minutes: A Modern View of the Origin of the Universe*, 2nd ed. (New York: BasicBooks, 1993), 154–55.

94. Warren Zev Harvey, "Grace or Loving-Kindness," in *Contemporary Jewish Religious Thought: Original Essays on Critical Concepts, Movements, and Beliefs*, ed. Arthur A. Cohen and Paul Mendes-Flohr (New York: The Free Press, 1987), 229–303; Rudolf Bultmann, *Theology of the New Testament*, vol. 1, trans. Kendrick Grobel (New York: Charles Scribner's Sons, 1951), 156–59, 262–69, 281–94, 329–36.

95. Brian Greene, *The Elegant Universe: Superstrings, Hidden Dimensions, and the Quest for the Ultimate Theory* (New York: Vintage Books, 1999), 17.

96. Ibid., 146. "String theory also requires extra space dimensions that must be curled up in a very small size to be consistent with our never having seen them. But a tiny string can probe a tiny space. As a string moves about, oscillating as it travels, the geometrical form of the extra dimensions plays a critical role in determining resonant patterns of vibration. Because the patterns of string vibrations appear to us as the masses and charges of the elementary particles, we conclude that these fundamental properties of the universe are determined, in large measure, by the geomet-

rical size and shape of the extra dimensions. That's one of the most far-reaching insights of string theory" (206).

97. Ibid., 169.

98. Ibid., 19.

99. Ibid., 183. Also see Gabriele Veneziano, "The Myth of the Beginning of Time," *Scientific American* (May 2004): 54–65.

100. Stephen Hawking, *A Brief History of Time*, updated and expanded Tenth Anniversary edition (New York: Bantam Books, 1998), 191.

101. Another "mysterious" phenomenon that is relevant here is what astronomers term "dark matter." See, for example, Martin Rees, *Our Cosmic Habitat* (Princeton, N.J.: Princeton University Press, 2001): "Astronomers have discovered that galaxies, and even entire clusters of galaxies, would fly apart unless they were held together by the gravitational pull of between five and ten times more material [dark matter] than we actually see. . . . We now strongly suspect that the dark matter cannot consist of anything that is made of ordinary atoms. The favored view is that it consists of swarms of particles that have so far escaped detection because they have no electric charge, and because they pass straight through ordinary material with barely any interaction. There is still boisterous debate about exactly what these mysterious and elusive entities could be; there are no firm candidates. . . . Dark matter is the No. 1 problem in astronomy today, and it ranks high as a physics problem, too" (71, 73, 75).

Notes to Chapter 5

1. Witold Rybczynski, *Home: A Short History of an Idea* (New York: Penguin Books, 1986).

2. Agnes Heller, *Everyday Life* (London, Routledge and Kegan Paul, 1984), 239.

3. William Earle, *Public Sorrows & Private Pleasures* (Bloomington: Indiana University Press, 1976), 157.

4. Gaston Bachelard, *The Poetics of Space*, trans. Maria Jolas (Boston, Mass.: Beacon Press, 1969), 6–7.

5. Ibid., 15.

6. I recognize, however, that the idea that a home is an alternative to nomadic existence is not universally shared, since there are nomadic cultures that combine the two.

7. Sigmund Freud, *The Uncanny*, in *Sigmund Freud vol. 14: Art and Literature* (Harmondsworth: Penguin, 1985), 368.

8. That the high-tech environments of hospitals are *not* conducive to making patients feel at home is a much discussed topic (problem) today. For an excellent treatment of the topic and how the "comfort-care" movement provides ways of dealing with the problem, see Timothy E. Quill, *Death with Dignity: Making Choices and Taking Charge* (New York: W. W. Norton, 1993). I discuss Quill's work in my *The Call of Conscience: Heidegger and Levinas, Rhetoric and the Euthanasia Debate* (Columbia: University of South Carolina Press, 2001), 230–238.

9. Thucydides, *History of the Peloponnesian War*, trans. Rex Warner (New York: Penguin Books, 1954), 2.43.

10. Ibid., 2.44.

11. Quintilian, *Institutio Oratoria*, trans. H. E. Butler (Cambridge, Mass.: Harvard University Press, 1922), 11.7–9.

12. Ibid., 11.9.

13. Ibid., 11.17.

14. Ibid., 11.18–20. The *impluvium* was the light-well in the center of the atrium with a cistern beneath it to catch the rainwater from the inward sloping roof. Thanks are due to Craig R. Smith for directing me to Quintilian's mnemonic system.

15. Robert Frost, *The Poetry of Robert Frost: The Collected Poems, Complete and Unabridged*, ed. Edward Connery Lathem (New York: Henry Holt, 1969).

16. My reading of Frost is much indebted to many conversations with Walter Jost and my reading of his "Lessons in the Conversation That We Are: Robert Frost's 'Death of the Hired Man'," *College English* 58 (April 1996): 397–422, wherein he offers a number of insights concerning "acknowledgment." What I have to say about this phenomenon and its relationship to rhetoric that is "new" has much to do with the ontological and phenomenological understanding of the matters developed in the first four chapters of this book.

17. Martin Heidegger, *Existence and Being*, trans. Douglas Scott, R. F. C. Hull, and Alan Crick (South Bend, Ind.: Henry Regnery, 1949), 357.

18. Akiko Busch, *Geography of Home: Writings on Where We Live* (New York: Princeton Architectural Press, 1999), 25–26.

19. Rybczynski, *Home: A Short History of an Idea*, 232.

20. Kenneth Burke, *A Rhetoric of Motives* (Berkeley: University of California Press, 1969), 19–29.

21. Abraham Joshua Heschel, *Man Is Not Alone: A Philosophy of Religion* (New York: Noonday Press, 1976), 193–195.

22. Jost, "Lessons in the Conversation That We Are," 420. He makes the same point in his *Rhetorical Investigations: Studies in Ordinary Language Criticism* (Charlottesville: University of Virginia Press, 2004), 182.

23. Busch, *Geography of Home*, 104–107.

24. Jost, *Rhetorical Investigations*, 182.

25. Stuart Kauffman, *At Home in the Universe: The Search for Laws of Self-Organization and Complexity* (New York: Oxford University Press, 1995), 29–30.

26. Martin Rees, *Before the Beginning: Our Universe and Others* (Reading, Mass.: Perseus Books, 1997), 28.

27. Le Corbusier (Charles-Edouard Jeanneret), *Toward a New Architecture*, trans. Frederick Etchells (New York: Dover, 1986), 107.

28. Ibid., 19.

29. Ibid., 123, 127.

30. Ibid., 241.

31. Ibid., 110–11.

32. Ibid., 19.

33. See, for example, Deuteronomy 29:18; Lamentations 3:65.

34. Isaiah 42:20; 48:8. Also see Abraham Joshua Heschel, *God in Search of Man: A Philosophy of Judaism* (New York: Noonday Press, 1955), 85–86.

35. Lawrence Kushner, *God was in this Place and I, I did not know: Finding Self, Spirituality, and Ultimate Meaning* (Woodstock, Vt.: Jewish Lights, 1991), 31–33.

36. Karsten Harries, *The Ethical Function of Architecture* (Cambridge, Mass.: MIT Press, 1997), 186.

37. James Howard Kunstler, *Home from Nowhere: Remaking Our Everyday World for the 21st Century* (New York: Simon & Schuster, 1996), 85.

38. Ibid., 81, 85.

39. In chapter 6, I present a detailed discussion and critical assessment of Levinas's philosophy of the caress.

Notes to Chapter 6

1. Louise Harmon, *Fragments on the Deathwatch* (Boston, Mass.: Beacon, 1998), 157–168.

2. Brian Greene, *The Elegant Universe: Superstrings, Hidden Dimensions, and the Quest for the Ultimate Theory* (New York: Vintage Books, 1999), 72.

3. I am well aware that putting the matter this way invites readers to think about the complexity of the "morality" of abortion. I leave it to them to think what they will about the matter.

4. Emmanuel Levinas, *Totality and Infinity*, trans. Alphonso Lingis (Pittsburgh, Pa.: Duquesne University Press, 1969), 221.

5. Emmanuel Levinas, *Otherwise than Being or Beyond Essence*, trans. Alphonso Lingis (Boston, Mass.: Kluwer, 1991), 57. In reacting to this point, one anonymous reviewer made the following noteworthy comment: "Freedom and non-freedom, and our approach to others, are not "givens" but are concepts that are wholly human constructions, even if they name constructs that exist prior to us. Think of the concept of gravity. Our beliefs about gravity include the belief that it exists even if we don't. But 'gravity' is not meaningful and capable of analysis apart from historical beings talking about it. Now, perhaps this is the author's point—that we should think about certain ontological categories of human existence as being every bit as empirical and 'out there' (extra-human) as we do gravity. It would be more persuasive if the author would make such an analogy." Okay.

6. Emmanuel Levinas, *Time and the Other*, trans. Richard Cohen (Pittsburgh, Pa.: Duquesne University Press, 1987), 58.

7. Emmanuel Levinas, *Existence and Existents*, trans. Alphonso Lingis (The Hague: Martinus Nijhoff, 1978), 21; Levinas, *Time and the Other*, 42.

8. Levinas, *Time and the Other*, 54.

9. Ibid., 69

10. Levinas, *Existence and Existents*, 24–25.

11. Ibid., 23.

12. Ibid., 30.

13. See my *The Call of Conscience: Heidegger and Levinas, Rhetoric and the Euthanasia Debate* (Columbia: University of South Carolina Press, 2001), 119–263.

14. Levinas, *Time and the Other*, 55.

15. Levinas, *Time and Infinity*, 144–145.

16. Ibid., 146.

17. "No matter how we may wish to view ourselves, despite all our fantasies of grandeur and dominion, all our fragile human successes, the real struggle once chemical evolution ended has always been against bacteria and viruses, against adversaries never more than seven microns wide. In the battle for species survival it has been our immune system, more than all of our other strengths and assets, more than our hands, our speed and agility, even more than our minds, that has sustained us and allows us to endure for whatever ends." Ronald Glasser, *The Body Is the Hero* (New York: Random House, 1976), 26.

18. Levinas, *Time and the Other*, 121.

19. Levinas, *Existence and Existents*, 45.

20. Fyodor Dostoevsky, *The Idiot*, trans. Constance Garnett (New York: Bantam [Classic Edition], 1981), 56–57.

21. William Barrett, *Irrational Man: A Study in Existential Philosophy* (New York: Doubleday, 1958), 140.

22. Levinas, *Time and the Other*, 74.

23. Ibid., 75.

24. Levinas, *Existence and Existents*, 91.

25. Emmanuel Levinas, "Ideology and Idealism," in *The Levinas Reader*, ed. Sean Hand (Cambridge: Blackwell, 1989), 247; Emmanuel Levinas, *Of God Who Comes to Mind*, trans. Bettina Bergo (Stanford, Calif.: Stanford University Press, 1998), xi.

26. Levinas, *Time and the Other*, 115.

27. Abraham Joshua Heschel, *Man Is Not Alone: A Philosophy of Religion* (New York: Noonday, 1951), 211.

28. Levinas, *Totality and Infinity*, 269.

29. Levinas, *Otherwise than Being*, 3–20.

30. David A. Cooper, *God Is a Verb: Kabbalah and the Practice of Mystical Judaism* (New York: Riverhead Books, 1997), 65.

31. Ibid., 67.

32. See, for example, Søren Kierkegaard, *Fear and Trembling* and *The Sickness unto Death*, trans. W. Lowrie (Princeton, N.J.: Princeton University Press, 1973); *Concluding Unscientific Postscript*, trans. D. F. Swenson and W. Lowrie (Princeton, N.J.: Princeton University Press, 1971). For an excellent discussion of Kierkegaard's

analysis of selfhood, see Calvin O. Schrag, *Existence and Freedom: Towards an Ontology of Human Finitude* (Evanston, Ill.: Northwestern University Press, 1961).

33. Emmanuel Levinas, *Ethics and Infinity*, trans. Richard A. Cohen (Pittsburgh, Pa.: Duquesne University Press, 1985), 97.

34. Emmanuel Levinas, *Collected Philosophical Papers*, trans. Alphonso Lingis (The Hague: Martinus Nijhoff, 1987), 21, 41.

35. Erving Goffman, *Interaction Ritual: Essays on Face-to-Face Behavior* (New York: Anchor Books, 1967), 5, 44.

36. Levinas, *Totality and Infinity*, 194–219; *Otherwise than Being*, 94; *Ethics and Infinity*, 87.

37. R. Buckminster Fuller, *Intuition* (New York: Anchor, 1973), 9–10.

38. Levinas, *Totality and Infinity*, 215.

39. Emmanuel Levinas, "Ethics of the Infinite" (interview with Richard Kearney), in *Dialogues with Contemporary Continental Thinkers: The Phenomenological Heritage*, ed. Richard Kearney (Manchester: Manchester University Press, 1984), 62–63; *Proper Names*, trans. Michael B. Smith (Stanford, Calif.: Stanford University Press, 1996), 72–74.

40. Levinas, *Collected Philosophical Papers*, 56.

41. Emmanuel Levinas, "Ethics and Politics," trans. Jonathan Romney, in *The Levinas Reader*, 82.

42. Emmanuel Levinas, "Useless Suffering," trans. Richard Cohen, in *The Provocation of Levinas: Rethinking the Other*, ed. Robert Bernasconi and David Wood (New York: Routledge, 1988), 165; Levinas, *Existence and Existents*, 95.

43. An interesting contrast to this way of thinking about morality is found in the related literatures of evolutionary ethics and evolutionary psychology. Here one finds discussions of the notion of "reciprocal altruism"—the "moral" process wherein being-for others is but a means to a selfish end: the promotion of the self's personal and genetic welfare. For an excellent work that deals with these literatures and the debate over reciprocal altruism, see Robert Wright, *The Moral Animal: Evolutionary Psychology and Everyday Life* (New York: Vintage Books, 1994). Although he has nothing to say about Levinas' philosophy, Wright's contribution to the debate does suggest that, as in the case of Charles Darwin's life, there is more to genuine morality (being-for others) than the "shameless ploy" of reciprocal altruism.

44. Emmanuel Levinas, *Alterity and Remembrance*, trans. Michael B. Smith (New York: Columbia University Press, 1999), 97. This statement can be read as a critique of Heidegger's ontology. We should recall, however, that Heidegger does recognize the "otherness" of Being.

45. Levinas, "Ethics as First Philosophy," trans. Sean Hand and Michael Temple, in *The Levinas Reader*, 82–83.

46. Levinas, *Collected Philosophical Papers*, 123–25.

47. Ibid., 23.

48. Levinas, *Ethics and Infinity*, 85–122; *Otherwise than Being*, 122–23, 144–65.

49. Levinas, *Ethics and Infinity*, 98.

50. Levinas, *Otherwise than Being*, 158.

51. Levinas, *Time and the Other*, 56.

52. Levinas, *Otherwise than Being*, 138.

53. Emmanuel Levinas, *In the Time of the Nations*, trans. Michael B. Smith (Bloomington: Indiana University Press, 1994), 109–13, 167–83; *Nine Talmudic Readings*, trans. Annette Aronowicz (Bloomington: Indiana University Press, 1990), 12–29.

54. Emmanuel Levinas, *Difficult Freedom: Essays in Judaism*, trans. Sean Hand (Baltimore, Md.: Johns Hopkins University Press, 1990), 281.

55. Emmanuel Levinas, "The Paradox of Morality" (interview with Tamra Wright, Peter Hughes, and Alison Ainley), trans. Andrew Benjamin and Tamra Wright, in *The Provocation of Levinas*, 169, 172.

56. Levinas, *Totality and Infinity*, 197–201, 246, 262, 303; *Time and the Other*, 126.

57. Levinas, "Useless Suffering," 158.

58. Levinas, *Of God Who Comes to Mind*, xi.

59. Levinas, "The Paradox of Morality," 174; *Collected Philosophical Papers*, 148.

60. Emmanuel Levinas, "The Trace of the Other," in *Deconstruction in Context: Literature and Philosophy*, ed. Mark Taylor (Chicago: University of Chicago Press, 1986), 348.

61. Levinas, *Existence and Existents*, 40.

62. Levinas, *Totality and Infinity*, 152.

63. Ibid., 154–58.

64. Levinas, *Nine Talmudic Readings*, 169.

65. Simone de Beauvoir, *The Second Sex*, trans. and ed. H. M. Parshley (New York: Vintage Books, 1989/1949), xxii. Also see Susannah Heschel, "Feminism," in *Contemporary Jewish Religious Thought: Original Essays on Critical Concepts, Movements, and Beliefs*, ed. Arthur A. Cohen and Paul Mendes-Flohr (New York: The Free Press, 1987), 255–59.

66. Levinas, *Totality and Infinity*, 265.

67. Levinas, *Existence and Existents*, 43; *Totality and Infinity*, 258, 265–66.

68. An anonymous reviewer to this manuscript reacted to my reading of Levinas in the following way: "Just because Levinas means to flatter women does not make his description any less insulting to feminists. It is well known that much of the oppression of women in the 19th and 20th centuries was done in the name of protecting women's 'superior' virtues." The point is well-taken. For an excellent critique of Levinas' presentation of "the Woman," see Luce Irigary, "Questions to Emmanuel Levinas: On the Divinity of Love," trans. Margaret Whitford, in *Re-Reading Levinas*, ed. Robert Bernasconi and Simon Critchley (Bloomington: Indiana University Press, 1991), 109–118. My reading of Levinas is informed by the belief that, if possible, "hermeneutic charity" should also play a role in interpreting his works.

69. Emmanuel Levinas, *Outside the Subject*, trans. Michael B. Smith (Stanford, Calif.: Stanford University Press, 1994), 138–39.

70. It is interesting to note that Levinas's take on rhetoric here can be aligned with the long disparaging conception of rhetoric as being the "harlot" of the arts. Levinas does not acknowledge this point and thus does not have anything to say about how it should be handled in light of his positive conception of "feminine alterity."

71. Levinas, *Totality and Infinity*, 71–72; *Difficult Freedom*, 8.

72. Fenelon, quoted in W. S. Howell (ed.), *Fenelon's Dialogues on Eloquence* (Princeton, N.J.: Princeton University Press, 1951), 23.

73. Henry W. Johnstone, Jr., *Validity and Rhetoric in Philosophical Argument: An Outlook in Transition* (University Park, Pa.: Dialogue Press, 1978), 129.

74. Levinas, *Totality and Infinity*, 197–209.

Notes to Chapter 7

1. Emmanuel Levinas, *Totality and Infinity*, trans. Alphonso Lingus (Pittsburgh, Pa.: Duquesne University Press, 1969), 171.

2. See, for example, ibid., 265–66.

3. Support for this point is based on my reading of Robert Wright's *The Moral Animal: Evolutionary Psychology and Everyday Life* (New York: Vintage Books, 1994), 327–79.

4. This is especially the case when the practice of rhetoric is aligned with "play," as it is in Richard A. Lanham, *The Motives of Eloquence: Literary Rhetoric in the Renaissance* (New Haven, Conn.: Yale University Press, 1976).

5. For an excellent work on the "pros" and "cons" of entertainment, see Neal Gabler, *Life the Movie: How Entertainment Conquered Reality* (New York: Alfred A. Knopf, 1999).

6. Beverly Pagram, *Home & Heart: Simple, Beautiful Ways to Create Spirit, Harmony & Warmth in Every Room* (New York: Rodale Press, 1998), 8.

7. James Howard Kunstler, *Home from Nowhere: Remaking Our Everyday World for the 21st Century* (New York: Simon & Schuster, 1996), 99–100.

8. For a discussion of how this dual function enables a house or other types of buildings to "speak" to us of "holy" things, see Karsten Harries, *The Ethical Function of Architecture* (Cambridge, Mass.: MIT Press, 1997), 180–200.

9. See Walter Fisher, *Human Communication as Narration: Toward a Philosophy of Reason, Value, and Action* (Columbia: University of South Carolina Press, 1987).

10. Judith Guest, *Ordinary People* (New York: Penguin Books, 1976), 25–26. For the Film version used here, see *Ordinary People*, dir. Robert Redford, Paramount Pictures, 1980 (videocassette).

11. Ibid., 89–90.

12. The phrase "rotten with perfection" is taken from Kenneth Burke's "Definition of Man" in his *Language as Symbolic Action: Essays on Life, Literature, and Method* (Berkeley: University of California Press, 1966), 3-24.

13. See, for example, Paul Watzlawick, Janet Helmick Beavin, and Don D. Jackson, *Pragmatics of Human Communication: A Study of Interactional Patterns, Pathologies, and Paradoxes* (New York: W. W. Norton, 1967).

14. Levinas, *Totality and Infinity*, 174.

15. Emmanuel Levinas, "Ethics of the Infinite" (interview with Richard Kearney), in *Dialogues with Contemporary Continental Philosophers: The Phenomenological Heritage*, ed. Richard Kearney (Manchester: Manchester University Press, 1984), 68.

16. Georges Gusdorf, *Speaking (La Parole)*, trans. Paul T. Brockelman (Evanston, Ill.: Northwestern University Press, 1965), 73.

17. When viewing this scene, I am always reminded of how in the Jewish religion all the mirrors are covered in a house of mourning so that family and friends will not concern themselves with how they look. Mourning the dead and paying our respects should not be fouled by egoism.

18. Although it should be noted that there is a hint of anti-Semitism on the part of Beth's family when her mother makes a reference to Conrad seeing a "Jewish doctor."

19. One anonymous reviewer's reading of this chapter caused him or her to worry about how my use of Levinas' metaphor of the "feminine" might generate misunderstanding: The "critique of Beth," noted the reviewer, "appears to be that she violated our expectations of women being appropriately feminine." No, the critique of Beth is that she violated an obligation that comes with human existence: the need for "the self" to be open-minded in order to caress the other in an appropriate way.

20. Levinas, *Totality and Infinity*, 171.

Notes to Chapter 8

1. Edmund D. Pellegrino and David C. Thomasma, *A Philosophical Basis of Medical Practice: Toward a Philosophy and Ethics of the Healing Professions* (New York: Oxford University Press, 1981), 209–210.

2. Neil Postman, *Amusing Ourselves to Death: Public Discourse in the Age of Show Business* (New York: Penguin Books, 1985).

3. Two reviewers (colleagues) of this chapter wondered if "teachers" (by which they meant "good" teachers) might find my discussion to be at times "self-indulgent" and "fairly obvious." Perhaps (at least those good teachers). But even these teachers, as *we* all know, are not always outstanding, or even up to par, in the classroom. My students constantly reminded me of this fact as they read evolving drafts of the chapter. What I have to say about teaching is related primarily to the collegiate setting.

4. Emmanuel Levinas, *Totality and Infinity*, trans. Alphonso Lingis (Pittsburgh, Pa.: Duquesne University Press, 1969), 171.

5. Abraham Joshua Heschel, *I Asked for Wonder: A Spiritual Anthology*, ed. Samuel H. Dresner (New York: Crossroad, 1997), 62–63.

6. Emmanuel Levinas, *Difficult Freedom: Essays on Judaism*, trans. Sean Hand (Baltimore, Md.: Johns Hopkins University Press, 1990), 275.

7. Jonathan Rosen, *The Talmud and the Internet: A Journey between Worlds* (New York: Farrar, Straus and Giroux, 2000), 14.

8. Ibid., 55.

9. Abraham Joshua Heschel, *God in Search of Man: A Philosophy of Judaism* (New York: Farrar, Straus and Giroux, 1955), 136.

10. For an in-depth analysis of these points, see Michael J. Hyde and Craig R. Smith, "Aristotle and Heidegger on Emotion and Rhetoric: Questions of Time and Space," in *The Critical Turn: Rhetoric and Philosophy in Postmodern Discourse*, ed. Ian Angus and Lenore Langsdorf (Carbondale: Southern Illinois University Press, 1993), 68–99.

11. Calvin O. Schrag, *The Self after Postmodernity* (New Haven, Conn.: Yale University Press, 1997), 139–140.

12. Ibid., 140.

13. Ibid., 141–142.

14. Calvin O. Schrag, *God as Otherwise Than Being: Toward a Semantics of the Gift* (Evanston, Ill.: Northwestern University Press, 2002), 138.

15. Ibid., 138.

16. I studied under Schrag throughout my master's and doctoral programs and I am still fortunate to have him as my teacher at the present time.

17. Hence, the title of Heschel's famous work, *God in Search of Man: A Philosophy of Judaism*.

18. Recall that this position is also especially crucial to Levinas. See, for example, his *Totality and Infinity*, trans. Alphonso Lingis (Pittsburgh, Pa.: Duquesne University Press, 1969), 194–216.

19. For an excellent collection of essays that deal with the matter of "altruism" from the perspective of "evolutionary ethics," see Matthew H. Nitecki and Doris V. Nitecki (eds.), *Evolutionary Ethics* (Albany: State University of New York, 1993).

20. Mark Edmundson, "On the Uses of a Liberal Education: As Lite Entertainment for Bored College Students," *Harper's Magazine* 295 (September 1997): 39–49. Further references to this essay will be cited by page number in the text.

21. Plato, *Apology* (40a), trans. Hugh Tredennick, in *The Collected Dialogues of Plato*, ed. Edith Hamilton and Huntington Cairns (Princeton, N.J.: Princeton University Press, 1961). Further references to this work will be cited in the text.

22. Plato, *Phaedo* (64a), trans. Hugh Tredennick, in *The Collected Dialogues of Plato*. Further references to this work will be cited in the text.

23. Abraham Joshua Heschel, *Man Is Not Alone: A Philosophy of Religion* (New York: Noonday Press, 1951), 296.

24. Levinas, *Totality and Infinity*, 171.

25. Martin Heidegger, *What Is Called Thinking?* trans. J. Glenn Gray (New York: Harper & Row, 1968), 15.

26. (New York: Doubleday, 1997). The book was made into a TV movie in 2001. I found the book to be much better than the movie.

27. See my *The Call of Conscience: Heidegger and Levinas, Rhetoric and the Euthanasia Debate* (Columbia: University of South Carolina Press, 2001), 260–261.

28. Laura Berman Fortgang, "Career Opportunities," *Winston-Salem Journal*, 5 March 1999, A2.

29. Sherwin B. Nuland, *How We Die: Reflections on Life's Final Chapter* (New York: Alfred A. Knopf, 1994), 268.

30. See my *The Call of Conscience*, 35–36, 137–139, 167, 252–254.

31. Zygmunt Bauman, *Mortality, Immortality, and Other Life Strategies* (Stanford, Calif.: Stanford University Press, 1992), 129–130.

Notes to Chapter 9

1. Cited in my *The Call of Conscience: Heidegger and Levinas, Rhetoric and the Euthanasia Debate* (Columbia: University of South Carolina Press, 2001), 218.

2. Emmanuel Levinas, "Useless Suffering," trans. Richard Cohen, in *The Provocation of Levinas: Rethinking the Other*, ed. Robert Bernasconi and David Wood (New York: Routledge, 1988), 158.

3. Kenneth Burke, *Language as Symbolic Action: Essays on Life, Literature, and Method* (Berkeley and Los Angeles: University of California Press, 1966), 44–62. The point I am making here would, of course, have less application to institutionalized religions that are exceptionally tolerant and open (e.g., Unitarians, Quakers).

4. See Jim Davenport, "6,000 Rally for Confederate Flag," Associated Press article posted on World African Network, 2000-01-10, 11:57:39: Wysiwyg://27/http://www. wanonline.com/news/news8693.html; and Jim Davenport, "Uncivil War: Confederate Flag Rhetoric Begins to Get Nasty," Associated Press article posted on World African Network, 2000-01-11, 11:07:51: wysiwyg://25/http://www.wanonline. com/news/news8711.html. Both of these articles have since been removed from the website.

5. I cover Heidegger's thinking about the issues here in *The Call of Conscience*, 57–64.

6. John Shelton Reed, "A Flag's Many Meanings," *Wall Street Journal*, Eastern edition, January 20, 2000, A22.

7. William L. Miller, *Arguing about Slavery: John Quincy Adams and the Great Battle in the United States Congress* (New York: Vintage Books, 1995), 8–24, 502–514.

8. Quoted in Miller, 134.

9. James H. Cone, *God of the Oppressed*, rev. ed. (New York: Orbis Books, 1997), 146–147.

10. Ibid., 147.

11. Quoted in Philip S. Foner, *The Life and Writings of Frederick Douglass* (New York: 1952), III, 244–245.

12. Mary Chesnut, *A Diary from Dixie*, ed. Ben Ames Williams (Cambridge, Mass.: Harvard University Press, 1949), 247.

13. Elizabeth Muhlenfeld, *Mary Boykin Chesnut: A Biography* (Baton Rouge: Louisiana State University Press, 1981), 52, 182–183.

14. Robert F. Durden, *The Gray and the Black: The Confederate Debate on Emancipation* (Baton Rouge: Louisiana State University Press, 1972), 162. Also see Anne Firor

Scott, *The Southern Lady: From Pedestal to Politics, 1830–1930* (Chicago: University of Chicago Press, 1970), 46–53.

15. Cited in Miller, *Arguing about Slavery*, 134–135.

16. Ibid., 132–133.

17. Speech quoted in Kenneth M. Stampp (ed.), *The Causes of the Civil War*, 3rd rev. ed. (New York: Simon & Schuster, 1991), 44–45.

18. Alice Fahs, *The Imagined Civil War: Popular Literature of the North and the South, 1861–1865* (Chapel Hill: University of North Carolina Press, 2001).

19. William C. Davis, *The Cause Lost: Myths and Realities of the Confederacy* (Lawrence: University Press of Kansas, 1996), 182–183.

20. Bell Irvin Wiley, *The Life of Billy Yank: The Common Soldier of the Union* (Baton Rouge: Louisiana State University Press, 1952), 44.

21. Stampp, *The Causes of the Civil War*, 201.

22. Miller, *Arguing about Slavery*, 20–21.

23. Richard M. Weaver, "Language Is Sermonic," in Richard L. Johannesen (ed.), *Contemporary Theories of Rhetoric: Selected Readings* (New York: Harper & Row, 1971), 175–179.

24. Miller, *Arguing about Slavery*, 22.

25. James M. McPherson, *What They Fought For: 1861–1865* (New York: Anchor Books, 1995), 50.

26. See Roy P. Basler (ed.), *The Collected Works of Abraham Lincoln*, 9 vols. (New Brunswick, N.J.: Rutgers University Press, 1953–55), 2:250.

27. See Steven A. Channing, *Crisis of Fear: Secession in South Carolina* (New York: Simon and Schuster, 1970), 264–265, 282, 286–287, 289, 293.

28. Commenting on the cotton gin's effects, Bruce Catton notes: "In 1800 the United States had exported $5,000,000 worth of cotton—7 percent of the nation's total exports. By 1810 this figure had tripled, by 1840 it had risen to $63,000,000, and by 1860 cotton exports were worth $191,000,000—57 percent of the value of all American exports. The South had become a cotton empire, nearly four million slaves were employed, and slavery looked like an absolutely essential element in Southern prosperity." *The Civil War* (New York: Houghton Mifflin, 1987), 8.

29. The quotation is from the "House Divided" speech, Springfield, Illinois, June 16, 1858, in Roy P. Basler (ed.), *The Collected Works of Abraham Lincoln*, 2:461–462.

30. Cited in Paul M. Angle (ed.), *Created Equal? The Complete Lincoln-Douglas Debates of 1858* (Chicago: University of Chicago Press, 1958), 128. Also see David Zarefsky, *Lincoln, Douglas and Slavery: In the Crucible of Public Debate* (Chicago: University of Chicago Press, 1990), 184–185.

31. Quoted in Stampp, 146–147.

32. Quoted in Angle (ed.), *Created Equal?* 235.

33. Zarefsky, *Lincoln, Douglas and Slavery*, 244.

34. Quoted in Wiley, *The Life of Billy Yank*, 109.

35. McPherson, *What They Fought For: 1861–1865*, 63.

36. Ibid., 67.

37. Miller, *Arguing about Slavery*, 512.

38. McPherson, 68.

39. Martin Luther King, Jr., *The Autobiography of Martin Luther King, Jr.*, ed. Clayborne Carson (New York: Warner Books, 1998), 219.

40. Ibid., 223–224.

41. Ibid., 227.

42. Ibid., 227–228.

43. Quoted in Robert Dreyfus, "Till Earth and Heaven Ring: The NAACP Is Back, and It Plans on Being Heard," *The Nation* (July 23/30, 2001): 15–16.

44. Ibid., 15.

45. http://www.scheritage.com/Whyarewedefendingtheflag.htm (pp. 1–2). Further references to this document will be cited in the text.

46. *NAACP News*, January 12, 2001: http://www.naacp.org.

47. Quoted in Sue Anne Pressley, "Flag War Isn't Over at Carolina Statehouse," *Washington Post* (January 16, 2001): A03.

48. After reading this sentence in a early draft of this chapter, my colleague Eric Watts, who is African American, circled the words "rebel yells" and wrote in the margins: "You know, from my perspective, such sounds are as painful as the cracking of a whip."

49. Brad Herzog, *States of Mind: A Search for Faith, Hope, Inspiration, Harmony, Unity, Friendship, Love, Pride, Wisdom, Honor, Comfort, Joy, Bliss, Freedom, Justice, Glory, Triumph, and Truth or Consequences in America* (Winston-Salem, N.C.: John F. Blair, 1999), 178.

50. John Dewey, *Theory of the Moral Life*, ed. Arnold Isenberg (New York: Irvington Publishers, 1980), 132–134.

51. Ibid., 132.

52. Robert Fripp, *Let There Be Life: A Scientific and Poetic Retelling of the Genesis Creation Story* (Mahwah, N.J.: HiddenSpring, 2001), 70.

53. Zygmunt Bauman, *Postmodern Ethics* (Cambridge, Mass.: Blackwell, 1993), 3.

Notes to Chapter Ten

1. Mary Shelley, *Frankenstein* (New York: Penguin Books, 1985), 170–172, 187. Subsequent references to this book will be cited in the text.

2. Clifford Stohl, *High-Tech Heretic: Reflections of a Computer Contrarian* (New York: Anchor Books, 2000), 6.

3. See, for example, Howard Rheingold, *The Virtual Community: Homesteading on the Electronic Frontier* (Reading, Mass.: Addison-Wesley, 1993).

4. Robert N. Bellah, R. Madsen, W. M. Sullivan, A. Swidler, and S. M. Tipton, *Habits of the Heart: Individualism and Commitment in American Life* (New York: Harper & Row, 1985), 162, 251. Also see James E. Katz, Ronald E. Rice, Sophia Acord, Kiku

Dasgupta, and David Kalpana, "Personal Mediated Communication and the Concept of Community in Theory and Practice," in *Communication Yearbook 28*, ed. Pamela J. Kalbfleisch (Mahwah, N.J.: Lawrence Erlbaum, 2004): 315–371.

5. See, for example, Ananda Mitra, "Trust, Authenticity, and Discursive Power in Cyberspace," *Communications of the ACM* 45 (March 2002): 27–29; Carolyn R. Miller, "Expertise and Agency: Transformations of Ethos in Human-Computer Interaction," in *The Ethos of Rhetoric*, ed. Michael J. Hyde (Columbia: University of South Carolina Press, 2004), 197–218; Barbara Warnick, "Online Ethos: Source Credibility in an 'Authorless Environment,'" paper delivered at the 11th Biennial International Conference of the Rhetoric Society of America, Austin, Texas, May 31, 2004; Daniel Terdiman, "Why Hoaxes Enliven the World of Web Diarists," *The New York Times* (July 29, 2004): E5.

6. Readers who are high on the learning curve of advancements in computer technology may thus find some of my examples to be rather "elementary." Such basic examples, however, better serve my purpose of disclosing the ontological relationship between acknowledgment and computer technology. The relationship is too easily overlooked when we become enthralled by all the new developments that can make our computers more "powerful" and "fun" to use. Joseph B. Walter, from Cornell University, provides an excellent bibliography of research in computer-mediated communication covering articles, chapters, and books. The bibliography dates back to the 1980s and is continually being updated. See http://www.people.cornell.edu/pages/jbw29/docs/471_Things_to_Read.html.

7. Theodore Roszak, *The Cult of Information: The Folklore of Computers and the True Art of Thinking* (New York: Pantheon Books, 1986), 104.

8. Hannah Arendt, *The Human Condition* (Chicago: University of Chicago Press, 1958), 289.

9. As I have argued elsewhere, both of these calls presuppose the workings of what Heidegger terms "the call of conscience." See my *The Call of Conscience: Heidegger and Levinas, Rhetoric and the Euthanasia Debate* (Columbia: University of South Carolina Press, 2001), 21–78.

10. Joan Stambaugh, *The Finitude of Being* (Albany: State University of New York Press, 1992), 56.

11. Sherry Turkle, *Life on the Screen: Identity in the Age of the Internet* (New York: Simon & Schuster, 1995), 263–264. For a fascinating study of the "dark side" of this phenomenon, see Carrie Anne Platt, "Starving for Acknowledgment: A Rhetorical Analysis of Pro Eating Disorder Websites" (Master's Thesis, Department of Communication, Wake Forest University, 2004).

12. Roland Barthes, *The Rustle of Language*, trans. R. Howard (New York: Hill and Wang, 1986), 54.

13. Jay D. Bolter, "Literature in the Electronic Writing Space," in *Literacy Online: The Promise (and Peril) of Reading and Writing with Computers*, ed. M. C. Tuman (Pittsburgh, Pa.: University of Pittsburgh Press, 1992), 35–36. Also see Barbara

Warnick, *Critical Literacy in a Digital Era: Technology, Rhetoric, and the Public Interest* (Mahwah, N.J.: Lawrence Erlbaum, 2001).

14. Richard Lanham, "Digital Rhetoric: Theory, Practice, and Property," in *Literacy Online: The Promise (and Peril) of Reading and Writing with Computers*, ed. M. C. Tuman (Pittsburgh, Pa.: University of Pittsburgh Press, 1992), 243. Also see his *The Electronic Word: Democracy, Technology, and the Arts* (Chicago: University of Chicago Press, 1993).

15. This story is taken from J. Anderson, "Blinded by the Byte," *Chicago Tribune* (April 10, 1992): sec. 5, 1–2. For an interesting contrast to this piece, see David Gelernter, "Computers and the Pursuit of Happiness," *Commentary* (January 2001): 31–35; Kim Vincente, *The Human Factor: Revolutionizing the Way People Live with Technology* (New York: Routledge, 2004).

16. Steven Levy, *Hackers: Heroes of the Computer Revolution* (New York: Dell, 1984).

17. Marshall McLuhan, *Understanding Media: The Extensions of Man* (London: Routledge, 1964), 5.

18. James Coates, "Information the First Line of Defense in the Silicon Trenches," *Chicago Tribune* (February 7, 1993): sec. 7, p. 8.

19. Turkle, *Life on the Screen*, 269.

20. Donna Haraway, *Simians, Cyborgs, and Women: The Reinvention of Nature* (New York: Routledge, 1991), 150.

21. William Gibson, *Neuromancer* (New York: Ace, 1984), 5–6.

22. Sherry Turkle, *The Second Self: Computers and the Human Spirit* (New York: Simon & Schuster, 1984), 198.

23. Gibson, 152.

24. Helen Schwartz, "Dominion Everywhere: Computers as Cultural Artifacts," in *Literacy Online: The Promise (and Peril) of Reading and Writing with Computers*, ed. Myron C. Tuman (Pittsburgh, Pa.: University of Pittsburgh Press, 1992), 105–106.

25. Michael Zimmerman, *Eclipse of the Self: The Development of Heidegger's Concept of Authenticity* (Athens: Ohio University Press, 1981), 75.

26. Mark Poster, *The Mode of Information: Poststructuralism and Social Context* (Chicago: University of Chicago Press, 1990), 16. Also see his *What's the Matter with the Internet?* (Minneapolis: University of Minnesota Press, 2001).

27. John Dewey, *The Public and Its Problems* (Chicago: Swallow Press, 1954), 184.

28. Nicholas Negroponte, *Being Digital* (New York: Vintage Books, 1995), 183, 231. Although Negroponte's book is a bit "dated" given the evolution of the computer revolution, it still remains a classic text that continues to speak to the present and the future of this revolution; thus, my use of it here.

29. Ibid., 227.

30. Ibid., 85.

31. Ibid., 217–218.

32. Ibid., 164–165. Negroponte writes: "For example, having heard from the liquor store's agent, a machine could call to your attention a sale on a particular Chardon-

nay or beer that it knows the guests you have coming to dinner tomorrow night liked last time. It could remind you to drop the car off at a garage near where you are going, because the car told it that it needs new tires. It could clip a review of a new restaurant because you are going to that city in ten days, and in the past you seemed to agree with that reviewer. All of these are based on a model of you as an individual, not as part of a group who might buy a certain brand of soapsuds or toothpaste" (165).

33. See, for example, Michael L. Dertouzos, *What Will Be: How the New World of Information Will Change Our Lives* (San Francisco, Calif.: HarperEdge, 1998), and his *The Unfinished Revolution: Human-Centered Computers and What They Can Do for Us* (New York: HarperCollins, 2001). For a discussion of the corporate and legal complications that can manipulate and thwart this progress, see Lawrence Lessig, *Free Culture: How Big Media Uses Technology and the Law to Lock Down Culture and Control Creativity* (New York: Penguin Press, 2004).

34. George Steiner, *Grammars of Creation* (New Haven, Conn.: Yale University Press, 2001), 313, 316–318.

35. Negroponte, 240.

36. Steward Brand, *The Clock of the Long Now: Time and Responsibility* (New York: Basic Books, 1999), 9.

37. For an excellent analysis of the problem, see Cass Sunstein, *republic.com* (Princeton, N.J.: Princeton University Press, 2001). Also see Felicia Wu Song, "Virtual Communities in a Therapeutic Age," *Society* (January/February, 2002), 39–45. Also see Platt's work (n. 11 above) on pro eating disorder websites.

38. Negroponte, *Being Digital*, 228–229.

39. Quoted in J. Burnett, *Early Greek Philosophy* (New York: World Publishing Co., 1969), 134.

40. Karl Jaspers, *Way to Wisdom*, trans. Ralph Manheim (New Haven, Conn.: Yale University Press, 1970), 130.

41. Søren Kierkegaard, *Concluding Unscientific Postscript*, trans. D. F. Swenson and W. Lowrie (Princeton, N.J.: Princeton University Press, 1971), 368.

42. Bill Henderson, "The Lead Pencil Club," in *Minutes of the Lead Pencil Club*, ed. Bill Henderson (Wainscott, N.Y.: Pushcart Press, 1996), 1.

43. Ibid., 8.

44. For an extended discussion of this point, see my *The Call of Conscience*, 204–219.

45. Michael Heim, "The Erotic Ontology of Cyberspace," in *Cyberspace: First Steps*, ed. Michael Benedikt (Cambridge, Mass.: MIT Press, 1991), 61. Also see D. F. Noble, *The Religion of Technology* (New York: Random House, 1997).

46. Jonathan Rosen, *The Talmud and the Internet: A Journey Between Worlds* (New York: Farrar, Straus and Giroux, 2000), 14.

47. Margaret Wertheim, *The Pearly Gates of Cyberspace: A History of Space from Dante to the Internet* (New York: W. W. Norton, 1999), 20, 43.

48. Mark Dery, *Escape Velocity: Cyberculture at the End of the Century* (New York: Grove Press, 1996), 8.

49. Wertheim, 25.

50. David Gelernter, "Judaism Beyond Words," *Commentary* (May 2002), 33.

51. Dery, 17.

52. Wertheim, 253–282.

53. Ernest Becker, *The Denial of Death* (New York: The Free Press, 1973), 6.

54. Abraham Joshua Heschel, *God in Search of Man* (New York: Noonday Press, 1955).

55. I am more than happy to leave it up to the reader to answer this question. The basic point that I would stress, however, is that communication technology *is* an outgrowth of our need to reach out to others. This need is rooted in the human condition. To the extent that one sees a religious dimension to this need, so be it.

56. Lindsey A. Randolph, "Advertising and Ethics: Nike's Quest to Become the Invited Guest," *The Philomathesian* 8 (Spring 2002): 8–10.

57. Calvin O. Schrag, "The Idea of the University and the Communication of Knowledge in a Technological Age," in *Communication Philosophy and the Technological Age*, ed. Michael J. Hyde (Tuscaloosa: University of Alabama Press, 1982), 102–103.

58. Ibid., 102–103. On this point, also see Albert Borgmann, *Holding On to Reality: The Nature of Information at the Turn of the Millennium* (Chicago: University of Chicago Press, 1999), esp. 203–208; David G. Brown (ed.), *Teaching with Technology: Seventy-five Professors from Eight Universities Tell Their Stories* (Bolton, Mass.: Anker, 2000); Eyal Press and Jennifer Washburn, "Digital Diplomas," *Mother Jones* (January/February 2001): 34–39, 82–83.

59. See Hubert L. Dreyfus, *On the Internet* (New York: Routledge, 2001), esp. 58–59, for an argument that emphasizes how computers hinder the educational benefits of such "risk." Dreyfus, however, admits no awareness of how computers can assist students suffering from communication apprehension.

60. During the discussion, students made much of how IM can limit acknowledgment and encourage social death. As one student noted: "It can be quite discouraging when you find that you are no longer on a 'friend's' 'buddy-list,' or that 'friends' are too often 'blocking' you from receiving their messages."

61. Negroponte, 193.

62. http://micro.magnet.fsu.edu/primer/java/scienceopticsu/powersof10/index.html.

63. I associate the "significance" of our insignificance with the fact that human being defines a dwelling place where the question of "the meaning and the truth of Being" can at least be raised and investigated.

64. Stohl, xiv, 33.

65. Ibid., 180–181.

66. Ibid., 181–182.

67. The PCL is but one of many projects that make up "The Wake Forest University Technology Initiative," which began taking form in 1995. For discussions and criti-

cal assessments of this initiative, see, for example, Jill J. McMillan and Michael J. Hyde, "Technological Innovation and Change: A Case Study in the Formation of Organizational Conscience," *Quarterly Journal of Speech* 86(2000): 19–47; Michael J. Hyde and Ananda Mitra, "On the Ethics of Constructing a Face in Cyberspace: Images of a University," in *Computers, Human Interaction, and Organizations: Critical Issues*, ed. Vicente Berdayes and John W. Murphy (Westport, Conn.: Praeger, 2000), 161–188; Brown, *Teaching with Technology*, esp. 41–43.

68. Kenneth Burke, *Language as Symbolic Action: Essays on Life, Literature, and Method* (Berkeley: University of California Press, 1966), 16.

69. Georges Gusdorf, *Speaking (La Parole)*, trans. Paul T. Brockelman (Evanston, Ill.: Northwestern University Press, 1965), 76, 125.

Notes to Chapter 11

1. Richard P. Feynman, *The Meaning of It All: Thoughts of a Citizen-Scientist* (Reading, Mass.: Perscus Books, 1998), 57.

2. Stephen W. Whicher (ed.), *Selections from Ralph Waldo Emerson* (Boston, Mass.: Houghton Mifflin Co., 1957), 306.

3. Ralph Waldo Emerson, *Nature* (Part 4, "Language"), in *The Essential Writings of Ralph Waldo Emerson*, ed. Brooks Atkinson (New York: The Modern Library, 2000), 15; *Essays: First Series* ("Heroism"), in *The Essential Writings*, 228.

4. Kenneth Burke, *Counter-Statement* (Berkeley: University of California Press, 1968), 167.

5. Cicero, *De oratore* (1.8.32), trans. H. Rackham (Cambridge, Mass.: Harvard University Press, 1942).

6. Leon Kass, "Death with Dignity and the Sanctity of Life," in *A Time to Be Born and a Time to Die*, ed. Barry S. Kogan (New York: Aldine de Gruyter, 1991),133. With Cicero in mind, we might also consider adding "risk" and "courage" to the list. For example, it certainly was risky and therefore courageous for Cicero to argue against Catiline and Marc Antony.

7. Robert Hariman, *Political Style: The Artistry of Power* (Chicago: University of Chicago Press, 1995), 121.

8. Ibid., 4.

9. Cicero, *De oratore* (33.118), trans. H. M. Hubbell (Cambridge, Mass.: Harvard University Press, 1942).

10. Georges Gusdorf, *Speaking (La Parole)*, trans. Paul T. Brockelman (Evanston, Ill.: Northwestern University Press, 1965), 74–75.

11. Cicero, *De oratore* (3.14.55).

12. Martin Heidegger, *Being and Time*, trans. Edward Robinson and John MacQuarrie (New York: Harper & Row, 1962), 256–273.

13. Michael C. McGee, "The 'Ideograph': A Link Between Rhetoric and Ideology," *Quarterly Journal of Speech* 66 (1980): 1–16. "An ideograph is an ordinary language

term found in political discourse. It is a high-order abstraction representing collective commitment to a particular but equivocal and ill defined normative goal" (13). Stephen A. Klien talks about an ideographic conception of the hero in his "Romantic Heroism and 'Public Character': Ethical Criticism of Performative Traditions in Public Discourse," in *Professing Rhetoric: Selected Papers from the 2000 Rhetoric Society of America Conference,* ed. Frederick J. Antczak, Cinda Coggins, and Geoffrey D. Klinger (Mahwah, N.J.: Lawrence Erlbaum Associates, 2002), 139–146.

14. An excellent case in point is David Zarefsky's *Lincoln, Douglas, and Slavery: In the Crucible of Public Debate* (Chicago: University of Chicago Press, 1990).

15. *The 9/11 Commission Report: Final Report of the National Commission on Terrorist Attacks Upon the United States* (Authorized Edition) (New York: W. W. Norton, 2004), includes a chapter on "Heroism and Horror," 278–323.

16. See Janny Scott, "Seeking Words When Words Are Not Enough," *The New York Times* ("New York Report," August 11, 2002), 23; John M. Murphy, "'Our Mission and Our Moment': George W. Bush and September 11th," *Rhetoric and Public Affairs* 6 (2003): 607–632. In introducing his analysis of Bush's "9/11 rhetoric," Murphy writes: "This is a speculative essay, an effort to explore a fascinating set of speeches. I invite responses in the hope that critics will begin to grapple with the rhetoric that infuses our increasingly bellicose and divided public sphere" (608). Although Murphy provides readers with a stunning piece of rhetorical criticism, I accept his invitation because he omits a specific discussion of the relationship that binds the rhetor as hero with the concern for true reality. Also see Gerard A. Hauser and Amy Grim (ed.), *Rhetorical Democracy: Discursive Practices of Civic Engagement* (Selected Papers from the 2002 Conference of the Rhetoric Society of America) (Mahwah: Lawrence Erlbaum Associates, 2004), esp. part 2 ("President's Panel: The Rhetoric of 9/11 and Its Aftermath"). Here we find seven short, yet insightful, essays on the topic by Francis A. Beer, Dana L. Cloud, Rosa A. Eberly, Mark Andrejevic, James Arnt Aune, Robert Hariman, and Thomas Farrell. These authors, however, also omit any consideration of the relationship that binds the rhetor as hero with the concern for true reality.

17. Richard Powers, "The Simile," *The New York Times Magazine*, September 23, 2001, 21.

18. Ibid., 21.

19. Ibid., 21–22.

20. Ibid., 22.

21. Ibid., 22.

22. Michael J. Hyde, *The Call of Conscience: Heidegger and Levinas, Rhetoric and the Euthanasia Debate* (Columbia: University of South Carolina Press, 2003), esp. 21–78.

23. Heidegger, 300.

24. Hyde, 46–57.

25. Quintilian, *Institutio Oratoria*, trans. H. E. Butler (Cambridge, Mass.: Harvard University Press, 1985), 2.1.10.

26. When considering this point, it is important to keep in mind that, from a phenomenological perspective, it is not essential that discourse be phonetically articulated in order to be language. For a more comprehensive assessment of the matter, see my *The Call of Conscience*, 34–78. Rhetorical scholars interested in epideictic discourse typically omit from their analyses an ontological appreciation of the matter. See, for example, Murphy; Dana L. Cloud, "The Triumph of Consolatory Ritual Over Deliberation Since 9/11," in *Rhetorical Democracy*, 75–80.

27. Hyde, 50–53.

28. Ernest Becker, *The Denial of Death* (New York: Free Press, 1973), 4–5.

29. William Barrett, *The Illusion of Technique: A Search for Meaning in a Technological Civilization* (New York: Anchor Press, 1978), 142–143.

30. For an expanded treatment of the relationship between rhetoric, home, and dwelling-place, see Michael J. Hyde, "Introduction: Rhetorically, We Dwell," in *The Ethos of Rhetoric*, ed. Michael J. Hyde (Columbia: University of South Carolina Press, 2004), xiii–xxviii.

31. See, for example, Colson Whitehead, "The Image," *The New York Times Magazine*, September 23, 2001, 21.

32. William Earle, *Public Sorrows & Private Pleasures* (Bloomington: Indiana University Press, 1976), 157.

33. Lawrence Kushner, *God was in this Place and I, I did not know: Finding Self, Spirituality, and Ultimate Meaning* (Woodstock, Vt.: Jewish Lights, 1991), 31–33.

34. A copy of Bush's National Cathedral address is archived at http://www.bushcountry.org/bush_speeches/president_bush_speeches_index.htm.

35. Howard Fineman, "Bush and God," *Newsweek*, March 10, 2003, 22–30.

36. Aristotle, *Rhetoric* (1367b37), trans. W. Rhys Roberts (New York: The Modern Library, 1954).

37. For a more detailed discussion of the rhetorical (epideictic) nature of the "face" and its use in narratives, see my *The Call of Conscience*, 187–254.

38. "President Bush's Address on Terrorism before a Joint Meeting of Congress," *New York Times*, September 21, 2001, B4.

39. Osama bin Laden, "Full text of Osama bin Laden, al Qaeda Statement and Islamic Jihad Statement," Agence France Presse, October 7, 2001, http://www.freerepublic.com/focus/fr/542287/posts.

40. Sissela Bok, *Lying: Moral Choice in Public and Private Life* (New York: Vintage Books, 1979), 97.

41. Ibid., 115.

42. Ibid., 33.

43. Don DeLillo, "In the Ruins of the Future: Reflections on Terror and Loss in the Shadow of September," *Harper's Magazine*, December 2001, 33.

44. Ibid., 34.

45. See Susan Sontag, "A Mature Democracy," *The New Yorker*, September 24, 2001, 32. Maher expressed his views on his ABC-sponsored TV show, "Politically Incor-

rect," September 26, 2001. Negative reaction to his comments led to the cancellation of the show. Of the two, Sontag was the most specific and detailed. She claimed that "the disconnect between last Tuesday's [9/11] monstrous dose of reality and the self-righteous drivel and outright deceptions being peddled by public figures and TV commentators is startling, depressing. The voices licensed to follow the events seem to have joined together in a campaign to infantilize the public. Where is the acknowledgment that this was not a 'cowardly' attack on 'civilization' or 'liberty' or 'humanity' or 'the free world' but an attack on the world's self-proclaimed superpower, undertaken as a consequence of specific American alliances and actions? How many citizens are aware of the ongoing American bombing of Iraq? And if the world 'cowardly' is to be used, it might be more aptly applied to those who kill from beyond range of retaliation, high in the sky, than to those willing to die themselves in order to kill others. In the matter of courage (a morally neutral virtue): whatever may be said of the perpetrators of Tuesday's slaughter, they were not cowards."

46. DeLillo, 38.

47. Abraham Joshua Heschel, *Man Is Not Alone: A Philosophy of Religion* (New York: The Noonday Press, 1951), 11.

48. Allan Gurganus, "Sherman's Ghost," *The New York Times Magazine*, September 23, 2001, 101.

49. Ibid., 101.

50. Quoted in Kenneth T. Walsh, "Leadership," *U.S. News & World Report*, Commemorative Issue ("One Year After 9-11: A Nation Changed") (2002), 65.

51. Robert M. Gates, *From the Shadows: The Ultimate Insider's Story of Five Presidents and How They Won the Cold War* (New York: Simon and Schuster, 1996).

52. *Le Nouvel Observateur* (France), Interview, January 15–21, 1998. Quoted in Phil Gasper, "Afghanistan, the CIA, bin Laden, and the Taliban," *International Socialist Review* (November–December, 2001): 29–31. For a more recent and expanded discussion of the matter, see George Crile, *Charlie Wilson's War: The Extraordinary Story of the Largest Covert Operation in History* (New York: Atlantic Monthly Press, 2003).

53. Ahmed Rashid, *Taliban: Militant Islam, Oil, and Fundamentalism in Central Asia* (New Haven, Conn.: Yale University Press, 2000).

54. Raul Mahajan, "The New Crusade: America's War on Terrorism," *Monthly Review* (February 2002): 22–23.

55. William J. Bennett, "What Is AVOT? An Open Letter from William J. Bennett." *AVOT Home Page*, 14 April 2002, http://www.avot.org/stories/storyReader$29.

56. Mahajan, 22–23.

57. Rabbi David Wolpe, "Don't Tell Me We Should Not Blame God," in *From the Ashes: A Spiritual Response to the Attack on America*, addresses collected by the Editors of Beliefnet (New York: Rodale, 2001), 38.

58. The philosopher and Talmudic scholar Emmanuel Levinas makes much of this point throughout his writings. For an extended discussion of the matter, especially

as it relates to the theory and practice of rhetoric, see my *The Call of Conscience*, 79–115.

59. Wolpe, 38–39.

60. Ibid., 39.

61. Ibid., 39.

62. Bok, 31.

63. A worthwhile answer to this question, especially with Jewish leaders such as Rabbi Wolpe in mind, must wait for another occasion. It seems to me, however, that the question requires a consideration of how answering it in a truthful manner might jeopardize Israel's relationship with the United States and, as a result, further expose Israel to the possibility of another Auschwitz.

64. David Zarefsky, "George W. Bush Discovers Rhetoric: September 20, 2001, and the U.S. Response to Terrorism," in *The Ethos of Rhetoric*, 153.

65. Still, Zarefsky does open a space for the kind of critique I am making by pointing out that the discussion of "why do they hate us" was the weakest part of Bush's speech and that it does not detract from a condemnation of terrorism to inquire into why there is rampant anti-Americanism and distrust of capitalism in certain parts of the world (143–144).

66. George Harper, "Why We Conquer," *Liberty* (June 2003): 21–30.

67. A copy of the full text is archived at: http://www.bushcountry.org/bush_speeches/president_bush_speeches_index.htm.

68. Harper, 30. Harper is also critical of how the media allowed itself to be manipulated by the Bush Administration. For related arguments, see Douglas Kellner "September 11, the Media, and War Fever," *Television and New Media* 3 (2002): 143–151; and Dina Roy, "The Media in a Time of War," *International Socialist Review* (May–June, 2003): 39–48.

69. Robert Hariman, "Public Culture and Public Stupidity Post-9/11," in *Rhetorical Democracy*, 96. Hariman's way of putting the matter encourages a question: How long do you think it will take before the American public (as a whole) accepts the findings of national and international investigators that weapons of mass destruction are not to be found in Iraq and that no definitive evidence exists that suggests that Iraq played a role in the events of 9/11?

70. Jacques Derrida, "Autoimmunity: Real and Symbolic Suicides," in Giovanna Borradori, *Philosophy in a Time of Terror: Dialogues with Jürgen Habermas and Jacques Derrida* (Chicago: University of Chicago Press, 2003), 134.

71. Ibid., 121.

72. George Will, "Sacrifices: Time for Americans to be told truth about the war," *Winston-Salem Journal*, April 8, 2004: A12. Also see Robert Dreyfuss and Jason Vest, "The Lie Factory," *Mother Jones* (February 2004):34–41; James Fallows, "Blind Into Baghdad," *The Atlantic* (January/February, 2004): 52–74; Kenneth M. Pollack, "Spies, Lies, and Weapons: What Went Wrong," *The Atlantic* (January/February, 2004): 78–92; Richard A. Clarke, *Against All Enemies: Inside America's War on Terror* (New York: Free Press, 2004). In this much publicized critique of the Bush ad-

ministration, Clarke never goes so far as to recommend that the president should disclose the whole truth about the United States' historical relationship with the terrorists. Clarke, in fact, too often dances around the issue. But he does have a number of things to say throughout his book that speak (albeit indirectly) to Bush's lack of genuine and heroic rhetorical leadership after 9/11. For example: "The nation needed thoughtful leadership to deal with the underlying problems September 11 reflected: a radical deviant Islamist ideology on the rise, real security vulnerabilities in the highly integrated global civilization. Instead, American got unthinking reactions, ham-handed responses, and a rejection of analysis in favor of received wisdom. It has left us less secure. We will pay the price for a long time" (287). I find this same point of view, developed in a more "rhetorically sensitive" way, in *The 9/11 Commission Report.*

73. Francis A. Beer, "Terrorist Rhetorics, Rhetorics of Democracies, and Worlds of Meaning," in *Rhetorical Democracy*, 74.

74. Cloud, 79.

75. Kenneth Burke, *Language as Symbolic Action: Essays on Life, Literature, and Method* (Berkeley: University of California Press, 1966), 16–24.

76. Jürgen Habermas, "Fundamentalism and Terror," in Borradori, *Philosophy in a Time of Terror*, 33.

77. Judith Shulevitz, "The Thrill," *The New York Times Magazine* (September 23, 2001): 28.

78. *Harper's Magazine* (April 2002): 33–40.

79. Ibid., 36.

80. Ibid., 40.

Notes to Conclusion

1. Paul Davies, *The Cosmic Blueprint: New Discoveries in Nature's Creative Ability to Order the Universe* (Radnor, Pa.: Templeton Foundation Press, 2004), 203.

2. Timothy Ferris, *The Whole Shebang: A State-Of-The-Universe(s) Report* (New York: Simon & Schuster, 1997), 312.

3. Lee Smolin, *The Life of the Cosmos* (New York: Oxford University Press, 1997), 118.

4. See Smolin, 87–88. Also see Martin Rees, *Our Cosmic Habitat* (Princeton, N.J.: Princeton University Press, 2001), who argues that such a "multiverse concept" is already a part of empirical science. As noted earlier in this book (chapter 2, note 20), however, Stephen Hawking's most recent mathematical theory on the nature of black holes does argue against the existence of parallel universes.

Index

ability to be, ix
Abraham, 31, 136, 157
absence, presence of, 58
academic egos, 166
accuracy (*justesse*), 259
acknowledgment, being of, 33; and
  communicative behavior, 1–2; and
  computer ads, 243–244; computerization of, 222–255; and creation, 7–10;
  as essence of teaching, 159–188, 246;
  fake, 234; as form of consciousness, xi,
  18; and heroes, 245; and hope, 7–10;
  as life-draining force, 2; and moral development of recognition, 3–5, 7, 56,
  235, 284, 290n. 4; negative, 2, 13, 36,
  48, 199, 230, 271; ontological significance of, x; paradox of, 26–28; positive, 1–2, 6, 36, 46, 48, 98, 104, 110,
  220, 271; question of, 1–14; and rhetoric, 5–7; test of, 18; and unacknowledged, 1; vitality of, 10. *See also* self-
  acknowledgment
Adam and Eve, xiii, 9, 22, 222, 284
Adams, John Hurst, 195
aesthetic distance, 6
aesthetics, 9, 90, 257
affirmation, xii, 37
"Afghan trap," 274
Afghanistan, 269, 273
African-Americans, 194, 210
agape, 165
ageism, 2, 13
agreements of judgment, 4
Albom, Mitch, *Tuesdays with Morrie*, 13,
  174–188, 247
Albright, Madeleine, 274–275

alienation, 51
Allah, 268, 274, 277
al-Qaeda, 268
alterity: *See* otherness
altruism, 166, 292n. 18
Amanpour, Christiane, 283
American Red Cross, the, 266–267
American values, 215
Anderson, Rob, xii
anger, 1
animalia metaphysica, 99, 110–111, 226–
  228, 239
annihilation anxiety, 180
anti-Semitism, 135, 310n. 18
anxiety, ix, xi, 1, 22, 44, 50–52, 83, 85,
  105, 109, 247, 280; and conscience, 50;
  and death, 2; sober, 53
apocalypse, 270–271
appropriateness, 12, 20, 70, 71, 74, 93–
  95, 97, 104, 107, 141–158, 203
arbitrariness, 62
architect, linguistic, 88
architectural design theory, xi, 12, 111
architectural emotion, 113
architecture, the ethical function of, 64,
  113
Arendt, Hannah, 227
argument, 6, 104, 109; in the making, 79;
  lines of, 101
Aristotle, 5, 63, 164, 266
Arnett, Ronald, xii
arrangement (*disposition*), 65
art, great works of, 61, 63
art of dying, 179
art of living, 179
artist, the great, 74